WOMEN AND HIV PREVENTION
IN CANADA

WOMEN AND HIV PREVENTION IN CANADA

Implications for Research, Policy, and Practice

Edited by
Jacqueline Gahagan

Women's Press
Toronto

Women and HIV Prevention in Canada: Implications for Research, Policy, and Practice
Edited by Jacqueline Gahagan

First published in 2013 by
Women's Press, an imprint of Canadian Scholars' Press Inc.
425 Adelaide Street West, Suite 200
Toronto, Ontario
M5V 3C1

www.womenspress.ca

Canadian Scholars' Press Inc./Women's Press gratefully acknowledges financial support for our publishing activities from the Government of Canada through the Canada Book Fund (CBF).

Library and Archives Canada Cataloguing in Publication

Women and HIV prevention in Canada : implications for research, policy, and practice / edited by Jacqueline Gahagan.

Includes bibliographical references.
Issued also in electronic formats.
ISBN 978-0-88961-486-4

1. HIV infections--Canada--Prevention--Case studies. 2. HIV-positive women--Services for-- Canada--Case studies. 3. Women--Health and hygiene--Canada--Case studies. I. Gahagan, Jacqueline C

RA643.86.C3W64 2013   362.19697'9200820971   C2012-908235-X

Text and cover design by Aldo Fierro
Cover image © Donna Boyko, *The Passion, The Spirit, The Fountain Within* (2011)

Printed and bound in Canada by Webcom

Canadä

MIX
Paper from
responsible sources
FSC
www.fsc.org   FSC® C004071

In memory of D.I.G.

TABLE OF CONTENTS

PREFACE

Despite the long-standing impact of HIV/AIDS on the lives of women in Canada, there is no comprehensive book on the subject that takes as its point of departure the lessons from the past two decades of HIV prevention efforts, with the aim of advancing our research, policy, and programmatic responses in a collaborative, multidisciplinary manner. This is particularly important as the epidemic continues to shift and change over time and as we continue to witness the gendered and differential impact of HIV/AIDS on the lives of men and women, and boys and girls. The rationale for this book emerged, therefore, as a result of reflecting on the burden of disease that HIV represents in the lives of women in Canada, as well as the recognition that the next generation of our efforts must emphasize upstream, primary, *and* secondary prevention intervention approaches to not only identify but also mitigate these burdens. To help illustrate these various impacts, this book draws from a diverse variety of health-related disciplines, methodologies, and theoretical and conceptual frameworks used to situate the tensions between HIV/AIDS as a complex public health issue and as a deeply gendered socio-political issue. The contributors to this book offer examples from their work in HIV/AIDS to demonstrate the ongoing need for a coordinated and collaborative approach to HIV/AIDS prevention for women, trans women, and girls in Canada from research, policy, and programming sectors.

This collection of readings will be of particular interest to upper-level undergraduate and graduate students in epidemiology and community health, sociology of health, nursing, health promotion, health service administration, social work, and health policy, among other social and behavioural sciences. The book is divided into a variety of chapters based on particular content issues that cover the epidemiology of women and HIV/AIDS in Canada, enhanced surveillance specific to women, pregnancy and fertility issues, housing as a determinant of health, HIV prevention and prisons, and new HIV prevention technologies, among other pressing primary and secondary HIV prevention issues for women. Each chapter offers a review of some key methodological, theoretical, and conceptual aspects embedded within a particular approach or study related to HIV prevention in Canada. A problem-based learning case study and a series of related questions are offered at the conclusion of the chapters as a means of further engaging the reader in the application of the key issues within and across policy, programming, and research sectors.

Within each chapter is housed a diverse array of current HIV/AIDS prevention examples from various perspectives, which are meant to serve as case studies from which readers are asked to determine, within and across disciplinary boundaries, how they would address the issues raised in an effort to mitigate the impact of HIV on the lives of women in Canada.

Introduction
WOMEN AND HIV IN CANADA: REFLECTIONS ON AN EPIDEMIC

Jacqueline Gahagan

More than two decades after its onset, the HIV/AIDS pandemic remains an enormous public health and deeply gendered social justice challenge in Canada and around the world. Despite our ongoing, collective efforts in preventing new HIV infections, the number of women living with HIV in Canada continues to rise. Women's vulnerability to HIV infection has, throughout the history of the epidemic, been shaped by a variety of interconnected determinants of health, including gender, income, education, unemployment, access to affordable housing, early childhood development (e.g., history of child abuse), physical environments (e.g., geographically isolated communities, prison environments, disadvantaged urban environments), access to health services, support networks, social environments (e.g., HIV/AIDS-related stigma and discrimination, racism), sexual violence, and culture, among others.

Gender as a social construct, gender-related expectations such as power inequalities between men and women, and issues of sexual and reproductive autonomy are examples of how such determinants of health intersect and influence HIV prevention efforts. Not only do these complex intersections determine women's health, broadly speaking, but they also serve to underscore the urgent need for novel approaches to the next wave of HIV prevention interventions that address underlying structural causes leading to HIV infection. There is little doubt that a greater understanding of the interplay between these factors will yield important innovation with respect to the development of multi-sectoral, transdisciplinary HIV prevention approaches, cutting across policy, research, programming, and front-line responses in Canada.

In reflecting on the epidemic in Canada and, in particular, on the consequences of HIV/AIDS for women, it is of little comfort to simply take stock of our successes where we can find them. Rather, as the numbers of women living with HIV in Canada increase, there is an urgent need for more action in the development of novel policy and prevention interventions that meet the complex primary and secondary HIV prevention needs of women, trans women, and girls. In the absence of effective microbicides or vaccines, we have largely continued to turn our attention to individual or micro-level behavioural interventions to prevent initial infection, as well as the onward transmission of the virus. The long history of the variable success of such interventions has fuelled other debates and questions about key HIV prevention issues. Who is becoming infected and why? Why do we see higher rates of infection within certain populations and lower rates in others? Whose needs are our HIV prevention efforts really meant to address? How are employment or housing policies useful in the prevention of HIV? How are the needs of socially or economically marginalized populations being represented in current HIV prevention interventions? Who is included in clinical trials for new HIV prevention technologies and medications? Who is absent? Who has access to the latest HIV prevention, care, treatment, and support innovations? How do these issues differ by one's age, sex, sexual orientation, gender, ethnicity, language, and other determinants of health?

These remain critical questions to grapple with in situating our collective moral compass as we determine the way forward in the next wave of prevention interventions for, with, and by women, trans women, and girls infected and affected by HIV in Canada. Consider, for example, how advances in highly active antiretroviral therapy (HAART) in the mid-1990s quickly became regarded as the "magic bullet" in getting ahead of the HIV epidemic. However, our hopes were dashed by the wide-ranging side effects from these new medications, and we are left wondering how to reframe our subsequent prevention efforts. Such examples serve to once again remind us of the need to understand the intersectionality of the various determinants of health that place women and men, and boys and girls at differential levels of risk for HIV infection in the first place. With this understanding also comes the need for a shift away from focusing solely on individual or micro-level health behaviours and a move toward understanding the broader structural or macro-level factors leading to HIV transmission and HIV-related health outcomes. To achieve this, a more complex analysis and evaluation of our efforts through a determinants of health framework in understanding the synergistic interplay of factors that increase the likelihood of becoming HIV positive is warranted. This is particularly relevant for women, trans women, and girls, given the widespread recognition of gender as a key determinant of health and, more specifically, gender-related expectations regarding sexuality and how these gendered expectations in turn serve to shape and impact our HIV prevention efforts.

The impetus for this book project emerged, in part, from a systematic review of the published qualitative evidence focused on HIV prevention for women in Canada, funded by the Canadian Institutes of Health Research (CIHR). Using a meta-ethnographic approach, this CIHR-funded synthesis identified where specific knowledge was lacking and where a greater understanding of both the implicit and explicit factors that contribute to HIV infection among women in Canada is needed. A key issue to emerge from this synthesis was the imperative of acknowledging HIV/AIDS as a key health priority cutting across sectors such as housing, justice, and education, and not simply within the formal and informal health sectors as discrete silos. A day-long session emerged as a knowledge dissemination process from this synthesis study. It was held at the 18th Annual Canadian Association for HIV Research (CAHR) Conference, where the idea for this edited volume of HIV prevention issues for women in Canada emerged. The resultant book, *Women and HIV Prevention in Canada: Implications for Research, Policy, and Practice*, provides not only an opportunity for sharing findings from a selection of key national projects related to women and HIV in Canada, but is also intended to help inform future directions in HIV prevention research, policy, and practice.

Recognizing the interconnectedness of the HIV prevention issues raised at the CAHR conference, the book stretches the boundaries of the epidemiological, social, and behavioural sciences through to the policy, programming, and practice approaches. This is done as a means of enabling the reader to further his or her understanding of one of the most cross-cutting health, social justice, and deeply gendered issues of our time: HIV/AIDS. Although the focus of the CAHR conference session was to highlight some key challenges and successes in HIV prevention for women in Canada, it soon became clear that the "teachable moments" from this session would yield appropriate material for upper-level undergraduate and graduate-level audiences with an interest in mitigating the impact of HIV among women, trans women, and girls living with and affected by HIV/AIDS in Canada. Given the complexities of HIV prevention among the diverse populations of women in Canada discussed at the CAHR session, it became clear that there is an urgent need for greater horizontality—working across sectors— in both our primary and secondary prevention efforts.

An additional key message to emerge from the CAHR conference session, and reflected throughout this book, is the need to reframe our collective understanding of the determinants of health that place women and men, and boys and girls in Canada at differential levels of risk for HIV infection and related health outcomes. Specifically, the call for a further shift away from focusing solely on individual-level "risk factors" and toward a greater recognition of the broader structural factors in HIV transmission and disease progression was clearly stated. This shift is seen to facilitate a more complex analysis of the issues that collectively, and not simply at the level of the individual, increase the differential likelihood of HIV infection for women, men, boys, and girls.

This book provides not only an opportunity to identify some key gaps and successes related to women and HIV prevention approaches in Canada, but is also meant to help shape and inform future directions in HIV prevention research, policy, and practice. Further, it sets out to engage the reader through a diverse variety of health-related disciplines, methodologies, and theoretical and conceptual frameworks in an effort to help illustrate the tensions between HIV/AIDS as a public health issue and as a gendered socio-political issue. The contributors to this book offer examples from their current work in the area of women and HIV/AIDS in Canada to help shed light on the pressing need for a more coordinated and collaborative approach to HIV/AIDS prevention for women in Canada. This volume also presents a unique opportunity to highlight some of the key needs and gaps in research, policy, and programming with the aim of advancing our transdisciplinary and collaborative efforts to augment our HIV prevention efforts for, by, and with diverse populations and communities of women in Canada.

ACKNOWLEDGEMENTS

It is with sincere gratitude that I acknowledge the following individuals for their enthusiasm, time, support and contributions to this book: Chris Archibald, Jessica Halverson, Jacqueline Arthur, Jocelyne Guay, and Kristen Beausoleil of the Public Health Agency of Canada; Wangari Tharao, Marvelous Muchenje, and Mira Mehes of Women's Health in Women's Hands; Mona Loutfy of the University of Toronto; Shari Margolese of Voices of Positive Women; Greta Bauer of the University of Western Ontario; Rai Reece of PASAN; Doris Peltier, Randy Jackson, Tracey Prentice, LaVerne Monette, Monique Fong, Krista Shore, Renée Masching, and the Voices of Women (VOW) Standing Committee; Saara Greene, Lori Chambers, Khatundi Masinde, and Chantal Mukandoli; Patricia Allard, Cécile Kazatchkine, and Alison Symington of the Canadian HIV/AIDS Legal Network; and San Patten of Patten and Associates.

I would also like to extend my sincere thanks to all those who participated in the research, policy, and programming work highlighted in this volume. Thank you to Shirley Wheaton, Eric Ross, and Carlye Stein for their very patient assistance with the formatting of the manuscript. Finally, I wish to thank Canadian Scholars' Press Inc./Women's Press for their support for this important book, especially Daniella Balabuk, Caley Baker, and my editor, James MacNevin, for believing in this project and for his expert guidance along the way.

Jacqueline Gahagan, PhD
Professor of Health Promotion
Head, Health Promotion Division
Director, Gender and Health Promotion Studies Unit
School of Health and Human Performance
Dalhousie University
Halifax, Nova Scotia

Chapter 1

THE CURRENT STATE OF WOMEN AND HIV IN CANADA: AN OVERVIEW OF HIV/AIDS EPIDEMIOLOGY IN CANADA

Chris Archibald and Jessica Halverson

OVERVIEW OF HIV IN CANADA

As part of its mandate to promote and protect the health of Canadians, the Public Health Agency of Canada (PHAC) produces data from a variety of sources to monitor trends in HIV and AIDS across the country. Surveillance data, which are based on the actual number of people who test positive for HIV and whose cases are formally reported, provides the foundation of epidemiological knowledge. Surveillance data are limited by the fact that they only capture those individuals who have been tested for HIV and whose HIV diagnosis has been reported to public health authorities. As such, the data may be impacted by testing options and testing availability, as well as testing behaviours among different populations. Routine surveillance data are also subject to other challenges, such as delays in reporting and under-reporting. To supplement these, PHAC also conducts targeted biological–behavioural surveillance studies among several at-risk populations, namely people who inject drugs, men who have sex with men, and Aboriginal peoples, with plans to expand to additional population groups. In addition, PHAC produces HIV estimates, which are generated using mathematical models that draw on surveillance and other data to arrive at the number of people living with HIV (prevalence) and the number of newly infected individuals in a given year (incidence). Taken together, surveillance data and national estimates provide a more comprehensive epidemiological snapshot. Current data indicate that the HIV epidemic in Canada shows no sign of abating (Yang et al., 2010).

Each year, the population of people living with HIV/AIDS in Canada continues to grow. At the end of 2008, an estimated 65,000 Canadians were living with HIV/AIDS, representing a 14% increase from the prevalence estimate for 2005. Prevalence figures rise in part due to treatment developments and improved health outcomes, but are also impacted by continued levels of new infections. PHAC estimated the national incidence for 2008 in the range of 2,300 to 4,300 infections per year, which was comparable to or even slightly higher than 2005 (estimated at 2,200 to 4,200 new infections) (Yang et al., 2010). Similarly, routine surveillance data demonstrate a plateau in the number of annual HIV case reports since 2002, at around 2,500 per year (PHAC, 2010a).

WOMEN WITHIN CANADA'S HIV EPIDEMIC

From 1985 through the end of 2009, a total of 11,403 women in Canada were diagnosed and reported as HIV positive, comprising nearly 18% of all historical HIV case reports. While accounting for less than 3% of cases in 1985, the proportion of cases among women grew slowly but fairly steadily over the next 20 years, peaking at nearly 28% in 2006.

PHAC's HIV and AIDS surveillance report through the end of 2009 (Figure 1.1) depicts this converging pattern over time.

Figure 1.1: Proportion of positive HIV test reports by sex, 1985–2009

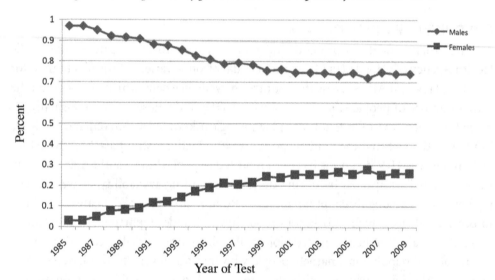

Source: Public Health Agency of Canada. (2010). *HIV and AIDS in Canada: Surveillance Report to December 31, 2009.*

A SNAPSHOT OF WOMEN LIVING WITH HIV IN CANADA

The profile of women affected by HIV is a diverse one, comprising a range of backgrounds and demographics.

Age

Of the positive HIV tests reported among adult women from 1985 through the end of 2008, nearly 75% were between the ages of 15 and 39 (PHAC, 2010b). Examining the most recent surveillance data from 2009, female HIV case reports broke down as follows: 2.2% were less than 15 years of age, 4.5% were 15–19, 25.2% were 20–29, 36.1% were 30–39, 22.2% were 40–49, and 9.8% were over the age of 50.

Surveillance data reveals a slightly different age distribution between the sexes, with women generally diagnosed at younger ages relative to men. Of all cumulative HIV case reports, 4% of female cases were within the age group of 15–19 years and 32.5% were within the age group of 20–29 years, whereas only 1% and 23.5% of male cases, respectively, fell within these same age groups. Among case reports in 2009, the highest proportions of HIV case reports among females were reported in the age groups of 20–29 and 30–39 years (25.2% and 36.1% respectively). By contrast, that same year, the largest proportion of HIV case reports among men was observed in the age group of 40–49 years (PHAC, 2010a).

The difference in age distribution of diagnosed cases of HIV by sex is perhaps most striking when examined as a proportion by age group, where the disproportionate impact of HIV on young women is clearly seen. As depicted in Figure 1.2, more than half of all HIV case reports in the age group of 15–19 years today are among women.

Figure 1.2: Proportion of positive HIV test reports that are female, by age group, 2009

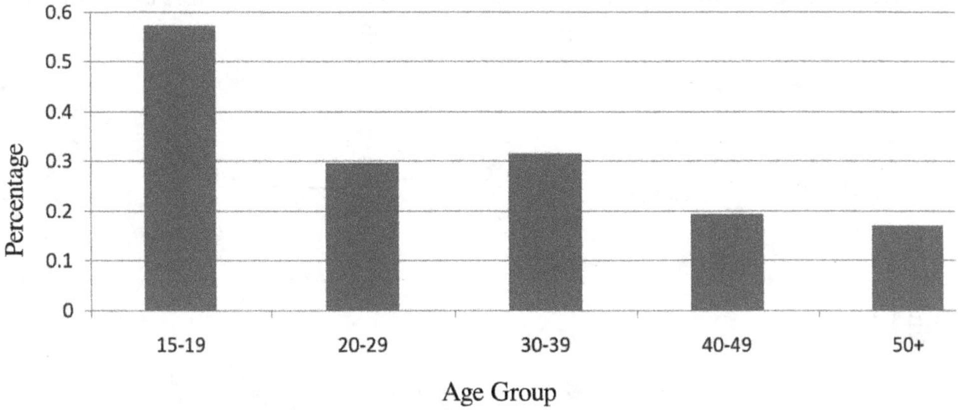

Source: Public Health Agency of Canada. (2010). *HIV and AIDS in Canada: Surveillance Report to December 31, 2009.*

Exposure Category

Historically, heterosexual contact has been the most frequently reported exposure category for all routine HIV case reports among women in Canada. In 2009, heterosexual contact accounted for 59.7% of case reports among women, and, more specifically, broke down into the following subcategories: origin from an HIV-endemic country (15%), sexual contact with a person at risk (21.6%), and no identified risk—heterosexual contact (23.1%).

In the beginning of the epidemic, injection drug use (IDU) played a significant, but minor, role in the transmission of HIV among women, as reported in routine surveillance data. From the mid-1980s to the mid-1990s, however, this exposure category grew significantly, such that IDU exceeded all other exposure categories. Peaking at over 50% in 1995, the IDU exposure category generally decreased over the next 10 years (PHAC, 2010b). In 2009, 35.4% of positive HIV test reports were attributed to IDU among women (PHAC, 2010a).

Available data reveal differences in patterns of reported exposure categories among women relative to men. One significant distinction is the role of IDU, with Canadian women experiencing a higher proportion of HIV cases attributed to this exposure category than men. Over the past decade, approximately 26–41% of all new HIV diagnoses reported among women were attributed to injection drug use, compared to approximately 14–21% for men. Surveillance data also reveals greater time-trend variation in reported exposure category for women as compared to men. For example, in the past decade, the proportion of each exposure category among adult male HIV case reports exhibited an overall plateau: the exposure category of men who have sex with men by far comprised the largest proportion of cases, and there was very little year-to-year fluctuation among the subsequent most-reported exposure categories, as illustrated in Figure 1.3.

Figure 1.3: Percentage of positive HIV test reports among adult males by exposure category, 2000–2009

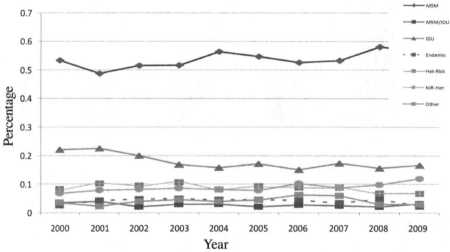

Source: Public Health Agency of Canada. (2010). *HIV and AIDS in Canada: Surveillance Report to December 31, 2009.*

By contrast, there are significant fluctuations in the exposure categories reported for adult female HIV cases over the last 10 years, and in particular the different heterosexual contact subcategories varied in the year-to-year proportion of cases they comprised. Figure 1.4 illustrates these variations.

Figure 1.4: Percentage of positive HIV test reports among adult females by exposure category, 2000–2009

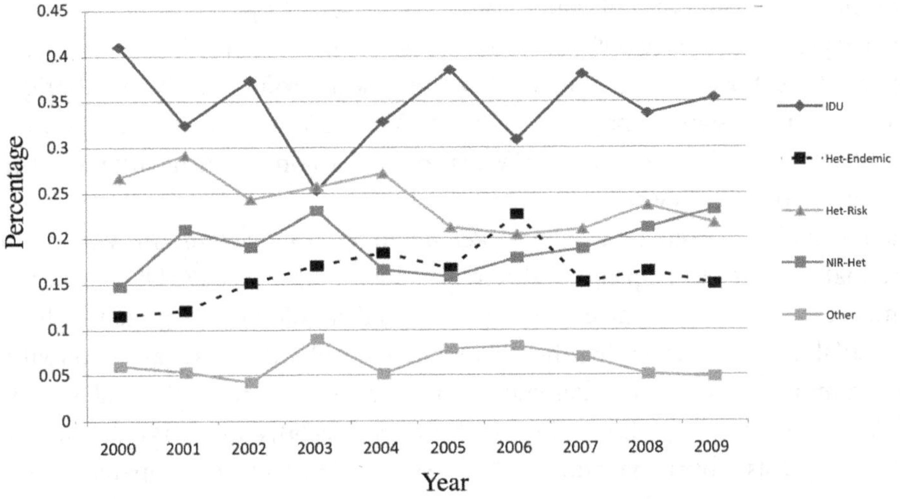

Source: Public Health Agency of Canada. (2010). *HIV and AIDS in Canada: Surveillance Report to December 31, 2009.*

Available data indicate that women who inject drugs may experience a higher risk of HIV infection than men. "I-Track," PHAC's national enhanced surveillance system that monitors risk behaviours associated with HIV and HCV among people who inject drugs, found that, at least in the sentinel sites studied in the Phase 1 report, women who inject drugs had a higher prevalence of HIV compared to men who inject drugs (PHAC, 2010e). Furthermore, women who inject drugs may also engage in more high-risk behaviours than men, such as borrowing or lending of used needles and higher numbers of sexual partners (Nelson et al., 2010).

The heterosexual contact–endemic subcategory stands out as another key exposure category in the HIV epidemic among women. Not only are women from HIV-endemic regions overrepresented in overall HIV case reports among women, but they also comprise the majority of HIV-positive tests reported within the heterosexual exposure HIV-endemic subcategory in recent years (PHAC, 2011).

Ethnicity

Due to a number of limitations in available data, the statistics on race/ethnicity may not be representative of all of Canada. In particular, it is important to note that two of Canada's largest provinces, Ontario and Quebec, do not provide race/ethnicity information on positive HIV test reports to the national level. Nevertheless, available data can help to indicate which population groups may experience greater vulnerability to HIV infection. Among women in Canada, two distinct racial/ethnic groups stand apart as being disproportionately affected by HIV: Aboriginal persons and Black persons.

Aboriginal persons

Aboriginal people continue to be overrepresented in Canada's HIV epidemic, and Aboriginal women in particular are significantly affected by HIV; from 1998–2008, women represented nearly 50% of all HIV case reports among Aboriginal people, compared to just over 20% among other ethnic/racial groups. Similarly, Aboriginal women comprise a significant proportion of HIV cases among all women in Canada. From 1998 through 2008, out of all HIV case reports among women with race/ethnicity information, 42.9% were Aboriginal.

Data on AIDS case reports can be broken down by specific community within the Aboriginal category to help reveal differences in the burden of AIDS between the communities. Although sample sizes are small and should be interpreted with caution, available data indicate that the sex breakdowns of AIDS cases are different for each community, with Inuit experiencing the highest proportion of females (40.9% of all AIDS case reports), followed by First Nations (29.9%), and Métis (19.2%). AIDS cases reported as Aboriginal, unspecified, were 27.4% female, compared to 9.1% among non-Aboriginal AIDS cases. These statistics indicate the major impact that HIV/AIDS has on Aboriginal women in Canada (PHAC, 2010d). Chapter 4 offers additional information on many of the challenges in meeting the HIV prevention needs of Aboriginal women.

Black persons

Available data indicate that women who self-identify as Black (which may include both immigrants and persons born in Canada) are also disproportionately affected by HIV. According to Statistics Canada, the Canadian population in 2006 (excluding Ontario and Quebec) was 1.0% Black, while out of all HIV case reports among women with race/ethnicity information in 2009, 14.3% were Black. By contrast, Black men comprised 6.0% of case reports among men. This trend was not unique to the year 2009: for the period 1998–2008, Black women comprised 18.8% of all HIV case reports among women with ethnic information, while Black men accounted for 6.6% of case reports among men during that same time period (PHAC, 2010b). Additional information on African, Caribbean, and Black women and HIV prevention can be found in Chapter 5.

Pregnancy and Vertical Transmission

Given that the majority of newly diagnosed HIV-positive women in Canada are of child-bearing age, it follows that perinatal exposure to HIV mirrors patterns similar to those observed among women in general. In particular, Black and Aboriginal infants are disproportionately affected. From 1984 through 2008, of all infants known to be perinatally exposed to HIV, Black infants accounted for 46.8% and Aboriginal infants accounted for 16.2% (PHAC, 2010c). According to data from the Canadian Perinatal HIV Surveillance Program, of the 75 infants confirmed to be infected with HIV in Canada during the years 2002–2009, 40 of those infants (53.3%) were Black and 17 of those infants (22.7%) were Aboriginal (PHAC, 2010a).

The number of infants perinatally exposed to HIV in Canada has increased over time. Nevertheless, the proportion of all HIV-exposed infants who become infected with HIV has decreased over the last decade. In 2001, 10.7% of all known perinatally exposed infants were confirmed as HIV positive; by 2009, that figure had dropped to 1.7%. Correspondingly, antiretroviral therapy coverage rates have steadily improved; data indicates that 91.5% of pregnant women known to be HIV positive received treatment in 2009 (PHAC, 2010a). These statistics indicate that pregnant women in Canada have gained improved access to screening and treatment; however, challenges remain, and many of these will be discussed in greater detail in Chapter 10.

GAPS AND DATA NEEDS

Surveillance data have significant limitations that must be taken into account when interpreting findings. When examining specific population groups in Canada, one of the greatest limitations is information on race and ethnicity. In particular, it is important to note that two of Canada's largest provinces, Ontario and Quebec, do not provide ethnic information on positive HIV test reports to the national level. Surveillance data has other inherent limitations, such as restricted category choices and reliance on self-reporting. Nevertheless, available data helps to indicate both the current and historical trends of HIV among women in Canada, and in particular to highlight those groups of women who experience heightened vulnerability to HIV infection.

CONCLUSION

The HIV epidemic in Canada has changed significantly since reporting first began in 1985, with women now comprising roughly 25% of all new HIV diagnoses and estimated new infections. The profile of women affected by HIV is a diverse one, consisting of a range of backgrounds and demographics. Available data indicate that women living with HIV in Canada have a significantly different profile than men living with HIV; they tend to be younger, are more likely to be exposed to HIV via heterosexual contact and injection drug use, and are also more likely to be a visible minority, especially Aboriginal or Black. These findings highlight the need for HIV prevention and related intervention strategies that are tailored, not only according to gender and/or sex, but also to the socio-demographic and behavioural diversity of women who are affected by HIV.

As HIV patterns among women in Canada continue to evolve, surveillance and research initiatives remain crucial to monitoring changing trends and to informing the development and implementation of effective prevention programs and policies.

PROBLEM-BASED LEARNING CASE STUDY

Several gaps in current surveillance data are noteworthy:

- Completeness of ethnicity data (Currently the two largest provinces, Ontario and Quebec, do not provide ethnicity data.)
- Better exposure information on heterosexual cases, including better definitions (There are currently three heterosexual subcategories.)

Problem-based learning example: The data presented suggest that women may be at risk for HIV infection through heterosexual sex with an infected male partner.

CRITICAL THINKING QUESTIONS

1. From an interdisciplinary perspective, what can be done with the data as presented to help inform HIV prevention strategies or policies for women in Canada?
2. How would this approach differ in working with diverse populations of women? Women who are street-involved? Women whose cultural beliefs may prevent them from presenting for HIV counselling and testing?

REFERENCES

Nelson, C., Martin, S., Tarasuk, J., Ogunnaike-Cooke, S., Fufe, M., Hennink, M., … Archibald, C. (2010, May). *A sex-based profile of IDU risk behaviours: Results from a national enhanced HIV surveillance system*. Paper presented at the 19th Annual Canadian Conference on HIV/AIDS Research, Saskatoon, Saskatchewan.

Public Health Agency of Canada. (2010a). *HIV and AIDS in Canada: Surveillance report to December 31, 2009*. Ottawa, ON: Surveillance and Risk Assessment Division, Centre for Communicable Diseases and Infection Control, Public Health Agency of Canada. Retrieved from www.phac-aspc.gc.ca/aids-sida/publication/survreport/2009/dec/index-eng.php

Public Health Agency of Canada. (2010b). HIV/AIDS among women in Canada. *HIV/AIDS Epi Updates, July 2010* (Chapter 5). Ottawa, ON: Surveillance and Risk Assessment Division, Centre for Communicable Diseases and Infection Control, Public Health Agency of Canada. Retrieved from www.phac-aspc.gc.ca/aids-sida/publication/epi/2010/5-eng.php

Public Health Agency of Canada. (2010c). Perinatal HIV transmission in Canada. *HIV/AIDS Epi Updates, July 2010* (Chapter 7). Ottawa, ON: Surveillance and Risk Assessment Division, Centre for Communicable Diseases and Infection Control, Public Health Agency of Canada. Retrieved from www.phac-aspc.gc.ca/aids-sida/publication/epi/2010/7-eng.php

Public Health Agency of Canada. (2010d). HIV/AIDS among Aboriginal Peoples in Canada. *HIV/AIDS Epi Updates, July 2010* (Chapter 8). Ottawa, ON: Surveillance and Risk Assessment Division, Centre for Communicable Diseases and Infection Control, Public Health Agency of Canada. Retrieved from www.phac-aspc.gc.ca/aids-sida/publication/epi/2010/8-eng.php

Public Health Agency of Canada. (2010e). HIV/AIDS among people who inject drugs in Canada. *HIV and AIDS Epi Updates, July 2010* (Chapter 10). Ottawa, ON: Surveillance and Risk Assessment Division, Centre for Communicable Diseases and Infection Control, Public Health Agency of Canada. Retrieved from www.phac-aspc.gc.ca/aids-sida/publication/epi/2010/10-eng.php

Public Health Agency of Canada. (2011). HIV/AIDS among people from HIV-endemic countries. *HIV/AIDS Epi Updates* (Chapter 13). Ottawa, ON: Surveillance and Risk Assessment Division, Centre for Communicable Diseases and Infection Control, Public Health Agency of Canada.

Yang, Q., Boulos, D., Yan, P., Zhang, F., Remis, R. S., Schanzer, D., & Archibald, C. P. (2010). Estimates of the number of prevalent and incident human immunodeficiency virus (HIV) infections in Canada, 2008. *Canadian Journal of Public Health*, *101*(6), 486–490.

Chapter 2
AN OVERVIEW OF DETERMINANTS OF HEALTH IMPACTING WOMEN AND HIV INFECTION IN CANADA

Jacqueline Arthur, Kristen Beausoleil,
Jocelyne Guay, and Jacqueline Gahagan

INTRODUCTION

Women's health is influenced by a complex interplay of factors and determinants of health that intersect to impact on women's health outcomes, including HIV infection. The various intersections among these factors, including those at the broader social and economic levels and those at the micro or individual levels, play a combined role in health (Public Health Agency of Canada [PHAC], n.d.). This chapter offers an overview of the various factors and determinants of health that impact on HIV infection among women in Canada.

The Determinants of Health

- Gender
- Biology and Genetic Endowment
- Education
- Social Status, Employment, and Income
- Social Environments and Social Support Networks
- Physical Environments
- Personal Health Practices and Coping Skills
- Healthy Child Development
- Health Services
- Culture and Race

GENDER

Unlike biological sex, gender refers to the socially determined roles, personality traits, attitudes, behaviours, values, and relative power and influence that society ascribes to the two sexes on a differential basis. "Gendered norms" influence the health system's practices and priorities, making health issues a function of gender-based social status (PHAC, n.d.). As a result, the social constructs of gender and sexuality (e.g., masculine and feminine roles, responsibilities, the gendered division of labour, status, and power) all play a role in HIV infection (Interagency Coalition on AIDS and Development [ICAD], 2003; United Nations Development Fund for Women [UNIFEM], 2001; World Health Organization [WHO], 2009). Emerging data on transgender populations suggest that they are at heightened risk of HIV infection due to the structural factors that reinforce a bi-gendered culture (Namaste, 1998, 2010). The intersecting nature of sex, gender, race, sexual orientation, age, class, and disability impacts how individuals negotiate health through intrapersonal, interpersonal, community, and institutional mechanisms. While gender is a determinant of health in its own right, its intersection with and influence on other determinants of health increases the vulnerabilities for women.

Gender has a profound impact on women's vulnerability to HIV, and gender inequality has been a "key driver" in the female HIV/AIDS epidemic worldwide (WHO, 2009). The two most common exposure categories for HIV transmission for women in Canada, heterosexual sex and injection drug use (IDU), involve risk behaviour related to the power relationships and inequalities between genders. Gendered roles of masculinity and femininity may support a stereotyped sexuality, whereby gendered norms associated with masculinity may encourage men to have multiple sexual partners (either concurrent or not), and encourage men to have sexual relationships with younger women (UNIFEM, 2001). Stereotypes around what constitutes "masculine" behaviour may result in men hiding sexual relationships with other men and also make them reluctant to access health services (ICAD, 2003; UNIFEM, 2001).

Conversely, gendered norms around femininity may encourage sexual innocence, ignorance, passivity, meekness, and submissiveness in women, resulting in women's increased vulnerability and dependence on sexual partners (ICAD, 2003; McPhedran & Bazilli, 2006; UNIFEM, 2001; Wingood & DiClemente, 2000; WHO, 2009). Gendered norms may also contribute to women's inability to negotiate safer sex practices and increase their risk of sexual assault. These gendered norms can be exacerbated when women are involved in survival or street-level sex work, as money further distorts the balance of power, causing unequal relationships between women and their clients. Gendered norms lie at the root of all of these behaviours, and they facilitate HIV exposure and transmission in women. Recent literature has also identified a strong association between requiring help injecting and HIV seroconversion in women who use injection drugs (O'Connell et al., 2005; Spittal et al., 2002; Tompkins, Sheard, Wright, Jones, & Howes, 2006; Wood et al., 2003); thus, an injection-dependent relationship exists between injection drug-using women and men, effectively limiting women's power and control over drug preparation, needles, and injecting.

BIOLOGY AND GENETIC ENDOWMENT

Biology and genetic endowment influence women's risk of HIV transmission, treatment outcomes, disease progression, and comorbidities. The risk of contracting HIV through penile-vaginal intercourse, for example, is greater for women than it is for men (Clow, 2005; Hope, 2008; Hope, Trull, McCoombe, McRaven, & Veazey, 2008; UNAIDS, 2008). Male-to-female HIV transmission has been shown to be two to four times higher than female-to-male HIV transmission (Canadian AIDS Society [CAS], 2000). Unprotected penile-anal intercourse is also considered to be of higher risk for HIV transmission than penile-vaginal intercourse; yet, penile-anal intercourse is rarely reflected in the literature in the context of heterosexual HIV exposure or sexually transmitted infections (STIs) (Bruckner & Bearman, 2005; DesMeules et al., 2004; Lescano et al., 2008). Some research shows that 5.6% of girls 15–17 years of age had had heterosexual anal intercourse, with the percentage increasing to 29.6% of women 20–24 years of age (Mosher, Chandra, & Jones, 2005). Data suggest, moreover, that condom use may not be consistent with anal sex (Lescano et al., 2008).

Impact of HIV Treatment on Women Living with HIV

Because women living with HIV are often under-represented in clinical trials of highly active antiretroviral therapy (HAART) (Boulassel, Morales, Murphy, Lalonde, & Klein, 2006; Squires, 2007), the full impact of treatment is unknown and may pose health risks to or impede the care of women living with HIV. One study comparing the side effects of HAART in women and men found that metabolic toxicities associated with treatment occur more frequently in women than men (Boulassel et al., 2006). Another study found higher levels of toxicity associated with nevirapine-based HAART in pregnant women living with HIV compared to those who took non-nevirapine-based HAART (Schalkwyk et al., 2008). These findings contributed to an international review of the drug for use in pregnant women living with HIV.

EDUCATION

Women with limited education, language skills, or both are hindered in their ability to access HIV prevention and treatment information and understand the information they receive (Atlantic Centre for Excellence in Women's Health, 2003; Gardezi et al., 2008; Tharao, Massaquoi, & Teclom, 2006; Williams, Newman, Sakamoto, & Massaquoi, 2009). When combined with abuse, lack of economic opportunity, and experiences with the child welfare system, limited education and language skills make certain groups of women, such as Aboriginal women, more vulnerable to sexual exploitation (Sikka, 2009) and, as a result, to infections such as HIV.

SOCIAL STATUS, EMPLOYMENT, AND INCOME

Low income and poverty can be associated with increased risk of HIV infection and disease progression (PHAC, 2010a). Women who are involved in less stable work and part-time jobs earn less than males and are required to do more unpaid labour than men (DesMeules et al., 2004; Spitzer, 2005). Unpaid labour and the unequal impact of poverty on women are manifest in dependent relationships, an inability to acquire stable housing (homelessness), and participation in survival sex work (Clow, 2005; Robertson, L., 2007; Csete, 2004).

Vulnerable Female Populations

Certain groups of women fall on the outer lower edges of the socio-economic hierarchy. Aboriginal women and racial minority women, for example, are faced with the double discriminatory effects of gender inequality and racial inequality, which impacts their socio-economic status (Newman, Williams, Massaquoi, Brown, & Logie, 2008; PHAC, 2009, 2010a). Studies show that male-to-female transgender persons also deal with multiple layers of discrimination and generally earn less than the overall population (Bauer et al., 2010; Scanlon, Bauer, Kaay, & Boyce, 2009).

Women involved in street-level sex work are one of the most vulnerable groups in Canadian society. Laws and social attitudes regarding sex work may prevent women involved in such work from accessing services, such as policing and health care, and may also subject them to acts of violence, robbery, or abuse (Betteridge, 2005; Csete, 2005; Mar & Betteridge, 2007). Street-level sex workers' desire to practise HIV prevention may be undermined by societal and personal factors, such as gendered power differentials, a history of sexual abuse, violence and discrimination, age, drug or alcohol dependencies, mental health issues, and homelessness. These factors can significantly diminish women's ability to negotiate condom use (Betteridge, 2005; Boivin, Roy, Haley, & du-Fort, 2005; Csete, 2005; Frappier, Paradis, & Roy, 2007; Mc-Keown, Reid, & Orr, 2004; McKeown, Reid, Orr, & Turner, 2006; Miller et al., 2002; Shannon, Bright, Duddy, & Tyndall, 2005; Shannon et al., 2008; Weber, Boivin, Blais, Haley, & Roy, 2004).

Income of Women Living with HIV

Women with low incomes or who live below the poverty line are at greater risk of disease progression from HIV to AIDS (Bauer et al., 2009; "Christina," 2008). Women living with HIV/AIDS face additional financial concerns related to travel to and from health services, treatment costs, time off from work, and fear of employment loss. Many single mothers living with HIV/AIDS have the added stress of ensuring adequate daycare support and coping with poverty (Barkey, Watanabe, Solomon, & Wilkins, 2009; Maggi & Daly, 2006). Single parents from Aboriginal and ethnic communities are especially vulnerable, because they make up a high number of people living in low income situations (DeMatteo, 2002).

According to a British Columbia study, risk factors for inadequate food security and hunger include being female, having a low income, having a low education, and being Aboriginal (Normen et al., 2005). Other risk factors include living with children, having a history of injection drug and alcohol use, and unstable housing (Normen et al., 2005). The study emphasizes the important role proper nutrition plays in the lives of women living with HIV, particularly in the case of single mothers with lower incomes.

SOCIAL ENVIRONMENTS AND SOCIAL SUPPORT NETWORKS

Social environments are largely created by gender and cultural norms that shape how women engage with society and how, in return, society engages with women. Gendered power dynamics ingrained in our social fabric are reflected in women's vulnerability to, or resilience against, HIV acquisition.

Violence and Abuse

A lack of social power makes women vulnerable to acts of men's violence. Research shows that the consequences of men's violence against women—whether sexual, emotional, or physical—include diminished self-esteem and sense of security, and damage to physical and emotional health. Men's violence against women also negatively impacts women's financial security and may result in women's self-blame and loss of the matrimonial home. Some studies strongly associate repeated physical and sexual violence with a positive HIV test report (Medjuck, 2009; Prentice, 2005).

The Vancouver Injection Drug User Survey (VIDUS) cohort reported that 68.6% of the 503 female participants had experienced sexual violence, with 53.4% revealing that the age of the first incident was 12 years or less. The prevalence of HIV among those who experienced sexual violence was higher than among those who had not, indicating that individuals who have experienced sexual violence are at greater risk of HIV infection (Braitstein et al., 2003). Similarly, the Cedar Project (2008) found that 69% of women had experienced some form of sexual abuse at least once in their lifetime. Other research on a cohort of women who use injection drugs in Vancouver found that "[y]oung [HIV] seropositive participants were more likely to be female, to work in the commercial sex trade, to have experienced sexual abuse, to have had more than 20 lifetime sexual partners, to inject heroin and speedballs at least daily, and to use crack cocaine at least daily" (Miller et al., 2002).

According to Statistics Canada (2005), Aboriginal women are three times more likely to experience intimate male partner violence than non-Aboriginal women. Twenty-four percent of Aboriginal women said that they experienced violence from a current or previous spouse or common-law partner in the five-year period leading up to 2004. This is significantly higher than the 7% of non-Aboriginal women in Canada who reported experiencing violence during the same period. According to the Native Women's Association of Canada (2008), "the ongoing effects of colonization in Canada have led to the dehumanization of Aboriginal women and girls and [the Native Women's Association of Canada] considers this to be a root cause of the violence [Aboriginal women] experience." One additional study on

Aboriginal women found a link between sexual violence and their initiation into sex work (Sikka, 2009).

Black women, including women who come from countries where HIV is endemic, may also experience heightened levels of violence. In many African and African-Caribbean cultures, for example, underlying issues of violence are never discussed within the family or community. The few girls or women who come forward often face stigma and reprisal from family for speaking out and seeking support (James, 2006).

Moreover, girls, young women, people living with disabilities, and lesbian, gay, bisexual, and transgender people are often targeted for physical and sexual victimization. Girls and women are disproportionately affected regardless of their country of origin, culture, social class, religion, or ethnic group. Their ability to practise HIV prevention may be affected by the aftermath of sexual violence (e.g., depression, loss of value, loss of sense of well-being) (James, 2006). Ultimately, men's violence against women and children, whether sexual or physical, has a direct impact on the ability of women and children to practise HIV prevention (James, 2006).

Fear of Disclosure

Studies show that some women are reluctant to disclose their status to their partners for fear of reprisals (i.e., abuse or abandonment) (Beauregard & Solomon, 2005; De-Matteo, 2002; Medjuck, 2009). Many African and Caribbean women living with HIV fear disclosing their status to their partners because of ethnocultural assumptions that link HIV/AIDS to promiscuity; thus, disclosure may lead to social stigma or physical harm and abandonment by a partner, who may in turn prevent them from seeking health services for fear of reprisal from community members (Beauregard & Solomon, 2005). In addition, fear of disclosure has kept many women from African and Caribbean communities from accessing health services and from establishing contacts with other HIV-positive women (Tharao et al., 2006).

Disclosure is considered one of the most difficult aspects of living with HIV in Aboriginal communities because of the resulting stigma, discrimination, and feelings of being ostracized (Prentice, 2004).[1] Discrimination against Aboriginal women living with HIV is compounded as gender discrimination adds to the stigma they experience (Prentice, 2004; Ship & Norton, 2002). An Aboriginal woman living with HIV/AIDS may be branded as promiscuous, a "bad mother," or "deserving of HIV/AIDS" if she discloses her HIV-positive test result to community members (Ship & Norton, 2002).

Social Exclusion

Social exclusion involves "disintegration from common cultural processes, lack of participation in societal activities, alienation from decision-making and civic participation, and barriers to employment and material resources" (Reid, 2003). It limits women's power and choices regarding health, health services, social capital, and equity. Examples of exclusion are particularly pervasive in the lives of women who already experience other forms of discrimination, such as heterosexism, homophobia, transphobia, or racism.

Women who have sex with women (WSW) are believed to be at increased risk of HIV due to their participation in behaviours that may result from social exclusion. Studies report that growing up in a heterosexist and homophobic environment can enhance WSW's isolation and exclusion, and may potentially foster risk behaviours such as injection drug use and sexual experimentation (Gilliam, 2001; Hughes & Evans, 2003; Remez, 2001; Saewyc et al., 2006).

Sex workers also face increased vulnerability to HIV as a result of factors linked to their social exclusion. For example, laws and society's attitudes stigmatize sex work, thereby limiting sex workers' access to services and health care for fear of discrimination. Further, difficult working conditions reduce sex workers' ability to negotiate and enforce safer sex behaviours. This has the effect of increasing sex workers' susceptibility to violence and coercion (Robitaille, 2010).

Being transgender has also been identified as a factor that increases women's HIV risk behaviour (Bauer et al., 2009). Trans women's vulnerability to HIV infection increases for those who also identify as Aboriginal, immigrant, young, or who are involved in sex work.

Racism and discrimination leave groups of people particularly vulnerable to HIV infection by excluding them from the social and economic mainstream, and by denying them the social supports needed to enhance and preserve life (Martin Spigelman Research Associates, 2002). Studies show that Black women's experience of racism intersects with other issues, such as gender, sexual orientation, and socio-economic status, and results in a level of social exclusion that elevates their risk of HIV infection and compounds their inability to cope with the disease (Gardezi et al., 2008; Robertson, S., 2007; Tharao et al., 2006). Thus, Black women's risk of HIV infection cannot simply be attributed to individual behaviour.

Aboriginal women also feel the effects of racism and social exclusion. The complex vulnerabilities that Aboriginal women face stem from the legacy of colonization and the multi-generational effects of social isolation, discrimination, entrenched poverty, and the residential school system (Prentice, 2005; Shannon et al., 2008).

Women's Support Groups
Support groups may be a source of resilience for women living with HIV, encouraging and inspiring them; such groups can even act as alternative communities (Beauregard & Solomon, 2005; Lawson et al., 2006; Ndlovu et al., 2009; Solomon & Wilkins, 2008). A Vancouver-based study of female sex workers who use illicit substances found that peer-driven interventions positively affect HAART adherence for this population (Deering et al., 2009). Another study reveals that seropositive mothers rely on the support of family,

friends, and professionals (DeMatteo, 2002). Other studies show that a supportive network is a valuable asset for women living with HIV (Beauregard & Solomon, 2005; Ndlovu et al., 2009). Respondents in these studies explain that feeling supported is important to helping them cope with the everyday experience of living with HIV/AIDS.

PHYSICAL ENVIRONMENTS
Unstable Housing and Homelessness
Studies illustrate the relationship between homelessness, low income and socio-economic status, and HIV risk behaviour (Shannon et al., 2005; Shannon, Bright, Gibson, & Tyndall, 2007). Urban areas with concentrated homeless populations encourage black market economies with ties to HIV risk behaviour, such as theft, sex work, and drug trafficking. However, even under poor socio-economic conditions, neighbourhoods can reduce HIV risk behaviour by addressing the underlying issues related to the physical environment by providing increased access to stable housing. As one study suggests, "stable housing could make a critical difference in a woman's ability to escape violence [and] remain safe" (Borwein et al., 2009).

Another study of street-involved women who inject drugs and who are involved in sex work in two Canadian cities (Montreal and Vancouver) found that more women involved in sex work had unstable housing than those who were not involved in sex work (Spittal et al., 2003). This same study also reported that the practice of borrowing used syringes was found to be independently associated with the sex trade. These types of studies clearly illustrate the relationship between homelessness, low income and socio-economic status, and HIV risk behaviour.

Another study examining housing insecurity and health among people living with HIV across Ontario found higher rates of homelessness among women living with HIV (12.7%) than among men living with HIV (5.6%) (Tucker, 2009; Tucker et al., 2009). One-third of the study's female respondents reported having been homeless at least once in their lifetime, and women living with HIV were more concerned about unstable housing than men living with HIV—this was especially true for HIV-positive women living with children (78% of women living with HIV in the cohort reported living with children). Women living with HIV also reported higher rates of depression and lower overall mental health scores than male participants.

By contrast, housing security has been shown to impact women's well-being. One study found that the quality of life of women from African and Caribbean communities was improved by living in affordable housing (Aryee, 2009). Certain factors have also been shown to shape the meaning and experience of "home" for women. For instance, one study that examined the housing needs and experiences of African and Caribbean mothers living with HIV in Toronto found that this group's housing experience was influenced by factors relating to racism, gender, and poverty. Findings from this study highlight the need for culturally appropriate supportive housing services for this group of women and their children (Greene et al., 2009).

Rural and Remote Environments

Women living in rural and remote areas may be unable to access accurate HIV risk information, care, or related services. Some studies have also found that women in rural or remote areas mistakenly associate HIV with "urban" populations or behaviours, which they perceive themselves as not belonging to or participating in (Atlantic Centre for Excellence in Women's Health, 2003; Bulman, 2005). Qualitative research conducted in the Maritimes suggested that isolation from urban centres has left many women with only a partial understanding of the facts surrounding HIV. Respondents in this study viewed HIV/AIDS as a disease affecting men who have sex with men (MSM), or as a disease affecting people living in other countries (Bulman, 2005).

Many Aboriginal people face unique risks and barriers to good health as a result of the geographic isolation of their communities.[2] Aboriginal people living in remote communities may believe that their location offers protection from HIV infection (Jackson & Reimer, 2008; Tenenbein, 2008). A study of 262 young street-involved Aboriginal women found that there were few differences in terms of HIV risk behaviour (e.g., participation in sex work, injection drug use) experienced by those living in a large urban centre (Vancouver, B.C.) versus those living in a smaller northern city (Prince George, B.C.) (Mehrabadi, Craib, et al., 2008). A study of the migration patterns of First Nations people from reserve communities to urban centres also indicates that issues associated with HIV/AIDS and related risk behaviours, including illicit drug use, are not limited to urban centres (Callaghan, Tavares, & Taylor, 2007). Aboriginal women who live in remote and isolated communities may also experience decreased access to health and social services (Jackson & Reimer, 2008), which may also contribute to the vulnerability of women at risk of and living with HIV/AIDS (Mehrabadi, Craib et al., 2008). Consequently, this group of women may experience two forms of isolation, with the first being diminished position within their communities as a result of discrimination linked to their positive HIV serostatus, and the second, limited access to services and support as a result of their remote geographic location.

Federal and Provincial/Territorial Prisons

Women in prison are at increased risk of HIV infection when compared with the general population. HIV prevalence among females in federal prisons is significantly higher than that in the general population, and HIV prevalence among females in federal prisons is higher than the HIV prevalence among males in federal prisons (Zakaria, Thompson, Jarvis, & Borgatta, 2010). Some women in prison continue to engage in many of the same risk behaviours that they engaged in prior to incarceration, such as drug use, needle sharing, unprotected sex, and sharing of tattooing equipment (Calzavara et al., 2007; Canadian HIV/AIDS Legal Network, 2008; Rehman, Gahagan, DiCenso, & Dias, 2004; Zakaria et al., 2010).

In 2007, the following three health education programs were available to individuals in federal prisons: the Reception Awareness Program, the Choosing Health in Prisons

Program, and the National HIV/AIDS Peer Education and Counselling Program (Zakaria et al., 2010). Findings from Correctional Service of Canada's 2007 National Inmate Infectious Diseases and Risk Behaviours Survey revealed that more women than men participated in these programs. However, in spite of higher participation rates among women, women in prison also reported that their access to these programs was limited by a lack of awareness, limited space, and competing clinical demands on nursing staff (Zakaria et al., 2010). In addition, while the vast majority of women in the survey cited no difficulty in accessing bleach to reduce infection risk in federal prisons for the purpose of harm reduction (72%), 28% of women nonetheless reported concerns relating to access.[3]

Other studies have also found that women in prisons face difficulty in accessing other harm reduction supplies and health services and/or programs, despite their availability (Burchell et al., 2003; Canadian HIV/AIDS Legal Network, 2007; McCoy, 2005; Rehman et al., 2004). Only 30% of women living with HIV (and/or HCV) reported receiving support from community-based organizations (DiCenso, Dias, & Gahagan, 2003). Moreover, while the majority of respondents described having had positive experiences in accessing community-based organizations while in prison, 34% reported having had problems (DiCenso et al., 2003). Access to educational material on reducing risk has also been reported as lacking in prisons (Canadian HIV/AIDS Legal Network, 2007; Rehman et al., 2004).

PERSONAL HEALTH PRACTICES AND COPING SKILLS

When women lack the power to make decisions about personal health practices and coping skills, they are more vulnerable to HIV infection. This is especially true for women struggling with sexual and reproductive health issues and issues around substance use.

Sexual Health

Women face increased risk of HIV infection when they lack the power to negotiate safer sex in intimate relationships. When coupled with the fear of male partner violence, it may impact women's ability to make choices, such as the ability to negotiate condom use. Moreover, women who do not perceive themselves to be at risk for HIV or other STIs may not be concerned with using condoms regularly (Williams et al., 2009). For example, condom use is much more common among younger generations. One survey revealed that people over the age of 40 years were less likely to use a condom (Adrien, Leaune, Dassa, & Perron, 2001). This may be explained by the fact that HIV prevention campaigns tend to target women in younger age groups.

National data on condom usage among sex workers vary (Jackson, Sowinski, Bennett, & Ryan, 2005; Mehrabadi, Craib, et al., 2008; PHAC, 2006; Shannon et al., 2005; Spittal et al., 2003; Weber, Boivin, Blais, Haley, & Roy, 2002). However, the majority of findings indicate that women involved in sex work are less likely to use a condom with their regular partners, which may contribute to sex workers' vulnerability to HIV. A recent study attributed sex workers' inability to negotiate condom use to fear of client aggression and to language barriers (especially for migrant sex workers) (Johnston, Fast, Moon, & Bungay, 2009). Nonetheless, a recent meta-analysis suggests that peer interventions can increase condom use among sex workers and their clients and may serve to empower sex workers to refuse clients without a condom (Logie & Newman, 2009).

Women need HIV prevention strategies that they can initiate themselves. The female condom currently exists but is often overlooked in preventing the spread of HIV infection. While there are disadvantages associated with the female condom, such as cost and aesthetics, it is the only effective non-pharmaceutical women-controlled barrier for preventing the acquisition or transmission of STIs including HIV (Kaler, 2004a, 2004b).

Substance Use

Substance use may increase women's vulnerability to HIV as a direct result of ways in which substances are administered (e.g., injecting drugs with contaminated needles), or more indirectly as a result of the physical, mental, and economic effects of dependency. Many women cite being introduced to substances through a spouse or common-law partner (Canadian Centre on Substance Abuse [CCSA], 2008). The literature also indicates that many people use substances as a mechanism for coping with childhood sexual, emotional, or physical abuse, and with stress, violence, isolation, neglect, and other mental health issues (CCSA, 2008; Cedar Project Partnership et al., 2008; DesMeules et al., 2004; Miller, Strathdee, Kerr, Li, & Wood, 2006; Poole & Dell, 2005; Spittal, 2006; Vancouver Area Network of Drug Users [VANDU] Women Care Team, 2009).

Being under the influence of substances can impair women's judgment and decision-making ability and cause them to choose behaviours that put them at risk for HIV infection. Alcohol may lower inhibitions around safer sex and condom negotiation (Anderson, 2002; First Nations Information Governance Committee, 2007; Gahagan & Rehman, 2004; Leonard, 2007). Similarly, crystal methamphetamine is said to lead to increased risk of HIV infection "through unprotected and uninhibited sex while under the influence" (CAS, 2004). The disorienting effect of other street drugs may also place women who use them at risk.

Injection drug use has been identified as a risk behaviour for HIV infection because it can put a user in direct contact with contaminated injection equipment and preparation paraphernalia. Injection drug use is the second most common HIV exposure category for females in Canada (PHAC, 2010b). According to the I-Track Study (PHAC, 2006), cocaine is the most commonly injected illicit drug in Canada. In 2009, the Canadian Centre on Substance Abuse estimated that between 75,000 and 125,000 Canadians use injection drugs; women were estimated to account for approximately one-third of those users (2009). Women are also more likely to share injection equipment than men (Bruneau et al., 2001).

The dependencies that addictions can create—and specifically dependencies related to drugs such as crack, cocaine, and heroin—can further exacerbate women's vulnerability to HIV infection. The need to support drug habits has been cited as a possible reason women enter sex work and engage in survival sex (British Columbia Centre of Excellence for Women's Health, 2010; O'Connell et al., 2005; Spittal et al., 2002).

Moreover, much of the literature available on women who use injection drugs suggests an overrepresentation of Aboriginal women in this population (PHAC, 2006; Spittal et al., 2003; Spittal et al., 2002). Nearly two-thirds of Aboriginal women with positive HIV test reports are exposed through injection drug use, with only one-third exposed via heterosexual sex; in contrast, approximately two-thirds of non-Aboriginal women with positive HIV test reports are exposed through heterosexual sex and one-third are exposed through injection drug use (PHAC, 2007, 2008).

HEALTHY CHILD DEVELOPMENT
Childhood Abuse

Some studies show that childhood physical, emotional, or sexual abuse may contribute to risk behaviours in later life, and thus increase vulnerability to HIV. Sexual violence in childhood was predictive of HIV risk behaviours, such as entering the sex trade at or before age 17, ever having been in the sex trade, and borrowing needles from a known HIV-positive person (Braitstein et al., 2003). Various studies have found that many women involved in sex work (or survival sex) and many women who use injection drugs have histories of abuse and sexual abuse (Bucharski, 2006; Cedar Project Partnership et al., 2008; Frappier et al., 2007; McKeown, Reid, Turner, & Orr, 2002; Mehrabadi, Craib, et al., 2008; Mehrabadi, Paterson, et al., 2008). In a study of street-level sex workers, 82% of participants reported a history of childhood sexual abuse by an average of four perpetrators, 72% of participants reported physical abuse, and 86% of participants reported current or past homelessness (Farley, Lynne, & Cotton, 2005). While this study indicates that a relationship exists between childhood abuse and sex work, it should be emphasized that not all women who are abused become involved in the sex industry and not all sex workers are or have been abused.

For many Aboriginal Peoples, the legacy of residential schools and cultural disruption has resulted in family breakdown and contributed to childhood sexual abuse and the overrepresentation of Aboriginal children in state care (Canadian Aboriginal AIDS Network [CAAN], 2009; Cedar Project Partnerhip et al., 2008; McKeown et al., 2002; Mehrabadi, Paterson, et al., 2008; National Clearinghouse on Family Violence, 2008). Aboriginal youths' current experiences are strongly impacted by a loss of culture, historical trauma, and the legacy of residential schooling. This issue is explored in greater depth in the *Population-Specific HIV/AIDS Status Report: Aboriginal Peoples* (PHAC, 2010a).

HEALTH SERVICES

Health services constitute a continuum of care that includes treatment and secondary prevention (Federal, Provincial and Territorial Advisory Committee on Population Health, 1999). The World Health Organization's report on gender inequity in health observes that women require more health services than men (2007). Nonetheless, many women in Canada face barriers to accessing mainstream health services. Barriers facing women include a lack of available information in languages other than English or French (Atlantic Centre for Excellence in Women's Health, 2003; Tebeje & Teffera, 2009; Tharao et al., 2006), logistical barriers, such as limited access to child care or child-friendly services for mothers accessing the health care system, and stigmatization by health professionals. Ultimately, these barriers to diagnostic care and treatment services increase women's vulnerability to HIV infection.

Women from visible minority groups and certain ethnocultural communities face additional barriers, including racism, a lack of cultural understanding among health professionals, and a lack of culturally appropriate health services and health information (Atlantic Centre for Excellence in Women's Health, 2003; Gardezi et al., 2008; Hawkins, Peltier, Barlow, Reading, & Weiman, 2009; Lawson et al., 2006; Women's Health in Women's Hands Community Health Centre, 2003). Studies show that Aboriginal women face particular challenges resulting from HIV-related discrimination, challenges in accessing current health information, and inadequate referral resources for HIV-positive women (Gahagan et al., 2009; Hawkins et al., 2009).

Immigrant women with little to no fluency in English or French may experience additional barriers to health information. Some community-based organizations offer translation services; however, many women from African and Caribbean communities do not use these services because of concerns regarding the confidentiality of their HIV-positive status (especially when the translator belongs to their community), as well as concerns regarding translation accuracy (especially when the translator is their partner) (Tharao et al., 2006). Thus, when women rely on community members or partners for translation, they run the risk of being stigmatized by their community or partner; but if they choose not to use translators, they may not receive adequate health information.[4]

A woman's sexual orientation may also affect her access to health services because health care providers may make false assumptions about risk activity based on sexual orientation. Research shows that some health care providers falsely assume that WSW (including women who self-identify as lesbian, bisexual, or two-spirit) are not at risk of HIV. This assumption does not account for the fact that many WSW have had or continue to have sexual contact with men, and it demonstrates a general lack of knowledge about WSW and their health care needs (Bell, Ompad, & Sherman, 2006; Hughes & Evans, 2003; Mathieson, Bailey, & Gurevich, 2002).

In fact, WSW may face increased vulnerability to HIV due to a number of factors related to their ability to cope and their comfort in accessing health services. WSW are reported to have higher rates of mental health issues and poorer coping strategies compared to heterosexual women (Hughes & Evans, 2003). Further, WSW report experiencing barriers to adequate health care as a result of the heterosexist and homophobic health care environment (Mathieson et al., 2002). Fear of discrimination by health care providers may prompt some WSW to avoid seeking care. In a study of 98 lesbian and bisexual women living in the Atlantic provinces, 38% of participants reported that they had gone without routine physical or mental health care at least once due to their sexual orientation (Mathieson et al., 2002).

Academic HIV/AIDS literature explains that the manner in which health care is delivered plays a role in the poor health outcomes experienced by certain groups of women (Singh, Gill, & Houston, 2005). Studies have shown that in order to reach particularly vulnerable female populations, such as street-involved women or women involved in survival sex, population-specific strategies, such as outreach programs, are needed to increase access to services (Rusch et al., 2008; Marshall, Charles, Hare, Ponzetti, & Stokl, 2005). A study in Vancouver's Downtown Eastside found that 14% of 126 women attending a weekly women-only community health clinic had not accessed sexual health care services (e.g., Pap smear, STI or HIV testing) in the past year (Rusch et al., 2008). These findings were notable because clients who presented with STIs were first-time program participants (Rusch et al., 2008).

Women living with HIV may also experience barriers around access to health services related to health care providers' insensitivity or ignorance about HIV/AIDS. Evidence also shows that women involved in commercial sex work are significantly affected by stigma and discrimination in their interaction with health care providers, and some evidence suggests that they may not disclose their high-risk activities to them (Bright et al., 2004; Rodrigues, Nguyen, Neff, Venne, & Boulianne, 2004; VANDU Women Care Team, 2009).

HIV Testing

Ensuring that people undergo HIV testing is a key component in reducing the spread of HIV and ensuring access to medical care for those who are HIV positive. At the end of 2008, an estimated 26% of the 65,000 individuals living with HIV in Canada were unaware of their infection (PHAC, 2008). Canadian literature indicates that women-specific barriers to HIV testing include the belief—of either the individual or the health care provider—that women are not at risk of HIV infection. Women-specific barriers to testing also include fear of HIV-related stigma and discrimination (Martin et al., 2005); fear of losing one's children by revealing HIV-related risk behaviours, such as illegal drug use (Bucharski, 2006); and fear of an HIV-positive test result (Bucharski, 2006). Some studies have found that certain groups of women experience additional and specific barriers to testing. For example, Aboriginal women in rural and remote locations and minority women have difficulty accessing diagnosis and testing services (Bornovalova, Gwadz, Kahler, Aklin, & Lejuez, 2008). Similarly, women engaged in sex work—especially migrant women—have noted challenges in accessing HIV education and testing (Johnston et al., 2009).

Some studies have also looked at women's experiences with HIV testing more generally. One study looked at HIV testing experiences for women who immigrated to Canada. Participants negatively described the HIV testing they received as part of the immigration medical examination (IME)—a required part of the immigration process (Rubin, Tharao, Ndlovu, & Muchenje, 2009). Another study revealed that women from countries where HIV is endemic were reluctant to learn their HIV status when going through the immigration process for fear that their children would be taken as a result (Tharao et al., 2006). Fear that one's children could be taken away was also identified as a significant barrier to HIV testing in a study of HIV-positive mothers of Aboriginal ancestry (Ship & Norton, 2002) and a study of young HIV-positive mothers (Jones & Sargeant, 2008).

CULTURE AND RACE

Canadian epidemiological data indicate that Aboriginal women and women from countries where HIV is endemic experience higher rates of HIV infection than women belonging to other groups. Evidence shows that factors linked to culture and race put women who belong to these ethnocultural groups at increased vulnerability to HIV infection. For women belonging to specific ethnocultural communities, culture may be experienced in two ways: first, via the customs, values, practices, and beliefs within their community; and, second, via the impact of the dominant culture on their lives as women within their community (Bucharski, 2006). Factors related to culture may have the effect of limiting women's access to health care. However, factors related to culture can also play a significant role in creating resilience to HIV/AIDS as women's strength and coping mechanisms may be rooted in their community values or linked to their culture.

The legacy of colonialism continues to have adverse effects on the socio-economic status of Aboriginal women because they are twice as likely as non-Aboriginal women to be poor, and more likely than non-Aboriginal women to live in an environment with substance use and intimate male partner violence (Prentice, 2004). These socio-economic conditions are strongly associated with a positive HIV test result in Aboriginal women because they set the stage for high-risk behaviours, such as sex work, injection drug use, and alcohol abuse (Csete, 2005; Prentice, 2004; Ship & Norton, 2002). Racist and sexist attitudes within mainstream society also put Aboriginal women at greater risk of sexual violence and sexual assault, thereby intensifying their vulnerability to HIV infection (Native Women's Association of Canada, 2007).

One study revealed that the integration of Aboriginal cultures into HIV testing approaches is key to gaining Aboriginal women's trust. Aboriginal women explained that culturally appropriate approaches such as "sensitivity to and knowledge of the issues that Aboriginal women may experience, inclusion of traditional teachings, practices and Aboriginal spirituality, an inviting physical environment and Aboriginal staff" were important to them (Bucharski, 2006, p. 736). This approach is important because culture can be a great source of strength and resilience for Aboriginal women, who draw on their own spirituality as a coping mechanism when caring for someone living with HIV/AIDS (Ship & Norton, 2002). In the words of the authors, "[Spirituality] is the glue that keeps [Aboriginal women] together" (Ship & Norton, 2002).

The Canadian Aboriginal AIDS Network (CAAN) delivered a position statement calling for action to support Aboriginal women, children, and families affected by HIV/AIDS. The statement recommends the revision of medical treatment formularies to reflect Aboriginal culture, and calls for an increase in culturally sensitive and gender-sensitive health care services (especially in the provision of HIV testing and counselling for Aboriginal women, which should include the integration of Aboriginal healing methods) (Prentice, 2004). There is some evidence that Aboriginal women do not use mainstream services because they fear discrimination. One study suggests that Aboriginal women associate mainstream HIV health care services with colonialism and racism, and therefore tend to avoid these services (Bucharski, 2006; Ship & Norton, 2002).

While this chapter recognizes that women who come from countries where HIV is endemic are diverse, studies suggest that certain cultural practices within specific ethnocultural communities can increase women's vulnerability to HIV and deter HIV prevention. For example, the patriarchal attitudes evident in many African and Caribbean cultures hold that women are expected to submit to male authority and privilege. Such attitudes can influence factors that lead to increased risk of HIV infection.

Polygamy—a patriarchal cultural and religious practice that permits a man to have more than one wife—increases women's HIV risk because risk of STI is greater among multiple partner marriages where condom usage may be limited (Medical Research Council, 2003; Newman et al., 2008; Tharao et al., 2006). Polygamy is illegal in Canada, though it has been documented within certain ethnocultural communities (Tharao et al., 2006; Williams et al., 2009).

Patriarchal attitudes may also constrain women's ability to negotiate condom use (Gardezi et al., 2008; Tharao et al., 2006). This is especially true within marriages (Newman et al., 2008). One study found that women of Jamaican descent identified marriage as a factor that increases women's vulnerability to HIV infection, because, according to the study's participants, there is no way to practise safer sex in marriage (Lawson et al., 2006). In the same study, women of Caribbean descent spoke about the vulnerability they experience and their lack of control over their own bodies. Women of Kenyan descent revealed similar findings, as participants explained how difficult it is for married women in their community to refuse sex without a condom.

Two culturally specific female genital-tract practices, female genital mutilation (FGM) and douching or vaginal drying, practised by some women of African and

Caribbean descent, put them at increased risk of HIV/AIDS (Tharao et al., 2006). Despite being internationally recognized as a violation of the human rights of girls and women (WHO, 2010), FGM[5] continues to be practised in some African communities in Canada. FGM involves narrowing the vaginal opening or sealing it, and the practice is linked to a cultural preference for premarital virginity and an emphasis on marital fidelity (Maillet, 2008). FGM is also motivated by beliefs about what is acceptable female sexual behaviour (WHO, 2010). This practice scars women's genital tracts, making it easier for infections to proliferate, including HIV. In addition, FGM and its emphasis on premarital virginity, combined with limitations in sexual education, may influence women's decision to engage in anal intercourse. Research suggests that women who wish to retain their virginity for marriage may practise anal intercourse as an alternative to vaginal intercourse (Bruckner & Bearman, 2005), thereby increasing their risk for HIV infection.

The second female genital-tract practice, douching or vaginal drying, involves cleansing the vagina and is used by women to remove signs of sexual intercourse. This practice dries the vaginal wall and increases friction during intercourse. The practice is most commonly seen in African and Caribbean communities in Canada, and is linked to strongly held ideas about cleanliness and purity (Tharao et al., 2006). Douching or vaginal drying results in increased friction during sex and may lead to tearing of the vaginal lining or of condoms, thereby increasing women's risk of HIV and other infections (Tharao et al., 2006).

Within certain ethnocultural communities in Canada, HIV/AIDS is seen primarily as an issue of moral impropriety (Newman et al., 2008). Specifically, there is a tendency among African and Caribbean communities in Canada to associate HIV with extramarital sex and promiscuity. This has an impact on women's ability to protect themselves against HIV, because many feel that they cannot ask their partner to use a condom for fear of being accused of sexual promiscuity (Lawson et al., 2006). In addition, speaking about sexual matters is considered taboo among some African and Caribbean communities in Canada. The "code of silence" around sexual matters, where people generally avoid discussing these subjects, makes it difficult to acknowledge HIV/AIDS within or outside of these communities (Gardezi et al., 2008; Lawson et al., 2006; Tharao et al., 2006).

African and Caribbean norms and values that prescribe the dynamics between women and their partners within their communities in Canada may impede HIV prevention or intervention strategies (Newman et al., 2008). Religious institutions also hamper HIV prevention efforts when they dictate certain behaviours that run contrary to public health messaging; for example, when religious institutions put restrictions on condom usage (Newman et al., 2008; Williams et al., 2009). Without the support of major cultural institutions, the ability of public health agencies to effect change and make headway in HIV prevention remains limited (Gardezi et al., 2008; Newman et al., 2008).

Homophobia among African and Caribbean communities can also result in men who have sex with men (MSM) engaging in and maintaining sexual relationships with women. This in turn poses a risk of HIV infection for the female partner (Lawson et al., 2006; Newman et al., 2008). The assumption that HIV/AIDS is a "gay disease" or that gay men are to blame for HIV/AIDS compounds the stigma felt by MSM in these communities. This stigma also thwarts HIV prevention efforts among both MSM and women involved with MSM in African and Caribbean communities.

SUMMARY

Women make up a diverse and complex segment of HIV/AIDS cases in Canada. Canadian surveillance data indicate that the proportion of women living with HIV/AIDS has increased over the last decade. Surveillance data reveal that the two most common exposure categories for women are heterosexual transmission and injection drug use. In the heterosexual exposure category, women are infected mainly through sexual contact with a person at risk. However, surveillance data do not give us a complete picture of the problem, because they do not explain why some women are more likely than others to engage in unprotected sex and share injection drug equipment. Surveillance data require complementary research to examine the complex interactions between the factors that make some women more likely to engage in risk behaviours. Research on these factors is conducted on the premise that if the root causes of the problem are better understood, the problem can be better addressed.

Research synthesized for this chapter shows that biology, gender, education, social status, employment and income, social environments and social support networks, physical environments, personal health practices and coping skills, healthy child development, health services, and culture and race are all determinants that influence women's health and their vulnerability to HIV infection. For some determinants of health, the link between the determinant and women's vulnerability to HIV infection is heavily supported by the evidence. For instance, research shows that poverty, housing insecurity, sexual violence and physical violence, sex work, and substance use are strongly associated with increased risk of HIV infection in women. For other determinants, the link between the determinant and women's vulnerability to HIV infection is less direct. This does not necessarily reflect the actual influence of the determinant, but rather highlights gaps where further research may be warranted.

Gender as a Key Determinant

While biology alone influences women's risk of HIV transmission, treatment outcomes, disease progression, and comorbidities, gender is recognized as a key determinant because of the way it interacts with and influences the other determinants. Research indicates that gendered roles of masculinity and femininity ultimately manifest in a gender power imbalance, which lies at the heart of gender-based inequities and disparities. Gender power imbalance can directly affect risk behaviours by limiting women's ability to negotiate safer sex in a number of ways. For instance, condom use is predominantly male-controlled, placing women at a disadvantage in negotiating safer sex. This is especially true for sexual relationships involving casual partners or for women involved in sex work because condom negotiation in these situations can be difficult, especially if the security of the individual is jeopardized.

Gender power imbalance is also manifest in relationships in which male partners use physical violence or emotional abuse to obtain sex, which act as causes and consequences of HIV infection in women. The high prevalence of drug use associated with sex work and among female youth at risk and increased risk of HIV infection is also grounded in gender power imbalance; research shows that injection-dependent relationships with men increase women's vulnerability to HIV infection.

Cultural attitudes about gender roles and sexual behaviour can also hinder women's ability to negotiate safer sex. For example, social norms in some ethnocultural communities condemn condom usage between women and their regular partners, even in cases where a woman may be aware that her husband lives with HIV or has other sexual partners.

The Effects of Intersecting Discrimination

In addition to gender, the social determinants of race and culture, sexual orientation, and stigmatizing attitudes about HIV/AIDS play a significant role in influencing women's vulnerability to HIV. This is especially true for women who are subject to multiple, compounding, and intersecting forms of discrimination. Intersecting discrimination is a contributing factor that helps explain why higher rates of HIV infection are seen among certain groups of women, including women from countries where HIV is endemic, Aboriginal women, lesbian women, women who are involved in sex work, women who use injection drugs, and women who live in poverty. As one example, the historical trauma of colonialism and racism continues to adversely impact the socio-economic status of Aboriginal women, making them more likely to engage in behaviours (e.g., street-based sex work, injection drug use) that increase their risk of HIV infection. Intersecting and stigmatizing attitudes about HIV/AIDS in the Aboriginal community further add to the challenges faced by Aboriginal women.

The Importance of Empowering Women

The research and responses to HIV/AIDS and women in Canada presented here highlight the importance of empowering women in order to redress gender power imbalances and discrimination. Research and evidence-based interventions show that women's participation in the design and delivery of interventions is effective, giving women a sense of ownership and direction in their lives. It is women's inclusion and active participation in a decision-making role within interventions that enhances their ability to control their lives, increases their leadership skills, and provides them with the tools to negotiate safer sex.

Gaps in the Research

Gaps in the research on women and HIV/AIDS in Canada remain. More must be learned about certain groups of women within diverse populations. For example, female youth at risk have been studied, but the inventory revealed that no research has been done on female youth from countries where HIV is endemic, even though efforts are underway to address their needs through specific interventions. In addition, few studies examine female youth from First Nations, Inuit, and Métis populations as separate populations, and no studies have been done on female youth who inject drugs. Further, no research projects specifically address First Nations, Inuit, and Métis women in prison, even though demographic data show that Aboriginal women are overrepresented in prison. Other groups of women that have been overlooked by researchers include older women, who are increasingly being diagnosed with HIV, and female sex workers who live and work outside Vancouver's Downtown Eastside.

Moreover, barriers to accessing appropriate gender-sensitive health services and information remain an issue for many women. HIV/AIDS-related stigma and discrimination, including sexism, transphobia, classism, historical colonialism, and racism, can limit access to health care, including HIV testing, care, and treatment, and reduce social and family support for women living with HIV/AIDS.

The evidence reviewed in this chapter shows that more research is required to identify and analyze culturally and gender-appropriate approaches to HIV/AIDS prevention, care, treatment, and support specific to certain groups of women, including female at-risk youth; women from countries where HIV is endemic; women who are involved in sex work; lesbian, bisexual, trans, and two-spirit women; Aboriginal women; women in prisons; women who use injection drugs; and older women.

The Canadian Response

In reviewing the Canadian response to HIV/AIDS among women, the research found that many organizations provide distinct prevention strategies aimed at distinct female populations. Some programs target women involved in sex work and focus on increasing their knowledge of HIV/AIDS, enhancing their capacity to empower themselves, and improving their access to health services. Several initiatives for women from countries where HIV is endemic provide support to women living with HIV/AIDS and endeavour to tailor services to them, including sexual health education workshops specifically designed to meet their cultural needs related to health care.

Other initiatives delivered to women as part of the Canadian response to HIV/AIDS aim to address the root causes of HIV/AIDS among women. Community-based organizations have worked to address key health needs of distinct female populations through culturally relevant services and peer support/counselling for women from countries where HIV is endemic and for Aboriginal women. Several projects have attempted to address issues related to the physical environments experienced by women in prison settings, disadvantaged urban environments, and remote communities by supporting peer-led activities tailored for these particular environments.

Other factors, such as violence against women (especially Aboriginal women) and disclosure of HIV status, have also been addressed by several projects that have dealt with issues of gender equality and the empowerment of women in heterosexual relationships. Nonetheless, gaps remain in the Canadian response to HIV/AIDS among women. For example, most projects treat Aboriginal women as a homogenous population, failing to recognize the differences between First Nations, Inuit, and Métis women. Projects have also overlooked the effects of intersectional discrimination and its marginalization of certain groups of women. In addition, while several projects address women's ability to negotiate safer sex, as well as their capacity to empower themselves, others do not take up these issues. However, it should be noted that these gaps may be attributed to the methodological limitations of the research, since certain projects may have been missed as a result of limited descriptors, and hence prevented a complete understanding of response activities.

The Importance of Partnership

Many of the projects reviewed as part of the *Population-Specific HIV/AIDS Status Report: Women* highlight the importance of partnerships among different sectors of society to effect change. The current Canadian response to HIV/AIDS in women involves a wide array of organizations and communities that have built networks across the country to encourage knowledge exchange for gender-relevant approaches to HIV/AIDS. It is important to continue strengthening organizations' capacity for evaluation and their capacity to collaborate with researchers to engage in community-based research to determine whether current programs, interventions, and activities adequately meet the prevention, care, treatment, and support needs of this population. Consequently, cross-sectoral and cross-jurisdictional activities to share best practices, to increase partnerships among a wider range of stakeholders, and to better use evidence in the development of strategies and interventions should be fostered and encouraged.

Future Developments

In recent years, women's health advocates have asked scientific communities to intensify their research into female-controlled barrier method contraceptives. Barrier methods offer the advantage of protection against pregnancy and some types of sexually transmitted diseases. Currently, the female condom remains the only available effective woman-controlled barrier against HIV infection for women, though it presents certain challenges for use. Ultimately, women need more affordable, more accessible, more reliable, more user-friendly, and more private (i.e., more easily hidden from a male partner) woman-controlled contraceptive barrier methods to give them the opportunity to protect themselves against the sexual transmission of HIV.

There are several microbicides currently being researched, which may prove promising for this purpose.

Canadian stakeholders involved in addressing HIV/AIDS among women have demonstrated a strong collective will to effect change. Stakeholders' unwavering dedication to increasing HIV/AIDS awareness and to reducing stigma and discrimination has contributed to a growing recognition that HIV/AIDS in women cannot be ignored. This chapter acknowledges the important role that stakeholders play in HIV/AIDS leadership, research, treatment, and prevention. Stakeholders must continue to build on their successes in their ongoing quest to get ahead of, and reverse the impact of, HIV/AIDS among women in Canada.

PROBLEM-BASED LEARNING CASE STUDY

Homeless female youth face unique HIV-related risks that are dependent upon a variety of determinants of health. Based on the material covered in this chapter, what are the key determinants of HIV risk that would need to be considered in developing prevention interventions for this population?

CRITICAL THINKING QUESTIONS

As described in this chapter, the determinants of health intersect to create and support vulnerabilities to and resiliencies against HIV infection among diverse populations of women and girls. In order to address them appropriately, action must be coordinated across multiple levels of government, community, researchers, and people living with or at risk of HIV/AIDS.

1. Identify and discuss the key determinants of health that would need to be considered in developing HIV prevention interventions for:
   a. Young homeless women
   b. Women who use injection drugs
   c. Women from HIV-endemic countries
2. Using the five principles of the *Ottawa Charter* (www.who.int/hpr/NPH/docs/ottawa_charter_hp.pdf) on public health and health promotion—*1. building healthy public policy, 2. creating supportive environments, 3. strengthening community action, 4. developing personal skills, and 5. reorienting health services*—consider which stakeholders might be responsible for addressing the specific determinants you identified above, and how those determinants might be addressed in a concerted effort.
3. Where does the role and responsibility of public health begin and end?
4. How can public health leverage better relationships with other governmental departments to address determinants of health that may fall outside of their scope of work?

NOTES

1 For further analysis of the Aboriginal community, consult the *Population-Specific HIV/AIDS Status Report: Aboriginal Peoples* (PHAC, 2010a).

2 Nearly half (47%) of all Aboriginal people in Canada live either on reserve or in a rural location, which includes remote and wilderness areas, small towns, villages, and other populated areas with a population of less than 1,000 (Statistics Canada, 2008).

3 Concerns cited included "maintenance issues" (such as dispensers that were empty, broken, and/or provided diluted bleach); "other inmates' behaviour" (such as other inmates hoarding and/or limiting access to bleach); having to request bleach; and lack of confidentiality when accessing bleach (Zakaria et al., 2010).

4 More information on these issues can be found in both the *Population-Specific HIV/AIDS Status Report: Aboriginal Peoples* (PHAC, 2010a) and the *Population-Specific HIV/AIDS Status Report: People from Countries Where HIV Is Endemic—Black People of African and Caribbean Descent Living in Canada* (PHAC, 2009).

5 FGM consists of "all procedures that involve partial or total removal of the external female genitalia, or other injury to the female organs for non-medical reasons" (WHO, 2010).

REFERENCES

Adrien, A., Leaune, V., Dassa C., & Perron, M. (2001). Sexual behaviour, condom use and HIV risk situations in the general population of Quebec. *International Journal of STD and AIDS, 12*(2), 108–115.

Anderson, K. (2002). *Tenuous connections: Urban Aboriginal youth sexual health and pregnancy.* Toronto, ON: Ontario Federation of Indian Friendship Centres.

Aryee, E. (2009, November). *Providing affordable housing and improving the quality of life of African-Canadian women living with HIV/AIDS in Ontario.* Paper presented at the 2009 Ontario HIV Treatment Network Conference, Toronto, Canada.

Atlantic Centre for Excellence in Women's Health. (2003). Made in Canada: Home grown research on Canadian women's health. *Canadian Women's Health Network, 5/6*(4/1), 14–17.

Barkey, V., Watanabe, E., Solomon, P., & Wilkins, S. (2009) Barriers and facilitators to participation in work among Canadian women living with HIV/AIDS. *Canadian Journal of Occupational Therapy, 76*(4), 269–275.

Bauer, G. R., Hammond, R., Hohenadel, K., Kaay, M., Scanlon, K., & Travers, R. (2010, June). *Social determinants of trans health in Ontario, Canada: The Trans PULSE Project Phase II.* Paper presented at the 21st Biennial Symposium of the World Professional Association for Transgender Health, Oslo, Norway.

Bauer, G. R., Hammond, R., Travers, R., Kaay, M., Hohenadel, K. M., & Boyce, M. (2009). "I don't think this is theoretical; this is our lives": How erasure impacts health care for transgender people. *Journal of the Association of Nurses in AIDS Care, 20*(5), 348–361.

Beauregard, C., & Solomon, P. (2005) Understanding the experience of HIV/AIDS for women: Implications for occupational therapists. *Canadian Journal of Occupational Therapy, 72*(2), 113–120.

Bell, A. V., Ompad, D., & Sherman, S. G. (2006). Sexual and drug risk behaviours among women who have sex with women. *American Journal of Public Health, 96*(6), 1066–1072.

Betteridge, G. (2005). Legal Network report calls for decriminalization of prostitution in Canada. *HIV/AIDS Policy & Law Review, 10*(3), 11–13.

Boivin, J., Roy, E., Haley, N., & du-Fort, G. G. (2005). The health of street youth: A Canadian perspective. *Canadian Journal of Public Health, 96*(6), 432–437.

Bornovalova, M. A., Gwadz, M. A., Kahler, C., Aklin, W. M., & Lejuez, C. W. (2008). Sensation seeking and risk-taking propensity as mediators in the relationship between childhood abuse and HIV-related risk behavior. *Child Abuse & Neglect: The International Journal, 32*(1), 99–109.

Borwein, A. M, Brandson, E. K., Palmer, A. K., Eyawo, O., Miller, C., Ding, E., ... Hogg, R. S. (2009). You're breaking my HAART: HIV and violence among a cohort of women on treatment in British Columbia, Canada. *The Canadian Journal of Infectious Diseases and Medical Microbiology, 20*(Suppl. B), 97B.

Boulassel, M. R., Morales, R., Murphy, T., Lalonde, R. G., & Klein, M. B. (2006). Gender and long-term metabolic toxicities from antiretroviral therapy in HIV-1 infected persons. *Journal of Medical Virology, 78*(9), 1158–1163.

Braitstein, P., Li, K., Tyndall, M., Spittal, P., O'Shaughnessy, M. V., Schilder, A., ... Schechter, M. T. (2003). Sexual violence among a cohort of injection drug users. *Social Science and Medicine, 57*(3), 561–569.

Bright, V., Shannon, K., Ranville, F., Hawkes, B., Tyndall, M. W., & Lai, C. (2004, May). *Health service delivery to female sex workers in Vancouver.* Paper presented at the 13th Annual Canadian Conference on HIV/AIDS Research, Montreal, Canada.

British Columbia Centre of Excellence for Women's Health. (2010). *Women-centred harm reduction: Gendering the national framework.* Vancouver, BC: British Columbia Centre of Excellence for Women's Health.

Bruckner, H., & Bearman, P. (2005). After the promise: The STD consequences of adolescent virginity pledges. *Journal of Adolescent Health, 36*(4), 271–278.

Bruneau, J., Lamothe, F., Soto, J., Lachance, N., Vincelette, J., Vassal, A., & Franco, E. L. (2001). Sex-specific determinants of HIV infection among injection drug users in Montreal. *Canadian Medical Association Journal, 164*(6), 767–773.

Bucharski, D. (2006). "You need to know where we're coming from": Canadian Aboriginal women's perspectives on culturally appropriate HIV counseling and testing. *Health Care for Women International, 27*(8), 723–747.

Bulman, D. E. (2005). A constructivist approach to HIV/AIDS education for women within the Maritime Provinces of Canada. *International Journal of Lifelong Education, 2*(6), 475–487.

Burchell, A. N., Calzavara, L. M., Myers, T., Schlossberg, J., Millson, M., Escobar, M., ... Major, C. (2003). Voluntary HIV testing among inmates: Sociodemographic, behavioral risk, and attitudinal correlates. *Journal of Acquired Immune Deficiency Syndrome, 32*(5), 534–541.

Callaghan, R. C., Tavares, J., & Taylor, L. (2007). Mobility patterns of Aboriginal injection drug users between on- and off-reserve settings in Northern British Columbia, Canada. *International Journal of Circumpolar Health, 66*(3), 241–247.

Calzavara, L., Ramuscak, N., Burchell, A. N., Swantee, C., Myers, T., Ford, P., … Raymond, S. (2007). Prevalence of HIV and hepatitis C virus infections among inmates of Ontario remand facilities. *Canadian Medical Association Journal, 177*(3), 257–261.

Canadian Aboriginal AIDS Network (CAAN). (2009). *Our search for safe spaces: A qualitative study of the role of sexual violence in the lives of Aboriginal women living with HIV/AIDS.* Vancouver, BC: CAAN.

Canadian AIDS Society (CAS). (2000). *Women and HIV/AIDS.* Retrieved from www.cdnaids.ca/womenandhivaids

Canadian AIDS Society (CAS). (2004). *Fact sheet: Crystal meth and HIV.* Retrieved from www.cdnaids.ca/web/backgrnd.nsf/cl/cas-bg-0087

Canadian Centre on Substance Abuse (CCSA). (2009). *Injection drug users overview.* Retrieved from www.ccsa.ca/Eng/Topics/Populations/IDU/Pages/InjectionDrugUsersOverview.aspx

Canadian Centre on Substance Abuse (CCSA). (2008). *Women overview.* Retrieved from www.ccsa.ca/Eng/Topics/Populations/Women/Pages/WomenOverview.aspx

Canadian HIV/AIDS Legal Network. (2007). *Hard time: Promoting HIV and hepatitis C prevention programming for prisoners in Canada.* Toronto, ON: Canadian HIV/AIDS Legal Network.

Canadian HIV/AIDS Legal Network. (2008). *HIV and hepatitis C in prisons* [Fact sheets]. Retrieved from www.aidslaw.ca/publications/interfaces/downloadFile.php?ref=1309

Cedar Project Partnership, Pearce, M. E., Christian, W. M., Patterson, K., Norris, K., Moniruzzaman, A., … Spittal, P. M. (2008). The Cedar Project: Historical trauma, sexual abuse and HIV risk among young Aboriginal people who use injection and non-injection drugs in two Canadian cities. *Social Science & Medicine, 66*(11), 2185–2194.

"Christina." (2008). HIV and me: Choosing motherhood. *The Positive Side, 16*(1), 1–4.

Clow, B. (2005). HIV/AIDS on rise for Canadian women: Prevention, treatment, care and support programs and policies do not address needs of girls and women. *Canadian Women's Health Network, 8*(1/2), 8.

Csete, J. (2004). Bangkok 2004. Not as simple as ABC: Making real progress on women's rights and AIDS. *HIV/AIDS Policy & Law Review, 9*(3), 68–71.

Csete, J. (2005). *"Vectors, vessels and victims": HIV/AIDS and women's human rights in Canada.* Toronto, ON: Canadian HIV/AIDS Legal Network.

Deering, K. N., Shannon, K., Sinclair, H., Parsad, D., Gilbert, E., & Tyndall, M. W. (2009). Piloting a peer-driven intervention model to increase access and adherence to antiretroviral therapy and HIV care among street-entrenched HIV-positive women in Vancouver. *AIDS Patient Care and STDs, 23*(8), 603–609.

DeMatteo, D. (2002). The "family" context of HIV: A need for comprehensive health and social policies. *AIDS Care, 14*(2), 261–278.

DesMeules, M., Stewart, D., Kazanjian, A., McLean, H., Payne, J., & Vissandjee, B. (2004). Women's health surveillance report: A multidimensional look at the health of Canadian women. *BMC Women's Health, 4*(Suppl. 1), 1–2. doi:10.1186/1472-6874-4-S1-S1

DiCenso, A., Dias, G., & Gahagan, J. (2003). *Unlocking our futures: A national study on women, prisons, HIV and hepatitis C.* Toronto, ON: Prisoners' HIV/AIDS Support Action Network.

Farley, M., Lynne, J., & Cotton, A. J. (2005). Prostitution in Vancouver: Violence and the colonization of First Nations women. *Transcultural Psychiatry, 42*(2), 242–271.

Federal, Provincial and Territorial Advisory Committee on Population Health. (1999). *Toward a healthy future: Second report on the health of Canadians*. Ottawa, ON: Health Canada.

First Nations Information Governance Committee. (2007). *First Nations Regional Longitudinal Health Survey (RHS) 2002/03; Results for adults, youth and children living in First Nations communities*. Ottawa, ON: Assembly of First Nations.

Frappier, J. Y., Paradis, A., & Roy, E. (2007). Relationships between sexual violence characteristics and prevalence of STI/HIV risk-related behaviours in street youth. *Journal of Adolescent Health, 40*(2, Suppl. 1), S15.

Gahagan, J., & Rehman, L. A. (2004). *Mind the sex gap: Bridging sexual and reproductive health and HIV prevention for young heterosexual males*. Retrieved from Atlantic Centre for Excellence in Women's Health website: www.cewh-cesf.ca/PDF/acewh/buddyStudy.pdf

Gahagan, J., Sweeney, E., Jackson, R., Mill, J., Dykeman, M., Prentice T., … Benton, A. (2009, April). *Challenges and barriers to health care HIV service delivery: The experience of Aboriginal women in Canada*. Paper presented at the 18th Annual Canadian Conference on HIV/AIDS Research, Vancouver, Canada.

Gardezi, F., Calzavara, L., Husbands, W., Tharao, W., Lawson, E., Myers, T., … Adebajo, S. (2008). Experiences of and responses to HIV among African and Caribbean communities in Toronto, Canada. *AIDS Care: Psychological and Socio-Medical Aspects of AIDS/HIV, 20*(6), 718–725.

Gilliam, J. (2001). Young women who have sex with women: Falling through cracks for sexual health care. *Issues at a Glance*. Washington, DC: Advocates for Youth.

Greene, S., Chambers, L., Ahluwalia, A., Masinde, K. I., Mukandoli, C., & O'Brien-Teengs, D. (2009). *A house is not a home: The impact of gender, race and stigma on the housing experiences of African and Caribbean mothers living with HIV*. Paper presented at the 2009 Ontario HIV Treatment Network Conference, Toronto, Canada.

Hawkins, K., Peltier, D., Barlow, K., Reading, C., & Weiman, C. (2009). *Sexual violence, HIV/AIDS and Aboriginal women: How Aboriginal women understand health and healing*. Paper presented at the 18th Annual Canadian Conference on HIV/AIDS, Vancouver, Canada.

Hope, T. (2008). *The virus beneath the skin: Genital tissue no foolproof barrier to sexual transmission of human immunodeficiency virus*. Paper presented at the 48th Annual Meeting of the American Society of Cell Biology, San Francisco, USA.

Hope, T., Trull, A., McCoombe, S., McRaven, M., & Veazey, R. S. (2008). *Analysis of the interaction of HIV with female genital tract tissue as a model to understand sexual transmission*. Paper presented at the 48th Annual Meeting of the American Society of Cell Biology, San Francisco, USA.

Hughes, C., & Evans, A. (2003). Health needs of women who have sex with women. *British Medical Journal, 327*(7421), 939–940.

Interagency Coalition on AIDS and Development (ICAD). (2003, May). *HIV/AIDS and gender issues*. Retrieved from www.icad-cisd.com/pdf/publications/Gender_Issues_EN_FINAL.pdf

Jackson, L., Sowinski, B., Bennett, C., & Ryan, D. (2005). Female sex trade workers, condoms and the public-private divide. *Journal of Psychology and Human Sexuality, 17*(1/2), 83–106.

Jackson, R., & Reimer, G. (2008). *Canadian Aboriginal people living with HIV/AIDS: Care, treatment and support issues.* Retrieved from Canadian Aboriginal AIDS Network website: www.caan.ca/pdf/CAAN_CTS_English_Final.pdf

James, L. (2006) *HIV prevention guidelines and manual: A tool for service providers serving African and African Caribbean communities in Canada.* Toronto, ON: Women's Health in Women's Hands Community Health Centre and African and Caribbean Council on HIV/AIDS in Ontario.

Johnston, C. L., Fast, D., Moon, S., & Bungay, V. (2009). Perceptions of risk among women who work in the indoor commercial sex industry in Vancouver, Canada. *Canadian Journal of Infectious Diseases and Medical Microbiology, 20*(Suppl. B), 26B–27B.

Jones, E. J., & Sargeant, S. (2008). *Barriers in access to primary health care for young HIV+ women: A qualitative research study.* Vancouver: YouthCO AIDS Society and Positive Women's Network.

Kaler, A. (2004a). The female condom in North America: Selling the technology of "empowerment." *Journal of Gender Studies, 13*(2), 139–152.

Kaler A. (2004b). The future of female-controlled barrier methods for HIV prevention: Female condoms and lessons learned. *Culture, Health & Sexuality, 6*(6), 501–516.

Lawson, E., Gardezi, F., Calzavara, L., Husbands, W., Myers, T., Tharao, W., … Wambayi, E. J. (2006). *HIV/AIDS stigma, denial, fear and discrimination: Experiences and responses of people from African and Caribbean communities in Toronto.* Toronto, ON: African and Caribbean Council on HIV/AIDS in Ontario and The HIV Social, Behavioural and Epidemiological Studies Unit, University of Toronto.

Leonard, L. (2007). *Women and HIV prevention: A scoping review.* Ottawa, ON: University of Ottawa.

Lescano, C., Houck, C. D., Brown, L. K., Doherty, G., DiClemente, R. J., Fernandez, M. I., … Silver, B. J., for the Project SHIELD Study Group. (2008). Correlates of heterosexual anal intercourse among at-risk adolescents and young adults. *American Journal of Public Health, 99*(1), 1131–1136.

Logie, C. H., & Newman, P. A. (2009). Peer interventions to promote empowerment and HIV risk reduction among sex workers: A systematic review and meta-analysis. *Canadian Journal of Infectious Diseases and Medical Microbiology, 20*(Suppl. B), 15B.

Maggi, J., & Daly, T. (2006). Gender matters: Understanding the emotional and social support needs of women with HIV/AIDS. *Research Bulletin: Time to Deliver on Gender and HIV/AIDS, 5*(2), 16–17.

Maillet, L. (2008, October). *When female genital mutilation crosses borders: Exploring factors to discontinue the practice among Canadian migrants.* Paper presented at the 136th Annual Meeting and Expo of the American Public Health Association (APHA), San Diego, USA.

Mar, L., & Betteridge, G. (2007). Subcommittee fails to recommend legal reforms needed to promote human rights of sex workers. *HIV/AIDS Policy & Law Review, 12*(1), 15–17.

Marshall, S. K., Charles, G., Hare, J., Ponzetti, J., & Stokl, M. (2005). Sheway's services for substance using pregnant and parenting women: Evaluating the outcomes for infants. *Canadian Journal of Community Mental Health 24*(1), 19–34.

Martin, R. E., Gold, F., Murphy, W., Remple, V., Berkowitz, J., & Money, D. (2005). Drug use and risk of bloodborne infections: A survey of female prisoners in British Columbia. *Canadian Journal of Public Health, 96*(2), 97–101.

Martin Spigelman Research Associates. (2002). *HIV/AIDS and health determinants: Lessons for coordinating policy and action*. Retrieved from Public Health Agency of Canada website: www.phac-aspc.gc.ca/aids-sida/publication/healthdeterminants/pdf/HIV-AIDS-and-Health-Determinants.pdf

Mathieson, C. M., Bailey, N., & Gurevich, M. (2002) Health care services for lesbian and bisexual women: Some Canadian data. *Health Care for Woman International, 23*(2), 185–196.

McCoy, L. (2005). HIV-positive patients and the doctor-patient relationship: Perspectives from the margins. *Qualitative Health Research, 15*(6), 791–806.

McKeown, I., Reid, S., & Orr, P. (2004). Experiences of sexual violence and relocation in the lives of HIV infected Canadian women. *International Journal of Circumpolar Health, 63*(2), 399–404.

McKeown, I., Reid, S., Orr, P., & Turner, S. (2006). Sexual violence and dislocation in women's acquisition of HIV in Manitoba. *Research Bulletin: Time to Deliver on Gender and HIV/AIDS, 5*(2), 8–9.

McKeown, I., Reid, S., Turner, S., & Orr, P. (2002). *Sexual violence and dislocation as social risk factors involved in the acquisition of HIV among women in Manitoba.* Winnipeg, MB: The Prairie Women's Health Centre of Excellence.

McPhedran, M., & Bazilli, S. (2006). Viruses of inequality: Women's health and human rights. *Centres of Excellence for Women's Health Research Bulletin, 5*(2), 20.

Medical Research Council (UK). (2003). *Polygamy in West Africa: What are the implications for sexual health?* London: Medical Research Council.

Medjuck, M. J. (2009). *"Shackled with HIV": HIV-positive women's experiences of gender-based intimate partner violence.* Retrieved from Positive Women's Network website: http://pwn.bc.ca/wp-content/uploads/files/Shackled_with_HIV_Medjuck.pdf

Mehrabadi, A., Craib, K. J. P., Patterson, K., Adam, W., Moniruzzaman, A., Ward-Burkitt, B., ... & Spittal, P. M. (2008). The Cedar Project: A comparison of HIV-related vulnerabilities amongst young Aboriginal women surviving drug use and sex work in two Canadian cities. *International Journal of Drug Policy, 19*(2), 159–168.

Mehrabadi, A., Paterson, K., Pearce, M., Patel, S., Craib, K. J., Moniruzzaman, A., ... & Spittal, P. M. (2008). Gender differences in HIV and hepatitis C related vulnerabilities among Aboriginal young people who use street drugs in two Canadian cities. *Women and Health, 48*(3), 235–260.

Miller, C. L., Spittal, P. M., Laliberte, N., Li, K., Tyndall, M. W., O'Shaughnessy, M. V., & Schechter, M. T. (2002). Females experiencing sexual and drug vulnerabilities are at elevated risk for HIV infection among youth who use injection drugs. *Journal of Acquired Immune Deficiency Syndromes, 30*(3), 335–341.

Miller, C. L., Strathdee, S. A., Kerr, T., Li, K., & Wood, E. (2006). Factors associated with early adolescent initiation into injection drug use: Implications for intervention programs. *Journal of Adolescent Health, 38*(4), 462–464.

Mosher, W. D., Chandra, A., & Jones, J. (2005). Sexual behavior and selected health measures: Men and women 15–44 years of age, United States, 2002. *Advance Data from Vital and Health Statistics, 362*, 1–56.

Namaste, V. (1998). *A needs assessment of transgender people and HIV/AIDS in Quebec, Canada: Sociological explanations of marginalization and risk.* Paper presented at the 12th International Conference on AIDS, Geneva, Switzerland.

Namaste, V. (2010). *Les trans et le VIH*. Presented to the Centre for Communicable Diseases and Infection Control, Public Health Agency of Canada, Ottawa, Canada..

National Clearinghouse on Family Violence. (2008). *Aboriginal women and family violence*. Retrieved from Public Health Agency of Canada website: www.phac-aspc.gc.ca/ncfv-cnivf/pdfs/fem-abor_e.pdf

Native Women's Association of Canada. (2007). *Culturally relevant gender based analysis: An issue paper*. Ottawa, ON: Native Women's Association of Canada.

Native Women's Association of Canada. (2008). *Voices of our sisters in spirit: A research and policy report to families and communities*. Ottawa, ON: Native Women's Association of Canada.

Ndlovu, U., Gillies, K., Binder, L., Ion, A., Tharao, W., O'Campo, P., … Carvalhal, A. (2009). *Stressors and ways of coping for women living with HIV in Toronto and Hamilton*. Paper presented at the 18th Annual Canadian Conference on HIV/AIDS Research, Vancouver, Canada.

Newman, P. A., Williams, C. C., Massaquoi, N., Brown, M., & Logie, C. (2008). HIV prevention for Black women: Structural barriers and opportunities. *Journal of Health Care for the Poor and Underserved, 19*(3), 829–841.

Normen, L., Chan, K., Braitstein, P., Anema, A., Bondy, G., Montaner, J. S., & Hogg, R. S. (2005). Food insecurity and hunger are prevalent among HIV-positive individuals in British Columbia, Canada. *Journal of Nutrition, 135*(4), 820–825.

O'Connell, J. M., Kerr, T., Li, K., Tyndall, M. W., Hogg, R. S., Montaner, J. S., & Wood, E. (2005). Requiring help injecting independently predicts incident HIV infection among injection drug users. *Journal of Acquired Immune Deficiency Syndromes, 40*(1), 83–88.

Poole, N., & Dell, C. A. (2005). *Girls, women and substance use*. Retrieved from Canadian Centre for Substance Abuse website: www.ccsa.ca/2005%20CCSA%20Documents/ccsa-011142-2005.pdf

Prentice, T. (2004). *HIV/AIDS and Aboriginal women, children and families: A position statement*. Ottawa, ON: Canadian Aboriginal AIDS Network.

Prentice, T. (2005). Alarming rates of HIV/AIDS for Canada's Aboriginal women: National response long overdue. *Canadian Women's Health Network, 8*, 11.

Public Health Agency of Canada. (n.d.). *Population health: What determines health?* Ottawa: ON, Centre for Health Promotion, Public Health Agency of Canada. Retrieved from www.phac-aspc.gc.ca/ph-sp/determinants/index-eng.php#What

Public Health Agency of Canada. (2006). *Enhanced surveillance of risk behaviours among injecting drug users in Canada: Phase 1 report*. Ottawa, ON: Centre for Communicable Disease and Infection Control, Public Health Agency of Canada. Retrieved from www.phac-aspc.gc.ca/i-track/sr-re-1/index-eng.php

Public Health Agency of Canada. (2007). *2004 Canadian sexually transmitted infections surveillance report*. Ottawa, ON: Centre for Communicable Disease and Infection Control, Public Health Agency of Canada. Retrieved from www.phac-aspc.gc.ca/publicat/ccdr-rmtc/07vol33/33s1/index-eng.php

Public Health Agency of Canada. (2008). *HIV/AIDS in Canada: Surveillance report to December 31, 2007*. Ottawa, ON: Centre for Communicable Disease and Infection Control, Public Health Agency of Canada. Retrieved from www.phac-aspc.gc.ca/aids-sida/publication/survreport/index-eng.php

Public Health Agency of Canada. (2009). *Population-specific HIV/AIDS status report: People from countries where HIV is endemic—Black people of African and Caribbean descent living in Canada.* Ottawa, ON: Centre for Communicable Disease and Infection Control, Public Health Agency of Canada. Retrieved from www.phac-aspc.gc.ca/aids-sida/publication/ps-pd/africacaribbe/index-eng.php

Public Health Agency of Canada. (2010a). *Population-specific HIV/AIDS status report: Aboriginal peoples.* Ottawa, ON: Centre for Communicable Disease and Infection Control, Public Health Agency of Canada. Retrieved from www.phac-aspc.gc.ca/aids-sida/publication/ps-pd/aboriginal-autochtones/index-eng.php

Public Health Agency of Canada. (2010b). *HIV/AIDS Epi Updates, July 2010.* Ottawa, ON: Centre for Communicable Disease and Infection Control, Public Health Agency of Canada. Retrieved from www.phac-aspc.gc.ca/aids-sida/publication/epi/2010/index-eng.php

Rehman, L., Gahagan, J., DiCenso, A. M., & Dias, G. (2004). Harm reduction and women in the Canadian national prison system: Policy or practice? *Women and Health, 40*(4), 57–73.

Reid, C. (2003). "We're not a part of society, we don't have a say": Exclusion as a determinant of poor women's health. In M. T. Segal, V. Demos, & J. J. Kronenfeld (Eds.), *Gender perspectives on medicine* (pp. 231–279). Bingley, UK: Emerald.

Remez, L. (2001). Levels of HIV risk behaviors are significantly elevated among women who have ever had sex with women. *Family Planning Perspectives, 33*(2), 91.

Robertson, L. (2007). Taming space: Drug use, HIV, and homemaking in Downtown Eastside Vancouver. *Gender, Place and Culture, 14*(5), 527–549.

Robertson, S. (2007). *Who feels it knows: The challenges of HIV prevention for young Black women in Toronto.* Toronto, ON: Black Coalition for AIDS Prevention.

Robitaille, P. (2010, March). Rebellion of the scapegoats: Inclusion and empowerment of sex workers in the fight against HIV. Paper presented at the 6th Canadian HIV/AIDS Skills Building Symposium, Montreal, Canada.

Rodrigues, I., Nguyen, N. M., Neff, K., Venne, T., & Boulianne, M. J. (2004, May). *Accessibility and use of health care services by sex workers in Laval.* Paper presented at the 13th Annual Canadian Conference on HIV/AIDS Research, Montreal, Canada.

Rubin, T., Tharao, W., Ndlovu, U., & Muchenje, M. (2009, November). *Immigrant women's experiences with immigration medical examination HIV testing.* Paper presented at the 2009 Ontario HIV Treatment Network Conference, Toronto, Canada.

Rusch, M. L. A., Shoveller, J. A., Burgess, S., Stancer, K., Patrick, D. M., & Tyndall, M. W. (2008). Demographics, sexual risk behaviours and uptake of screening for sexually transmitted infections among attendees of a weekly women-only community clinic program. *Canadian Journal of Public Health, 99*(4), 257–261.

Saewyc, E., Skay, C., Richens, K., Reis, E., Poon, C., & Murphy, A. (2006). Sexual orientation, sexual abuse, and HIV-risk behaviors among adolescents in the Pacific Northwest. *American Journal of Public Health, 96*(6), 1104–1110.

Scanlon, K., Bauer, G., Kaay, M., & Boyce, M. (2009, November). *Social determinants of trans health in Ontario: Trans Pulse Project.* Paper presented at the 2009 Ontario HIV Treatment Network Conference, Toronto, Canada.

Schalkwyk, J. E., Alimenti, A., Khoo, D., Maan, E., Forbes, J. C., Burdge, D. R., ... Money, D. M. (2008). Serious toxicity associated with continuous nevirapine-based HAART in pregnancy. *BJOG: An International Journal of Obstetrics and Gynaecology, 115*(10), 1297–1302.

Shannon, K., Bright, V., Duddy, J., & Tyndall, M. W. (2005). Access and utilization of HIV treatment and services among women sex workers in Vancouver's Downtown Eastside. *Journal of Urban Health, 82*(3), 488–497.

Shannon, K., Bright, V., Gibson, K., & Tyndall, M. W., for the Maka Project Partnership. (2007). Sexual and drug-related vulnerabilities for HIV infection among women engaged in survival sex work in Vancouver, Canada. *Canadian Journal of Public Health, 98*(6), 465–469.

Shannon, K., Kerr, T., Allinott, S., Chettiar, J., Shoveller, J., & Tyndall, M. W. (2008). Social and structural violence and power relations in mitigating HIV risk of drug-using women in survival sex work. *Social Science and Medicine, 66*(4), 911–921.

Ship, S. J., & Norton, L. (2002). HIV/AIDS and Aboriginal women in Canada. In C. Amaratunga & J. Gahagan (Eds.), *Striking to the heart of the matter: Selected readings on gender and HIV* (pp. 47–63). Halifax, NS: Atlantic Centre for Excellence in Women's Health.

Sikka, A. (2009). *Trafficking of Aboriginal women and girls in Canada*. Retrieved from Institute on Governance website: www.iog.ca/publications/2009_trafficking_of_aboriginal_women.pdf

Singh, A. E., Gill, J., & Houston, S. (2005) New resources on screening for HIV in pregnancy. *Alberta RN, 61*(8), 11.

Solomon, P., & Wilkins, S. (2008). Participation among women living with HIV: A rehabilitation perspective. *AIDS Care, 20*(3), 292–296.

Spittal, P. M. (2006). Drastic elevations in mortality among female injection drug users in a Canadian setting. *AIDS Care, 18*(2), 101–108.

Spittal, P. M., Bruneau, J., Craib, K. J. P., Miller, C., Lamothe, F., Weber, A. E., ... Schecter, M. T. (2003). Surviving the sex trade: A comparison of HIV risk behaviours among street-involved women in two Canadian cities who inject drugs. *AIDS Care, 15*(2), 187–195.

Spittal, P. M., Craib, K. J., Wood, E., Laliberte, N., Li, K., Tyndall, M. W, ... Schecter, M. T. (2002). Risk factors for elevated HIV incidence rates among female injection drug users in Vancouver. *Canadian Medical Association Journal, 166*(7), 894–899.

Spitzer, D. L. (2005). Engendering health disparities. *Canadian Journal of Public Health, 96*(Suppl. 2), S78–S96.

Squires, K. E. (2007). Gender differences in the diagnosis and treatment of HIV. *Gender Medicine, 4*(4), 294–307.

Statistics Canada. (2005, July 14). Family violence in Canada: A statistical profile. *The Daily*, 3–5.

Statistics Canada. (2008). *Population by age groups, sex and Aboriginal identity groups, 2006 counts, for Canada, provinces and territories—20% Sample data*. Catalogue no. 97-558-XWE2006002. Ottawa, ON: Statistics Canada.

Tebeje, M., & Teffera, H. (2009, November). *Reaching vulnerable women in priority areas in the Greater Toronto Area: Voices of Positive Women's Community Connections Project*. Paper presented at the 2009 Ontario HIV Treatment Network Conference, Toronto, Canada.

Tenenbein, S. (2008). Your best protection is your behaviour. *Bloodlines, 8*, 37–39.

Tharao, E., Massaquoi, N., & Teclom, S. (2006). *Silent voices of the HIV/AIDS epidemic: African and Caribbean women research study (2002–2004).* Toronto, ON: Women's Health in Women's Hands Community Health Centre.

Tompkins, C. N. E., Sheard, L., Wright, N. M. J., Jones, L., & Howes, N. (2006). Exchange, deceit, risk and harm: The consequences for women of receiving injections from other drug users. *Drugs: Education, Prevention, and Policy, 13*(3), 281–297.

Tucker, R. (2009). *Positive Spaces Healthy Places: Key findings.* Paper presented at the satellite session "Women and HIV Prevention in Canada: The Past, the Present and the Future: Implication for Research, Policy and Practice," at the 18th Annual Canadian Conference on HIV/AIDS Research, Vancouver, Canada.

Tucker, R., Greene, S., Monette, L., Rourke, S., Sobota, M., Koornstra, J., … The Positive Spaces Healthy Places Study Team. (2009). *The need for stable and affordable housing among women living with HIV in Ontario: The Positive Spaces Healthy Places Study.* Presented at the 2009 Ontario HIV Treatment Network Conference, Toronto, Canada.

UNAIDS. (2008). *Women and girls.* Retrieved from www.unaids.org/en/PolicyAndPractice/Key-Populations/WomenGirls/default.asp

United Nations Development Fund for Women (UNIFEM). (2001). *Turning the tide: CEDAW and the gender dimensions of the HIV/AIDS pandemic.* Retrieved from www.genderandaids.org/downloads/topics/TurningTheTide.pdf

Vancouver Area Network of Drug Users (VANDU) Women Care Team. (2009). *"Me, I'm living it": The primary health care experiences of women who use drugs in Vancouver's Downtown Eastside.* Vancouver, BC: The British Columbia Centre of Excellence for Women's Health.

Weber, A. E., Boivin, J. F., Blais, L., Haley, N., & Roy, E. (2002). HIV risk profile and prostitution among female street youths. *Journal of Urban Health: Bulletin of the New York Academy of Medicine, 79*(4), 525–535.

Weber, A. E., Boivin, J. F., Blais, L., Haley, N., & Roy, E. (2004). Predictors of initiation into prostitution among female street youths. *Journal of Urban Health, 81*(4), 584–595.

Williams, C. C., Newman, P. A., Sakamoto, I., & Massaquoi, N. A. (2009). HIV prevention risks for Black women in Canada. *Social Science and Medicine, 68*(1), 12–20.

Wingood, G. M., & DiClemente, R. J. (2000). Application of the theory of gender and power to examine HIV-related exposures, risk factors, and effective interventions for women. *Health Education & Behavior, 27*(5), 539–565.

Women's Health in Women's Hands Community Health Centre. (2003). *Racial discrimination as a health risk for female youth: Implications for policy and healthcare delivery in Canada.* Toronto, ON: The Canadian Race Relations Foundation.

Wood, E., Spittal, P. M., Kerr, T., Small, W., Tyndall, M.W., O'Shaughnessy, M. V., & Schecter, M.T. (2003). Requiring help injecting as a risk factor for HIV infection in the Vancouver epidemic: Implications for HIV prevention. *Canadian Journal of Public Health, 94*(5), 355–359.

World Health Organization (WHO). (2007). *Unequal, unfair, ineffective and inefficient gender inequities in health: Why it exists and how we can change it.* Final Report to the WHO Commission on Social Determinants of Health, Women and Gender Equity Knowledge Network. Geneva: WHO.

World Health Organization. (2009). *Gender inequalities and HIV.* Retrieved from www.who.int/gender/hiv_aids/en/

World Health Organization. (2010). *Female genital mutilation* [Fact sheet]. Retrieved from www.who.int/mediacentre/factsheets/fs241/en

Zakaria, D., Thompson, J. M., Jarvis, A., & Borgatta, F. (2010). *Research report: Summary of emerging findings from the 2007 National Inmate Infectious Diseases and Risk-Behaviours Survey.* Ottawa, ON: Correctional Service of Canada.

Chapter 3
ADVANCING OUR KNOWLEDGE: FINDINGS OF A META-ETHNOGRAPHIC SYNTHESIS

Jacqueline Gahagan, Christina Ricci, Randy Jackson, Tracey Prentice,
Judy Mill, and Barry Adam

INTRODUCTION

Although significant strides have been made in HIV policy and prevention in Canada, there has been an overall absence of syntheses of qualitative research in relation to our prevention efforts. While it is generally recognized that quantitative data focusing on, for example, HIV infection rates among women in Canada can provide information critical for targeted secondary intervention efforts, qualitative research findings are often more challenging to synthesize for the purposes of informing policy and prevention efforts. Specifically, the utility of undertaking such syntheses of our qualitative prevention efforts is reflected in our subsequent ability to illuminate the intersecting contextual determinants of health that underlie infection rates.

The purpose of our synthesis was therefore to focus specifically on the qualitative HIV prevention research conducted in Canada with the aim of unpacking gender-based and Indigenous prevention strategies and responses. To better understand these issues, our synthesis provided the opportunity to examine, assess, and interpret current qualitative knowledge in an effort to identify HIV prevention gaps and implications for future research and prevention programming. This chapter offers an overview of the key findings to emerge from our synthesis of the published qualitative HIV prevention literature from 1996 (when new HIV treatments were first introduced) to 2008. Key outcomes of this synthesis provided contextually rich comparisons of experiences across select populations of women and allowed for the development of recommendations where research findings may not be well integrated in current approaches, and suggestions of future research areas in need of consideration. Clearly, given the rising rates of HIV infection among women in Canada, specifically Aboriginal women, additional clarification on how to frame the next wave of prevention efforts is warranted. Further, as the Federal Initiative on HIV/AIDS argues, Aboriginal peoples and women are among "the most vulnerable individuals and groups in society ... [T]his reality demands a national HIV/AIDS response that addresses human rights, determinants of health and gender dimensions of the epidemic" (Health Canada, 2009).

Despite the call for prevention efforts to focus on human rights and determinants of health, previous research related to women's HIV-related experiences suggests that additional steps are needed to understand the system-wide effects of poverty, unstable housing, violence, post-traumatic stress, and addictions, particularly injection drug use, on the likelihood of HIV seroconversion. Recognizing these intersecting issues, our meta-ethnographic review aligned with several of the thematic areas identified by the Canadian Institutes of Health Research and Canadian Institutes for Health Research Knowledge Transfer strategic plan, and was informed by both gender-based and Indigenous research perspectives.

This synthesis project also directly responds to the demands put forward in the *Blueprint for Action on Women & Girls and HIV*:

> Women and girls of all cultural backgrounds and life experiences are effectively absent from the HIV/AIDS research agenda and research decision-making at all levels ... The long and brutal legacy of colonization of Aboriginal people [in Canada and] globally has created an HIV epidemic in urban, rural and isolated Aboriginal communities that impedes access to prevention and education in these communities. Susceptibility of Aboriginal peoples to HIV and barriers to treatment are compounded for women and girls through the living legacy of the colonization process. (2006, p. 2)

META-ETHNOGRAPHIC OVERVIEW

This synthesis included the following steps: (1) an initial scoping exercise to search the research literature using agreed-upon inclusion criteria; (2) a quality appraisal of relevant studies meeting the search criteria for inclusion in a synthesis of HIV prevention research; and (3) a main interpretative review guided by a meta-ethnographic approach that is informed by both a gender-based perspective and an Indigenous approach to research. This final stage involved the integration of themes from across the studies that met both the inclusion and the quality criteria.

Scoping Review Considerations

As we have seen over the course of the epidemic, HIV prevention is a domain in which public and human rights policy (e.g., *R. v. Cuerrier* [Elliot, 1999]), professional and community intervention (e.g., social marketing campaigns), individual behaviour (e.g., decisions related to the use of condoms), and socio-cultural context (e.g., ethnicity, social status) intersect, converge, or collide. The research team was particularly interested in both Aboriginal and non-Aboriginal women's experiences of prevention (our topical parameter) efforts in Canada and how this might inform future public policy and/or practice in the prevention field to be useful and meaningful to the populations involved.

For the purpose of this synthesis study, population parameters for inclusion were limited to studies involving women (either HIV negative or HIV positive) of any race/ ethnicity or nationality living in Canada. With respect to Aboriginal Peoples, given shared socio-historical experience (e.g., colonialization), the population parameter for Aboriginal Peoples included Inuit, Métis, and First Nations (both Status and non-Status as defined by the Canadian Constitution). Within the synthesis were reports of qualitative studies conducted according to both the topical and population parameters from 1996 (when effective new treatments were introduced) to the time the review was conducted (spring/summer 2008). All study reports received were entered into an electronic database, noting both retrieval date and publication time frames.

The research team, including three research assistants, met regularly via teleconference and had access to a secure, password-protected online forum for discussion between meetings as well as for posting results of the data collection process. The search strategy was divided between the three research assistants by year (1996–1999, 2000–2003, 2004–2008). In preparation for this process and in the development of our search terms, the Project Coordinator met with the Social Sciences and the Health Sciences reference librarians at Dalhousie University, as well as a librarian with meta-analysis expertise. This information was provided to the research team during several teleconferences devoted to developing the list of search terms. The basic search terms used in every search included: HIV + AIDS + prevention + Canada + Aboriginal (Inuit, Métis, and First Nations) + women + girls + female. Additional search terms included the Public Health Association of Canada's (PHAC) Determinants of Health, which include: income and social status; social support networks; education and literacy; employment/working conditions; social environments; physical environments; personal health practices and coping skills; healthy child development; biology and genetic endowment; health services; gender; and culture (PHAC, n.d.).

The following Social Science databases were systematically searched: SocIndex, Sociological Abstracts, Social Services Abstracts, Academic Search Premier (EBSCO), Research Library, and CBCA Full-text Reference. The following Health Sciences databases were also systematically searched: PubMed, Cinahl, Embase, and Web of Science. It should be noted that there were unexpected challenges that arose in utilizing the databases. Some had not updated their search terminology and/or are American, so the search strategy had to be refined to include the following keywords: "Indian," "Indigenous," "Indigenous people," "Native [American]," "American Indian," and "Eskimo," as well as truncated versions of the key words.

In addition to the electronic database search, backward and forward chaining search strategies were utilized. Backward chaining refers to follow-up of references listed in the database-retrieved literature, whereas forward chaining refers to searching relevant citations contained in retrieved electronic databases. Additional search strategies included hand searches of relevant journals, books, HIV prevention study reports, and edited volumes, as well as author searching to determine what individuals have produced other than completed works in the same topic area.

Scoping Review Strategies

The initial scoping review yielded approximately 150 articles. Given the volume of data and management of information, two strategies were employed. First, where supported by licensing agreement, search results were transferred into EndNote (a reference manager support program) and, second, given the need for comparative appraisal and the need to draw inferences across studies, full citations were loaded into the Excel data management system to facilitate and enable comparisons efficiently.

Three widely used appraisal methods were employed to assess the relative merit and inform decision making with respect to inclusion of retrieved literature into this proposed meta-ethnography: individual Professional Judgment, the Critical Appraisal Skills Programme, and Comparative Appraisal, each of which is briefly outlined below.

Professional Judgment. Based on professional qualitative skill and/or organizational knowledge and experience relative to the area of HIV prevention, each team member will "rely solely on their own expertise to form a judgment about the quality" of each retrieved research report using a process similar to peer review processes (Dixon-Woods et al., 2007, p. 43). Individual research team member's decision making with respect to this area will be recorded in a virtual electronic database that will serve to house the project.

Critical Appraisal Skills Programme (CASP). Developed by the Milton Keynes Primary Care Trust (2002), CASP is "a widely used tool that has been employed in previous syntheses of qualitative studies to inform decisions about exclusion of poor-quality papers" (Dixon-Woods et al., 2007, p. 43). This tool directs the reader of retrieved literature to ask questions in three broad areas, including methodological rigour, overall credibility of presented findings, and relevance of findings to the main focus of the synthesis. This assessment tool has been developed for those unfamiliar with qualitative research and its theoretical perspectives. This tool presents a number of questions that deal very broadly with some of the principles or assumptions that characterize qualitative research.

Comparative Appraisal. Following individual appraisals, a comparative appraisal will be conducted, which will "allow [the research team] to create cross-study summaries and displays of key elements included in reports and prepare [the team] for integrating findings in these reports" (Sandelowski & Barroso, 2007, p. 79). All information gathered during the course of appraising via professional judgment and CASP will be entered into tabular format (e.g., an Excel spreadsheet). This will facilitate further analysis, such as "meta-study inferences and, thereby, provide [a beginning] interpretative context" toward the final meta-ethnographic synthesis (Sandelowski & Barroso, 2007, p. 79). Inferences will be directed toward facilitating the emergence of themes upon which the main interpretative review will be based.

Finally, it is also important to note that our methodology did consider sources of information outside of peer review academic journals. Recognizing that some of the most promising programs are less likely to be disseminated through peer review channels, the research assistants contacted experts in the field outside of academia. The research team was specifically looking for information about effective strategies and approaches for HIV prevention for women in Canada.

The first step in this process was to search organization websites for relevant information; fact sheets were excluded and the focus remained on locating reports and articles related to qualitative research on HIV prevention and Aboriginal and non-Aboriginal women in Canada. In addition to searching the websites, all organizations were contacted directly by email for any other relevant material they might be able to provide.

Once the list was complete and duplicate organizations were removed, the research assistants contacted a total of 97 community organizations. These organizations were located across Canada, with a mandate to work with HIV/AIDS and/or women. There was an immediate positive response from organizations. Many organizations were pleased to learn that more research was being conducted, and if they did not have any material they could share, they forwarded contacts they thought could assist us in our search. Those with materials on hand sent us documents or directed us to appropriate Web links. The methodology for collecting grey literature was limited to searching the Internet for organizations and searching their websites for any affiliate organizations and related materials. Similar to the peer-reviewed articles, the research assistants independently screened each website and document to ensure they pertained to HIV prevention and women. The most common reason why material was excluded was that it did not focus on women or HIV prevention, or that the information provided was a fact sheet and not a qualitative research study.

After reviewing both academic literature and grey material, a total of 38 articles met our search criteria. After the relevant articles were identified, a number of research team members met face-to-face on two different occasions to develop and then finalize the codebook. The codebook identified 10 themes that would frame and guide discussion for the final paper, as follows: Determinants of Health, Risk Settings, Perceptions/Attitude/Knowledge, HIV Transmission, HIV Risk, Targeted Approaches, Ethnocultural Populations, Programming Implications/Prevention, Policy Implications Prevention, and Living with HIV: Support and Barriers. Several sub-themes were identified within each main theme.

RESULTS

As stated previously, there were a total of 38 qualitative studies on HIV prevention related to Canadian women published between 1996 and 2008 included in this synthesis. Although for the purposes of our synthesis we adopted a definition of HIV prevention that included both primary prevention (e.g., preventing the occurrence of the initial HIV infection) and secondary prevention (e.g., preventing the onward transmission of the virus), there is some debate in the studies about where HIV prevention efforts should be directed. Repeated reading of the qualitative studies by the research team revealed that, although each study tells a unique story about HIV prevention from the perspective of the individual women or groups of women included in these studies, embedded in the synthesis were recurrent themes specific to the influence of gender, culture, ethnicity, and identity on HIV prevention. The identification of themes, inconsistencies, and gaps helps contribute to our understanding of the challenges in developing appropriate HIV prevention programming and policy to better meet the needs of the diverse populations of women in the Canadian context.

The studies varied greatly in terms of their specific focus (i.e., HIV prevention in relation to injection drug use/culture/sexual orientation/secondary prevention), participant characteristics, and methodologies. Specific populations of women included: young women, women living with HIV/AIDS, Aboriginal women, Black women, Asian women, lesbian women, bisexual women, sex workers, mothers living with HIV/AIDS, women who use drugs, immigrant and refugee women, and women in prison. Service providers were also included, such as nurses, HIV/AIDS prevention workers, social workers, and doctors.

The age of participants across the various studies ranged from 14 to approximately 60 years (several studies did not specify the upper age limit of participants). Methods used included one-on-one interviews with women, key informant interviews, focus groups, and document review for discourse analysis. Most studies used an exploratory, descriptive approach and conducted thematic analysis. The use of participatory action research (PAR) techniques and community advisory committees were described in several of the research studies. For example, in the study by Shannon et al. (2008), a team of survival sex workers were hired, trained, and supported to play a key role in the research project, from conceptualization to implementation and dissemination. Discussion group topic guides were developed through a collaborative process between sex workers and researchers, and all groups were co-facilitated by a sex worker. Similarly, the study by Gardezi et al. (2008) involved working with a Community Advisory Committee (CAC). The CAC advised on community needs, recruitment of participants, research instruments, interpretation of study results, dissemination of findings, and future actions.

Although the synthesis focused on studies that recruited women, many studies also included men. Unfortunately, several studies with mixed male and female participants did not include a gender-based analysis or provide sex-disaggregated results. Gender-based and sex-based analysis of these studies could have resulted in valuable information contributing to the existing body of research on women and HIV/AIDS in Canada and how men's and women's HIV prevention needs differ. Many of the studies explored the impact of one variable on HIV prevention (e.g., ethnicity), but did not discuss specifically how social determinants of health, such as gender and culture, may intersect and overlap to create layered barriers to HIV prevention, care, and treatment, or the need for integrated policies and programs.

Finally, geographic location varied across Canada. The majority of the research studies included in this project took place in Ontario, British Columbia, and Alberta. It is noteworthy that the Yukon Territories, Northwest Territories, Nunavut, Prince Edward Island, and Newfoundland were not represented in this synthesis. While the research was conducted in rural, remote, and urban areas, the majority of studies took place in urban settings, often focusing on large metropolitan centres such as Vancouver and Toronto.

THEMES

The studies that met the scoping review criteria and quality appraisal assessment were entered into Atlas.ti. They were coded using the coding structure developed by the research team, which was situated within the conceptual frameworks of participatory action research (PAR), gender-based analysis (GBA), and Indigenous approaches to research. The data were then coded into domain areas, which allowed for a deeper understanding of, for example, challenges with safer sex practices such as condom use, as well as by properties and dimensions, such as underlying causes or reasons for such challenges in safer-sex adherence, for example, gender-based beliefs about sexual autonomy. Further, a comparative method was employed to understand variations in the findings within and across the studies included in this synthesis. The following sections provide the key themes that emerged from the synthesis of the qualitative literature on HIV prevention among Aboriginal and non-Aboriginal women in Canada: ongoing sexism and discrimination experienced by women in HIV research, programming, and policy; women's inclination to rank HIV low in their hierarchy of needs/priorities; competing social roles ("woman," partner, caregiver, mother, daughter, IDU, sex trade worker, etc.); women's perceived passive role in sexual relationships with male partners, which may lead to a lack of power to negotiate safer sexual practices; safety concerns related to sexual abuse or family violence; existing service barriers embedded within the formal health care system; unique secondary prevention considerations around finding peer support and family considerations; prenatal testing; and the interconnectedness of women's formative years and their HIV risk.

Many of the women in the reviewed literature spoke of the historical, cultural, socio-emotional, and physical wounds that have affected their health, language, identities, self-respect, and very survival as women (Benoit, Carroll, & Chaudhry, 2003). Violence, poverty, discrimination, racism, oppression, social isolation, stigma, substance abuse, trauma, and violence were also commonplace in the lives of many women. Through this synthesis, it became clear that much research and front-line work is still needed to ensure that gender and gender-based analysis remain integral aspects of primary and secondary HIV prevention interventions. Examples of gender-appropriate interventions are: female-centred programs; services offered in existing health/women's centres; both female and male involvement in initiatives; relationship-based HIV prevention negotiation skills training; empowerment-based programs; and female-controlled technologies, such as microbicides and female condoms (Health Canada, 2003).

Culture and Ethnicity

Culture and ethnicity were the focus of the majority of the articles included in this synthesis. Specifically, 40% of included studies focused on HIV prevention relevant to Aboriginal women. An additional 13% looked at HIV prevention issues as experienced by African and Caribbean women, one study looked at the experiences of Asian youth, and the remainder of the studies focused on Caucasian populations. Although many studies did not specifically investigate the impact of culture or ethnicity on their population, in many cases study populations were disaggregated by ethnicity, or ethnicity was discussed as it evolved out of the interviews or focus group discussions. In general, the findings indicated that HIV prevention services were usually not culturally tailored or sensitive, and if programs did consider ethnicity, they often ignored the diversity within ethnic groups (Flicker et al., 2008).

ABORIGINAL WOMEN

The Tension between a Western Biomedical Approach to HIV and Traditional Aboriginal Approaches to Health and Illness

Several of the studies described Aboriginal women's experiences of grappling with a disconnect between their traditional or cultural understanding of illness and healing and the Western biomedical approach to HIV put forth by most mainstream Canadian health care services (Benoit et al., 2003; Bucharski, Brockman, & Lambert, 1999; Clarke, Friedman, & Hoffman-Goetzb, 2005; Larkin et al., 2007; McKay-McNabb, 2006; Mill, 1997, 2000; Mill, Lambert, Larkin, Ward, & Harrowing, 2008; Ship & Norton, 2001; Wardman & Quarts, 2006). Specifically, there was a lack of focus on holistic approaches to health and well-being (body, mind, spirit, and nature). Many participants in these studies described healing or health in terms of journeys (healing path), connections to nature and spirituality (Tree of Life, the Creator), traditional medicine models (the medicine wheel), or in reference to community-based traditional healers or Elders (Mill, 1997).

Women's experiences with HIV-related services were characterized by a lack of Aboriginal health practitioners and a lack of focus on Aboriginal-specific issues. For example, in McKay-McNabb's (2006) study of Aboriginal women living with HIV, many of the women described needing to relate HIV to their traditional understanding of health and healing before they could move forward with their personal acceptance of their new HIV-positive identity. This finding was echoed in other studies, which documented how participants found their connection to their Aboriginal spirituality helpful in accepting their diagnosis. Some women described their HIV diagnosis as a catalyst for renewing their interest in Aboriginal cultural and healing traditions. However, it should be noted that not all of the women included in these studies felt connected to these aspects of their Aboriginal heritage.

For some, there was a strong feeling that they had become HIV positive for a reason (Mill, 2000). Specifically, being a strong person and therefore being able to learn from living with HIV could serve as a catalyst for facing other issues, such as addictions. Indeed, the dominant biomedical approach to HIV remains focused on individual risk behaviours and the empowerment of women in isolation from broader political, economic, and structural factors that influence initial HIV infection. In fact, some women included in the studies conceptualized HIV as payment for past mistakes, exemplifying a sense of individual fatalism and discrediting the influence of social issues. Some women expressed their belief that they deserved to be HIV positive on the basis of their previous behaviour. One woman said: "Like, I did it, I deserved it." Some women presented fatalistic views about their illness, believing that they had always known they would become HIV positive (Mill, 2000).

A focus on the treatment of existing symptoms rather than the prevention of broader risks or social factors that mitigate risk behaviours continues to stymie HIV prevention efforts. In terms of programming, the expressed Aboriginal belief that a disease must exhibit physical symptoms of illness before treatment is sought may contribute to Aboriginal women being diagnosed later and having poorer HIV treatment outcomes. HIV prevention strategies, especially the promotion of HIV testing, must consider this culturally influenced belief and its interaction with the dominant biomedical approach in an effort to address HIV prevention for Aboriginal women through culturally competent education approaches for individuals, communities, and health practitioners. This synthesis also revealed the need for more holistic approaches to health and HIV that value and embrace the interplay between culture, context, health promotion, and disease prevention paradigms, including the involvement of community leaders, fathers, and family members.

For example, Aboriginal leaders identified the importance of including fathers and family members in prenatal care. Prenatal classes that were geared toward married couples and the nuclear family did not deal with issues and concerns of single parents and therefore failed to meet the emotional, physical, and spiritual needs of many Aboriginal women (Bucharski, Brockman, & Lambert, 1999). Aboriginal leaders also called for the involvement of Elders in the delivery of services. It should be noted, however, that while Aboriginal staff were viewed as being beneficial for building trust with some clients, others felt that working with non-Aboriginal staff would not be a major concern for many clients, especially if service providers were both open-minded and non-judgmental (Wardman & Quarts, 2006). However, the degree to which community is involved may vary from context to context. As such, health professionals must remain open-minded about the degree to which a population may adhere to traditional values and beliefs (Mill, 2000).

The Legacy of Colonialism and Residential Schools on HIV Vulnerability

Mill (1997) describes Aboriginal women's HIV risk as being shaped by their relationships, formative years, self-esteem, and need to engage in survival strategies. These themes are repeated in much of the literature on the impact of gender and HIV risk. Women, especially women from cultural minority groups, experience the highest burden of HIV due to social, economic, and political marginalization. The reality that Aboriginal women in Canada are experiencing higher rates of HIV than non-Aboriginal women speaks to the cumulative impact of culture and gender on HIV vulnerability. Findings from this synthesis relayed stories of women's understanding of how their community and culture was detrimentally impacted by colonialism and, specifically, residential schools. Some Aboriginal women attributed the high prevalence of sexual abuse to the loss of the traditional role of Aboriginal men as protectors of women, resulting from colonization, the socialization experiences in residential schools, and other assimilation practices. It is therefore not surprising that these experiences profoundly affected women's mental health and well-being (Bucharski, Reutter, & Ogilvie, 2006).

Understanding how HIV risk and HIV/AIDS affect Aboriginal populations necessarily raises the issues of the legacy of disadvantage that resulted from European contact and colonialism. This legacy continues to impact negatively on the physical, mental/emotional, social, and spiritual health of Aboriginal peoples, families, and communities. Residential schooling, multi-generational abuse, and forced assimilation in tandem with widespread poverty, racism, sexism, and loss of culture, values, and traditional ways of life have given rise to a range of pressing social problems that include alcoholism, substance abuse, high suicide rates, violence against women, and family violence (Ship & Norton, 2001). These findings point to the need for a gender-based analysis of HIV risk. However, it must be noted that gender alone cannot fully account for the higher infection rates in young Aboriginal women (or young men): factors related to colonialism, racism, poverty, and geographical location (e.g., rural or urban) are also salient. A response to the HIV/AIDS epidemic in Aboriginal communities must begin with an understanding of the unique social, cultural, and economic issues facing Aboriginal peoples.

Embedded in these narratives are common themes that run from childhood to adulthood, including an absence and loss of love, security, esteem, family, friends, home, and education. Aboriginal women's experiences were layered on individual and community histories characterized by trauma, turbulent childhoods, violence and abuse, and physical relocation (McKeown, Reid, & Orr, 2003; Mill et al., 2008; Ship & Norton, 2001). The life histories of these women revealed many common characteristics, such as unstable family situations, frequent moves, and strained interfamilial relationships (Mill, 1997). Many reported experiencing physical violence in childhood, inflicted by family members. As a result, many ran away from their home situation, citing sexual abuse as the main reason (McKeown, Reid, & Orr, 2003). Some children were apprehended by the Child and Family Services government agency and placed in foster care. Reasons included neglect, abandonment, alcohol abuse of parent(s), and physical/sexual abuse. In discussing her experience of living in a foster home, one woman explained, "I cried for years wondering when my mom and dad were going to come and pick me up. They never did" (McKeown, Reid, & Orr, 2003).

Acknowledgement of how the legacy of colonialism intersects with current racism and sexism to marginalize and negatively impact Aboriginal women's health is important in providing culturally competent, accessible, safe, and supportive environments within which HIV prevention work can occur. However, it is essential that culture and gender are not only presented as challenges to health, but also seen as sources of strength and resiliency that can inform HIV prevention strategies. It is important to note that although several of the participants felt they were raised in a "white man's world," some of the Aboriginal beliefs that they had learned as children persisted and were evident in their adult worldview. These participants were often unaware that their beliefs were grounded in their Aboriginal culture.

The Influence of Stigma and Racism ✗

Several authors discussed how the primary source of information on HIV within Aboriginal communities is based on seroprevalence research, which fails to situate HIV in the context of the broader social determinants of health. In a joint study, Health Canada and the University of Manitoba (1998) warned that HIV research that focuses solely on the increasing infection rates in Aboriginal communities can reinforce negative stereotypes and discrimination against Aboriginal people, both within their community and among non-Aboriginal Canadians. The concern is with accepting that Aboriginal populations are more susceptible to HIV without exploring why and without challenging the social conditions that increase risk. In addition, there is also a risk of supporting stereotypes, perpetuating "othering," and adding to the stigma and discrimination already disproportionately experienced by Aboriginal Canadians (Larkin et al., 2007).

In terms of non-Aboriginal youth, there is a tendency to associate contracting HIV with poor decision making and to resist the idea that social processes have any bearing on the construction of individual risk. Whether talking about "people in Africa," "poor people," or "city or urban dwellers," young people often perceive HIV to be something that happens to people elsewhere (Larkin et al., 2007). In contrast, Aboriginal youth worried more about HIV/AIDS, which they recognized as a real and persistent problem in their community (Larkin et al., 2007). Many of these youth also talked about the powerful contribution of intercommunity stigma to HIV risk and silence. Others talked about how the stigma is "contagious," and as a result, entire families can be treated as outcasts (Flicker et al., 2008).

The issue of denial was of particular concern to youth who identify as lesbian. While reflecting on her presentation to a coming-out group for lesbian youth, one

young woman revealed how denial experienced by young people who are HIV positive is mirrored in the attitudes toward HIV risk among lesbians (Travers & Paoletti,
1999). The denial and invisibility of HIV among young lesbians raised heightened
concerns about romantic or sexual partners. Young gay men were more likely to eventually encounter other HIV-positive peers, while young HIV-positive lesbians (given
the low seroprevalence among this group) were likely to experience longer term isolation and marginalization within their peer group. This was evident in the comment
of one young woman who worried about the inability of lesbians to accept that HIV
is a reality in their community (Travers & Paoletti, 1999).

Larkin et al. (2007) and Flicker et al. (2008) interviewed youth to explore how
they understood HIV/AIDS risk. Many of the Aboriginal youth in these studies spoke
of colonialism, racism, and the overrepresentation of their community in the HIV
epidemic. Unlike their non-Aboriginal peers, many of these youth saw HIV as a real
issue that directly affects their community, as a genuine threat and a death sentence.
While some of the Aboriginal youth brought up colonialism and its relationship to
substance abuse and sexual abuse, others held their community responsible for the
high prevalence of HIV without relating HIV to the determinants of health. Larkin
et al. (2007) perceived the youth's discourse of self-blame as a possible reflection of
the negative portrayals of Aboriginal populations in mainstream society. Despite
the existence of internalized racism expressed by some youth, the majority of the
youth described gaining an important sense of identity and support through their
connection to their culture and community and felt that culturally specific HIV resources and services were greatly needed. Many youth felt that it was important for
the Elders in their communities to learn more about HIV/AIDS so that they could
take a leadership role in alleviating stigma. Some youth suggested a youth conference
and an intergenerational connection where Elders and youth could learn and work
together to fight this problem in their communities (Flicker et al., 2008). Further
youth engagement in stigma reduction and public education around HIV prevention
are needed to help lessen the impact of racism and discrimination and to shift the
focus to comprehensive prevention for all.

Insufficient, Inappropriate, and/or Inaccessible Services

Many Aboriginal women expressed a desire for integrated health care services that
respected traditional Aboriginal approaches to health and that also offered opportunities for them to have input into service planning and delivery. Some of the common barriers to HIV-related and other formal health care services described in these
studies included a lack of culturally appropriate available services; fear of HIV testing
and a lack of knowledge regarding testing and treatment options; non-existent or
inconsistent HIV-related services in rural or remote locations; past negative experiences interacting with health practitioners; a lack of confidentiality when accessing
Aboriginal-specific or HIV-specific health services in small communities; and, lastly,

services were not always open to family members, which was especially problematic for women with children.

Limited HIV-related services in small or remote communities, as well as a lack of culturally specific health services in urban communities, represent significant barriers to HIV prevention, education, care, treatment, and support for Aboriginal women. For some HIV-positive women, living in urban and metropolitan centres far from their home communities was necessary to help ensure anonymity. There is also a perception that there is greater acceptance of HIV-positive women in larger cities (Ship & Norton, 2001). The lack of sustainable infrastructure and financial resources for women-specific prevention has been linked to a lack of support for sustainable community-based authority and governance in HIV/AIDS in Canada (Canadian HIV/AIDS Legal Network, 2005).

Many Aboriginal people also reported "feeling helpless" and "weary" of trusting health care providers with mainstream, non-Aboriginal-specific policies. In their own or other Aboriginal people's negative experiences, this resulted in discriminatory treatment (Bucharski, Reutter, & Ogilvie, 2006). Many also expressed a desire for female physicians, due in part to the high rate of family violence, physical and sexual abuse issues, and risk behaviours in their earlier or current lives (Benoit et al., 2003). In this same study, participants were in search of culturally appropriate services that (1) offered support and a safe refuge from the inhospitable urban decay around them; (2) provided staff who understood Aboriginal women's historical wounds and were aware of the lingering racism and sexism that continue to negatively affect their health, language, identity, and self-respect; (3) endorsed a philosophy that promoted preventive health care and incorporated traditional Aboriginal medicine into modern health care practices; and (4) welcomed Aboriginal women's families, especially their children (Benoit et al., 2003). Women also identified the value of peer support and appreciated the opportunity to meet with other mothers who shared similar life situations (Benoit et al., 2003).

Suggested approaches to addressing these issues included partnering to create integrated health and social services in an effort to better address women-specific health and well-being needs and assuage women's concerns about accessing HIV-specific services for fear of lack of confidentiality; more public education to reduce stigma and potentially improve testing and treatment uptake; inclusion of traditional healers and Elders in the development and delivery of HIV-related strategies and programs; the provision of health service models that are open to family members; and consideration of on-reserve and off-reserve issues and the unique barriers experienced by people living in rural or remote communities.

LACK OF FOCUS ON AFRICAN AND CARIBBEAN WOMEN'S HIV-RELATED NEEDS

Despite the fact that Black women in Canada represent a significant group affected by the HIV epidemic, researchers and policy-makers have largely ignored their unique needs (Tharao & Massaquoi, 2002). Fewer Black women access prevention, treatment, support, and care services for HIV in Canada than other women; however, they are overrepresented in recent epidemiological statistics, especially among women being diagnosed during prenatal testing. There are very few prevention programs and educational resources targeted specifically to Black women. This suggests that many Black women may have limited knowledge of HIV/AIDS, its modes of transmission, and how it can be prevented. Most significantly, this may result in a lack of understanding of their own risk of infection (Tharao & Massaquoi, 2002). Findings indicate the need for greater sensitivity on the part of service providers and also the need for more services delivered by and for African and Caribbean communities (Gardezi et al., 2008).

Layering of Various Forms of Marginalization

Increasing rates of HIV infection among African and Caribbean women in Canada have been attributed to the layering of various forms of marginalization. For example, fewer economic opportunities for visible minorities and discrimination related to the unequal transferability of accredited skills and education results in women being more likely to be financially dependent on men. Racism negatively affects employment, housing, education, and other opportunities; further, a diagnosis of HIV has a detrimental impact on immigration status and/or ability to sponsor family members, making individuals unwilling to find out their status (Mitra, Jacobsen, O'Connor, Pottie, & Tugwell, 2006; Newman, Williams, Massaquoi, Brown, & Logie, 2008; Tharao & Massaquoi, 2002;).

African and Caribbean women's economic disadvantage and the increased risk for HIV infection remains a significant prevention issue. Due to the economic marginalization of African and Caribbean women, a positive HIV test result may be regarded as yet another issue in a long list of daily hurdles, with many individuals preferring not to know their HIV status (Tharao & Massaquoi, 2002). In other words, compared to HIV, other issues seem to be more important for Black Canadians in their daily life, including intergenerational conflict, problems encountered by Black youth in the school system, unemployment, racism, and immigration and settlement issues (Gardezi et al., 2008).

Community-Based Sexual Norms

All of the studies included in this synthesis on African and Caribbean women's HIV-related needs discussed existing sexual norms that perpetuate male control in sexual relationships and create an environment conducive to possible gender-based violence (Gardezi et al., 2008; Mitra et al., 2006; Newman et al., 2008; Omorodion, Gbadebo, & Ishak, 2007; Tharao & Massaquoi, 2002). These norms were described as being culturally reinforced social roles, leading to sexualized and gendered identities for African and Caribbean women. Specifically, Gardezi et al. (2008) and Omorodion and colleagues (2007) described how sex, sexuality, and physical and psychological health are generally not discussed in many African and Caribbean homes or communities. Additionally, there was a noted lack of information or concern regarding HIV or STIs among the women interviewed in the two aforementioned studies. This situation was attributed to limited education opportunities, leading to misinformation about the epidemic. Traditional cultural practices that increase risk of infection, such as genital mutilation and vaginal cleansing, were also discussed by women as contributing to HIV risk.

Lack of Culturally and Linguistically Appropriate Resources and Services

Many of the African and Caribbean women included in these studies expressed that their needs were not met by the North American systems of health care delivery, which are based primarily on a biomedical, monocultural model embedded with cultural, linguistic, racial, gender, and class barriers. For example, Tharao and Massaquoi (2002) and Newman et al. (2008) describe how policy on HIV testing in pregnancy was announced without culturally appropriate and language-specific resources for Black women. Additionally, services often do not have the funds to provide culturally and linguistically appropriate resources. African and Caribbean women also spoke of the mistrust of HIV prevention services:

> The history of Black people is very interlinked to discrimination. You know you have colonization, you have slavery ... and I have actually heard women say, "You didn't care about me before, so why should I believe you care about me now, that you're going to be doing these things for me?" (Newman et al., 2008, p. 836)

Among Black African participants, there was strong evidence that discussions of sex, sexuality, and physical and psychological health issues were not part of their everyday experience (Gardezi et al., 2008). This silence and secrecy can result in a tendency, noted particularly among men, not to seek medical care until a health condition is acute and, as a result, likely to yield worse health outcomes. It also impedes access to information about HIV or sexual health, discourages people from seeking treatment, and contributes to the ongoing denial of HIV as affecting African and Caribbean communities in Canada (Gardezi at al., 2008).

While HIV prevention strategies focused on women's experiences are clearly important, men are an undeniable component of Black women's vulnerability to HIV infection (as well as being vulnerable themselves). Men can play a significant role in lowering Black women's HIV risk (Newman et al., 2008). An HIV prevention discourse dominated by messages for men (especially men who have sex with men) was also implicated in a disconnect between Black women and prevention messages. Cultural disconnects were also attributed to what was seen as the prevailing discourse around risk groups, particularly gay men and drug users, which led many Black women to exempt themselves from current HIV prevention messages (Newman et al., 2008).

Young people's perceptions of the influence of religion on sexual activity reinforced findings in the literature showing the link between religiosity and sexual behaviour. Young people with strong religious convictions indicated that sexual networking between members of the same faith influenced the sexual activities they engaged in. Patterns of sexual behaviour were the outcome of conceptualizations of sex as "sinful" and the belief that premarital sex and condom use contravened religious doctrines and laws (Omorodion et al., 2007). The influence of religion on health-related beliefs, specifically prohibition against condoms, was documented as an example of community-held beliefs, values, and norms that can interfere with HIV prevention.

A more nuanced understanding of socio-cultural issues that increase the risk of infection for Black women is needed to address the multiple challenges in developing appropriate prevention approaches. Some of the challenges result from a lack of understanding of the cultural values, beliefs, and practices of Black women. To accurately assess the risk of HIV infection for African and Caribbean women, an understanding of these practices is essential (Tharao & Massaquoi, 2002). Many Black women emphasized the need for "spokespersons," such as celebrities or religious leaders, to draw attention to HIV in their communities and also emphasized the need for community development measures to provide venues for discussion and action. Further, it was noted that information about HIV may not be reaching their communities, perhaps because the distribution channels, language, images, and cultural appropriateness of the messages are not geared to the needs of diverse Black Canadian audiences (Gardezi et al., 2008).

Confidentiality and Stigma

Concerns about confidentiality extended to a fear of using a translator or interpreter from their own community to help with accessing health services (Newman et al., 2008). A "politics of blame" was described to explain the stigma, denial, discrimination, and fear related to HIV that women felt existed in their community. Fear of not being treated with respect when seeking or receiving HIV information, as well as multiple intersecting forms of discrimination, emerged as a powerful context for understanding HIV risk and prevention among Black women (Newman et al., 2008). Reluctance to access health services for fear of encountering a racist perception that African or Caribbean people are carriers of HIV and other diseases remains problematic in HIV prevention approaches (Gardezi et al., 2008). Commonly believed images, stereotypes, and attitudes about the disease itself, compounded by constant anxiety about what others think or feel about African or Caribbean people, may determine whether individuals seek and/or access services (Tharao & Massaquoi, 2002).

Fear of stigmatization for the community as a whole, as opposed to personal stigma, was a deterrent for testing. HIV prevention strategies traditionally address issues of personal safety, personal choice, and individual rights. For women who are raised in communally oriented societies, the well-being of the family and the community may trump the rights of the individual. Successful strategies and programs for many communities must be adjusted in order to address this reality. Individual strategies should be complemented with community-level strategies to modify cultural values, beliefs, norms, and practices that may increase risk of HIV infection (Tharao & Massaquoi, 2002).

The suggestion that it would be "better not to know" one's HIV status because the stress of knowing would lead to physical decline needs to be attended to in subsequent HIV prevention strategies. The association of HIV with rapid decline and death is strong, with terms such as "dead and walking" used to describe community perceptions of HIV-positive people. This makes it difficult for HIV-positive individuals to disclose their status to distant family members back home and reassure them that they are healthy (Gardezi et al., 2008). HIV prevention opportunities were identified in strategies that capitalize on existing community institutions and strengths. The church was regarded as a powerful cultural institution that could be tremendously effective in supporting HIV prevention. The widespread reach of the church was regarded as an important resource for disseminating HIV/AIDS information (Newman et al., 2008).

ASIAN WOMEN (YOUTH-FOCUSED)

Our document-scoping review resulted in only one article specific to Asian women's HIV-related needs in Canada. The article by Kwong-Lai Poon and Trung-Thu Ho (2002) consisted of a qualitative analysis of the cultural and social vulnerabilities to HIV infection among gay, lesbian, and bisexual Asian youth. This study identified the following themes as creating vulnerabilities to HIV for Asian youth living in Canada: (1) the lack of sex education at home, (2) homophobia in Asian families, (3) unresponsive health and social service providers, (4) lack of social support, (5) negative stereotypes, (6) ideal standards of beauty, and (7) negative perceptions of safer sex practices among Asian lesbian and bisexual women.

AGE

The predominant theme to emerge from the research based on young women and HIV prevention was that young women are ill equipped to discuss sex and safety with their sexual partners (Beazley & Schmidt, 1996; Cleary, Barhman, MacCormack, & Herold, 2002; DiCenso et al., 2001). The primary recommendation from the reviewed literature was to teach youth how to discuss and negotiate safer sex. Providing youth with accurate, practical information about sex from informed, non-judgmental teachers and service providers was seen as a necessary step to curb misinformation and lack of information regarding available services. Additional recommendations included ensuring that accessible anonymous testing and counselling are available to youth and actively involving both genders in HIV prevention discussions and initiatives.

Youth also talked about difficulty accessing appropriate sexual health services. Both males and females indicated barriers such as clinic locations, hours of operation, or insufficient time for appointments. In rural communities, the issue of location provided additional challenges. Transportation to and from clinics was a barrier, given that many students do not have access to a car or public transportation (DiCenso et al., 2001). In rural communities, both male and female students expressed concern about confidentiality when using any of the sexual health services, given the high risk of being seen in the local drug store or sexual health clinic (DiCenso et al., 2001).

In some cases, physicians' offices were not seen as the most appropriate venue to receive information. For example, a few young women commented that physicians had not fully informed them about contraceptives, an omission that left them with misunderstandings about the proper use and possible side effects of birth control pills (Beazley & Schmidt, 1996). In other instances doctors would not share information unless a parent was present. One 15-year-old girl stated:

> When I asked my doctor about birth control pills, he said he wouldn't give it [information] to me unless he talked to my mother. I think that was his way of scaring me into talking to her about it. Well, it didn't work. (Beazley & Schmidt, 1996, p. 3)

It is important to note that even the most articulate, educated, skilled young women were not able to have discussions with partners who were unwilling to engage. Participants reported that partners who inhibited the communication process did not want to talk about sexual health issues, sexual histories, and/or to sexually self-disclose (Cleary et al., 2002).

> And sometimes he would say things like, "Well, is that really necessary for us to talk about" because he hated talking about the past. Obviously, you don't want to talk about the past with someone new … but he would be like, "Do we have to talk about this? I don't want you to get upset blah blah blah." (Cleary et al., 2002, p. 126)

Assumptions were also used to avoid potentially awkward discussions about condom use. In the study by Cleary et al. (2002), instead of initiating conversations related to condom use, young women assumed that their partners would know that they needed to use a condom. In other cases, the men seemed to assume that the women would be taking care of the contraception. It was evident that many of the participants did not think that there were any substantive risks involved in having a sexual relationship with their partner. Most used unfounded assumptions in making their own decisions on condom use and contraception. Under these circumstances, they felt quite safe (Cleary et al., 2002).

Students explained that sex education classes did not provide them with useful information: little was taught beyond the basic "plumbing" of sexual health and the focus was on the negative consequences of unhealthy sexual decisions (DiCenso et al.,

2001). Although most students had been taught the various forms of birth control, very few could identify forms other than the pill and condoms. Students didn't consider teachers to be the best sexual health educators, and they often feared that teachers would tell their parents or give them poor grades if they learned they were sexually active (DiCenso et al., 2001). Both male and female adolescents said they would like to be able to talk to their parents about sex (DiCenso et al., 2001). Youth also talked about being bored with traditional sexual health education approaches and thought the current strategies were outdated and unrealistic (DiCenso et al., 2001; Flicker et al., 2008).

Although both urban and on-reserve youth said they prefer peers who are living with HIV/AIDS to educate them about the disease, many of these youth said they would like to learn from the Elders in their communities about sexual health education and other diseases. As mentioned above, many youth felt that it was important for the Elders to learn more about HIV/AIDS so that they could take a leadership role in alleviating stigma.

Both men and women over 35 years of age resisted the use of condoms because they felt they belonged to a generation that grew up not seeing the need for safer sex. As a result, long-standing patterns of unprotected intercourse with sexual partners was a strong barrier to the adoption of safer sex (Nadeau, Truchon, & Biron, 2000). Similarly, for married men and women, the implied "safety" within marital relationships and the unequal gender-power relations between men and women were regarded as obstacles to condom use (Newman et al., 2008).

SEXUAL ORIENTATION AND IDENTITY

Overall, our synthesis found a very limited focus on the HIV/AIDS-related information and prevention service needs of lesbian, bisexual, and transgender women. Kwong-Lai Poon and Trung-Thu Ho (2002) interviewed 15 gay, lesbian, and bisexual Asian youth to investigate cultural and social barriers to HIV prevention and identified multiple barriers to sexual health education and resources related to unresponsive and/or homophobic family members and service providers. Travers and Paoletti (1999) found that age-specific, barrier-free, well-advertised services were urgently needed for HIV-positive lesbian, gay, and bisexual youth to prevent social isolation and despair. Service providers can play a significant role in enhancing quality of life for these youth. First and foremost, services must be youth-specific and barrier-free. Misinformation, shame, self-blame, denial, social isolation, and fear can be reduced through individual and group counselling supports. Finally, there is an important role for community supports including peer-based programming (Travers & Paoletti, 1999). It is important for counsellors to consider that youth may have little, if any, life experience in coping with adverse life events, or the death of family members or friends. These factors may make the helplessness associated with fear of dying from AIDS particularly acute for HIV-positive lesbian, gay, and bisexual youth.

Counselling supports should thus focus on building hope through assisting youth in sorting through residual conflicts or difficulties related to sexual identity formation, familiarizing them with current treatment methods, and providing the requisite skills for living with HIV infection (Travers & Paoletti, 1999).

DRUG USE

Six studies in our synthesis focused on the HIV prevention or care needs of women who use drugs (Elwood-Martin et al., 2005; Harvey et al., 1998; Jackson et al., 2002; Shannon et al., 2008; Ship & Norton, 2001; Strike, Challacombe, Myers, & Millson, 2002). These studies contained a wealth of information regarding the contexts within which women who use drugs must navigate in their HIV prevention efforts. The authors described the need for harm reduction initiatives (i.e., needle exchange programs) to be complemented and supported by larger policy shifts (i.e., harm reduction services in prisons) and revised drug laws based on human rights principles and evidence-based evaluation data (Harvey et al., 1998; Kwong-Lai Poon & Trung-Thu Ho, 2002; Strike et al., 2002). Jackson et al. (2002) described individual behavioural-level issues that impact HIV risk, such as women being less likely to use condoms with regular sexual partners, and uncovered the important contribution that peers can make in promoting healthy behavioural choices. Shannon et al. (2008) explored how addiction, interpersonal relationships, violence, local policing, and sex work all influence one another in relation to HIV risk within Vancouver's Downtown Eastside. HIV prevention strategies that move beyond an individual, behavioural focus to include structural and environmental interventions are recommended as a way to create environments that will enable and sustain effective HIV prevention (Shannon et al., 2008).

Many of the respondents who indicated that they have in the recent past shared a needle spoke of how this occurred when they ran out of needles and the needle exchange was closed, or they had some unexpected access to drugs and were without a needle. Several spoke of sharing needles while incarcerated (Jackson et al., 2002). In the study by Ship and Norton (2001), all of the Inuit women interviewed were aware of the risks of HIV from unprotected sex and sharing needles. The notion of negotiated risk, particularly in resource-limited settings, offers an important insight into the provision of HIV prevention within a harm reduction framework.

Participants offered several recommendations to enhance the profile and availability of harm reduction. The key component of these recommendations was focused around augmenting education to all sectors of the community to make them more aware of the need for these services. It was felt that there is a general lack of awareness around how harm reduction services can fit with existing philosophies and treatments of addictions (Wardman & Quarts, 2006). Participants suggested that educational efforts should be offered in a participatory fashion to capture the experiences of those who would be affected by the integration of harm reduction services. In addition, it was suggested that combining harm reduction education with other health promotion initiatives might provide an easier point of entry for HIV prevention strategies. Participants also strongly emphasized the diversity of groups in need of prevention education campaigns (Wardman & Quarts, 2006).

The value of community leaders must not be underestimated, as their support is crucial for delivering harm reduction services. In addition to elected leadership, the support and trust of community Elders, who can also play a key role in advocating for these services, must be gained (Wardman & Quarts, 2006). Changing community members' attitudes and beliefs around harm reduction was seen as vital in gaining widespread acceptance of harm reduction approaches to service provision. Community education efforts could be facilitated by existing media, which are often used for communication in First Nations communities (Wardman & Quarts, 2006).

WOMEN LIVING WITH HIV/AIDS

Five articles included in our synthesis explored the HIV-related needs of women living with HIV/AIDS. The primary focus of these articles was to discuss the social and psychological impact of HIV on women's lives and their care, treatment, and support needs. The primary themes discussed were parenting challenges, the significance of the diagnosis event, and barriers to support-service use (Antle, Wells, Goldie, DeMatteo, & King, 2001; Heath, 1999; McKeown et al., 2003; Metcalfe, Langstaff, Evans, Paterson, & Reid, 1998). According to Metcalfe et al. (1998), women disclosed an interest in support groups or peer meetings, integrated care with other social and health services, and the need for female-friendly environments where children were welcome. Heath (1999) discussed how larger social/structural issues, such as unemployment, poverty, and lack of housing, child care, information, and support, contributed to HIV-positive women's isolation and inability to access local resources. Recommendations included peer-based support, woman-friendly services, female staff, child care and education for communities, and service providers.

Participants across diverse populations and cultures indicated experiencing various levels of social isolation. For mothers living with HIV/AIDS, a lack of emotional and social support was reported. In addition, as a consequence of multiple stigmas and barriers to services, First Nations women living with HIV/AIDS and their children have little, if any, emotional and social support. Life becomes a daily struggle for most HIV-positive women who are unable to provide for basic needs— food, clothing, shelter, and transportation—for themselves and for their children. Unable to afford expensive treatments, HIV-positive women must often make difficult choices between purchasing medications for themselves and basics for their families. As this single HIV-positive mother described:

> Your first priority is your child. All the money that you get if you live on welfare or have a job goes to your child, to your child's well-being.

> Sometimes you get a little bit for yourself ... money, time out or chance
> to sit and share with other women. (Ship & Norton, 2001, p. 27)

For the women in Vancouver's Downtown Eastside, there are very few places where Aboriginal women can go and sit with their children in a safe, non-judgmental environment. There are even fewer support systems available for children to learn how to cope with the fact that their mothers are living with HIV or AIDS (Benoit et al., 2003).

Many families expressed significant concern about discrimination, particularly toward their children, should they disclose their HIV status (Antle et al., 2001). As such, it is important that professionals understand the complex dynamics in families living with HIV/AIDS (Antle et al., 2001). For example, social workers in a range of settings could become more proactive in reaching out to families living with HIV. Those working with adults who are HIV positive need to include a child and family focus, inquiring about potential children, helping to evaluate the impact of HIV/AIDS on these children, and addressing the extra demands of parenting (Antle et al., 2001). Families need to know that they are not alone. Social workers need to recognize and prepare for the ways in which HIV/AIDS touches their lives, their clients' lives, and their clients' families and children (Antle et al., 2001).

Many women live in secrecy due to the multiple forms of stigma associated with HIV/AIDS. However, they also suffer from gender discrimination because, as women, they carry the additional stigma of being branded as "promiscuous," "a bad mother," and "deserving of HIV/AIDS" (Shannon et al., 2008). Reluctance to disclose the seropositive status of a loved one is also related to fear of rejection, fear of emotional and physical harm to children, fear of discrimination, and/or simply needing time to come to grips with the reality of living with HIV/AIDS (Ship & Norton, 2001).

Isolation of caregivers is a consequence of the continuing stigma attached to HIV/AIDS in Aboriginal communities and the resulting dilemmas of disclosure. Lack of services, counselling, and supports for the caregiver, the loved one living with HIV/AIDS, and, in some cases, the family, particularly those living in Aboriginal communities and smaller urban centres, serves to reinforce their isolation (Ship & Norton, 2001). Counselling and support for caregivers are almost nonexistent. Many caregivers find it difficult to accept the HIV diagnosis of a loved one. Caregivers need time and support in working through their complex and often contradictory feelings and to undergo a grieving process, much like those diagnosed with HIV/AIDS.

Participants also stated that they experienced a lack of acceptance of people living with HIV/AIDS, not only from society at large, but, more painfully, from their family members and from members of their community. The shame, stigma, and discrimination associated with the disease leads to the perception among some women that an HIV diagnosis is something they would be better off not knowing. This in turn can serve to limit access to and uptake of HIV testing services, timely diagnosis, and early access to treatment for those who are found to be infected. This may also be an important issue in relation to secondary prevention of HIV, where those who are living with HIV but don't know their HIV status may see no need to take precautions to prevent the onward transmission of the virus.

While some participants have endured hardships and persevered, sought the support they needed and have begun to develop their new identities as women living with HIV/AIDS, other participants continue to struggle to deal with the risk factors that are a part of their everyday life. According to McKay-McNabb (2006), it is important to understand that Aboriginal women who are affected by HIV/AIDS also go through developing a new identity when they have a family member or loved one living with HIV/AIDS. Each of the Aboriginal women interviewed shared experiences unique to her life and her individual stages of identity that truly revealed what it was like to walk along the path to healing with HIV/AIDS (McKay-McNabb, 2006).

Several HIV-positive women indicated encountering problems with male partners after an HIV diagnosis. Four women described verbal, psychological, or physical abuse that either followed or was aggravated by disclosure of their HIV status to their partners. Two of the women described difficulties in accessing HIV-related support services because of opposition from their partners. It was found that heterosexual men are more prone to denying their own or their partner's HIV status than women (Gardezi et al., 2008).

Lesbians with HIV continue to be a hidden and isolated population, and despite attempts to include greater numbers of HIV-positive lesbians in research, they are reluctant to come forward. Those who did, however, spoke poignantly about HIV-related stigma among lesbians and the resulting social marginalization and isolation. It is likely that because lesbians primarily contract HIV from sharing needles or from sex with men, social stigma is further intensified, adding to their sense of isolation (Ship & Norton, 2001).

Almost all of the participants mentioned the importance of a strong support system to assist HIV-positive individuals to adapt to and accept their diagnosis. Women expressed a need to become involved in a support group exclusively for HIV-positive women. They felt that involvement in a women's support group would give them an opportunity to express their feelings more openly (McKeown et al., 2003). Several of the participants were surprised by the amount of support that was available once they knew where to find it and were able to ask for it. For the most part, most found it very helpful to talk with other Aboriginal men and women who were HIV positive. Although most of the participants had at least one family member, such as a parent or sibling, who provided support following their diagnosis, several felt that their families had not provided the support they needed at the time of their diagnosis (Mill et al., 2008).

HIV/AIDS SERVICE PROVIDERS: TESTING AND COUNSELLING

Several articles included in our synthesis focused on issues related to providing HIV prevention education, testing, counselling, care, treatment and/or support to women from the perspective of service providers (Worthington & Myers, 2003; Strike et al., 2002; Beazley & Schmidt, 1996; Spittal et al., 2003; Hilton et al., 2001; Mitra et al., 2006). These studies illustrate some of the key issues that arise between service providers and service users that can serve as either barriers or facilitators to HIV prevention for women. Worthington and Myers (2003) outline how women described patient–provider power dynamics during HIV testing as being potentially stigmatizing and disempowering. Spittal et al. (2003) describe how a group of needle exchange workers had to "bend" inefficient service delivery policies to better meet the needs of their clients. Hilton, Thompson, Moore-Dempsey, and Hutchinson (2001) describe the specialized education and support needs of outpost nurses who engage, retain, and treat marginalized women who are at high risk of acquiring HIV and other health and safety issues. Further, they also describe the challenges of connecting marginalized women to the mainstream health care system and influencing colleagues to be responsive to their unique needs. Olivier and Dykeman (2003) discuss the commonalities between the HIV prevention work completed by both nurses and social workers and suggest the need for greater collaboration in areas of service delivery, policy development, advocacy, and professional development.

Many practitioners linked decisional conflict to HIV-related stigma that women feared from their social network. There is the fear of the negative consequences of testing: fear of alienation and ostracism, fear that their partners may leave if they find out they tested, and fear of being isolated from the community. Others linked HIV stigma to institutional discrimination, noting that specific populations of women fear how their test results will affect their immigration status or their being able to afford all required medications and related treatments if they do not have a health plan (Mitra et al., 2006).

Despite varying levels of distrust of the health system, health care providers were seen by some as an important resource for providing HIV prevention information. Key informants explained the importance of making HIV/AIDS education as accessible as possible through their own family doctors' offices or in health clinics. Health care providers were specifically acknowledged as conduits for imparting HIV information to Black youth, particularly immigrant youth, who were described as vulnerable due to lack of exposure to HIV education and being protected by their families (Newman et al., 2008). However, in the study by Beazley and Schmidt (1996), physicians were not the preferred source of reproductive health information for young women, who felt that physicians either did not take enough time to fully inform them or used inaccessible medical terminology. As such, the women interviewed in this study offered two key suggestions for physicians. First, within their offices and communities, they must provide accurate and non-judgmental information in language that is accessible to young women. Second, they must do so before adverse outcomes of sexual intercourse are experienced (Beazley & Schmidt, 1996). Several other considerations were raised in relation to physicians, including the possibility of experiencing stigma from physicians, the need to switch to a new physician once a patient is found to be HIV positive, and the paternalistic attitudes of some physicians in dictating what patients ought to do about their HIV status, rather than discussing options with patients (Newman et al., 2008).

Overall, physicians must make their practices more accessible and user friendly. Specifically, young women will benefit more when their doctors: (1) provide office environments that encourage frank, clear, and confidential discussions; (2) listen actively to their young female patients; (3) present caring, accurate, and non-judgmental messages; and (4) discuss societal influences that negatively affect their adolescent patients. More user-friendly practices could help young women gain confidence in their own sexual decision-making skills, have better control over their sexual behaviours, and become proficient in the use of various options for the prevention of pregnancy and STIs (Beazley & Schmidt, 1996).

Although the key principles of the ideal HIV testing situation constitute the groundwork for culturally appropriate testing, the women also identified additional strategies that relate specifically to their Aboriginal culture. In addition to incorporating and respecting cultural practices, programs must also respect both the age and literacy levels of clients. For instance, youth tend to prefer messages that are blunt and that use appropriate, accessible language (Wardman & Quarts, 2006). Key informants offered specific suggestions for mainstreaming HIV prevention education and testing information into general health education programs, thereby allowing for a greater integration of HIV/AIDS into the existing health discourse of women's health. This could include discussions of HIV testing within the context of a general health checkup (Newman et al., 2008).

DISCUSSION
Overarching Themes and Gaps
One of the predominant messages that emerged from this synthesis was the importance of women's day-to-day lived reality, including the social and structural contexts that shape their individual and collective HIV risk. The importance of tailored programming and policy cannot be overstated and was reflected to some degree in each article included in this synthesis. When women are regarded and treated as a homogenous group with identical HIV prevention needs, the ensuing prevention interventions lack the specificity to address the unique constellation of social determinants of health among the diverse populations and communities of women in Canada. More research, funding, and support are needed to allow for tailored policy and programming responses that can address the impact of overlapping, intersecting, and multi-sectoral social determinants of health on HIV risk.

HIV-related service providers, specifically nurses, front-line AIDS service organization workers, harm reduction workers, peer support workers, and social workers, need to be valued and supported in their roles to avoid burnout and promote ongoing training and collaboration (Antle et al., 2001; Gardezi et al., 2008; Heath, 1999). Integrated care holds promise for improving accessibility to, and knowledge of, existing resources for HIV prevention among the diverse populations of women in Canada. Confidential programs and services, including anonymous HIV testing and counselling, must be made accessible to all. Community-wide education to promote available services, increase general knowledge regarding HIV/AIDS, and decrease social stigma continues to be one of the primary recommendations to come out of the literature.

A major limitation found in this body of literature was the varying level of descriptive detail provided in the published journal articles. For example, several studies included both male and female participants, but did not provide sex-disaggregated information in their results or discussion sections (Clarke et al., 2005; Kwong-Lai Poon & Trung-Thu Ho, 2002; Larkin et al., 2007; Mill et al., 2008). Without this information, we are unable to ascertain how gendered issues surrounding HIV prevention differ for men and women. Other studies did not report on the age, ethnicity, or physical location of participants. Several articles that focused on Aboriginal women took a pan-Aboriginal approach, without discussing diversity among Aboriginal women in Canada. Without detailed information on participant characteristics, we are unable to garner relevant information for priority setting, fund allocation, and policy or programming decision making.

A second limitation was a lack of positioning of individual study findings within a larger structural, macro-level context of HIV prevention for the purpose of making connections between studies. One of the strengths to be derived from contextualized HIV prevention research is the insight that can come from creating links between macro-level factors and micro-level factors, thereby shifting the discourse from individual risk behaviours to risk environments. Few articles discussed how larger social issues such as housing, poverty, racism, and settlement impact HIV prevention for women. Additionally, only one study mentioned women-controlled HIV prevention technologies (i.e., microbicides). Lastly, it is important to note that many of the articles did not specifically set out to address HIV prevention.

Given the long history of strained researcher–community relations, particularly within many Indigenous communities, there may be resistance to disseminating through mainstream "peer review" networks. For example, it is likely that HIV interventions and prevention strategies conducted by and for Indigenous peoples without the assistance of academic researchers may not be disseminated through academic peer review outlets. In our search strategy, studies were limited to those written in English and published in peer-reviewed journals. This may be problematic for cultures that might resist "writing down" or sharing Indigenous knowledge. As such, the written record of the Western academy may not provide the full picture of these lessons.

Recognizing that not all of the most promising HIV prevention approaches are disseminated through peer-review channels, the research team contacted experts in the field for suggestions and recommendations for other kinds of documents, specifically program reports, agency evaluations, and other types of community-based or government reports that would help us learn more about effective strategies and approaches for HIV prevention with Aboriginal and non-Aboriginal women in Canada. However, the information gathered did not meet our literature search inclusion criteria and were removed from our analysis and discussion. It is important to take these limitations into consideration in subsequent reviews in order to identify what is currently being implemented by community-level HIV/AIDS organizations and to help identify best or wise practices in HIV prevention efforts in Canada beyond what is housed in academic, peer-reviewed journals.

Recommendations

Shifting the discourse away from a biomedical focus largely concerned with individual HIV risk behaviours to "risk contexts" acknowledges the complexity of the social, political, and economic determinants of HIV prevention. This in turn serves to create a robust understanding of the intersecting contexts of HIV risk, resulting in a more comprehensive approach to HIV prevention for women. We argue that this approach needs to be more widely adopted as a framework for government-led and community-based HIV prevention programming and policy in Canada.

It is clear from this synthesis that problems arise when trying to translate a framework of determinants of health into effective HIV prevention programs and policies. The *Federal Initiative to Address HIV/AIDS in Canada* (PHAC, 2004) and the *Blueprint for Action on Women and Girls and HIV* (2006) have identified women among the most vulnerable to HIV in Canada. Both have expressed the need for a national HIV/AIDS response that addresses human rights, determinants of health, and gendered dimensions of the epidemic. Despite widely accepted endorsements of the importance of these approaches in shaping HIV prevention policies and programs, more needs to be done to address and lessen the burden of HIV among women in Canada, specifically minority women. This gap may be partially due to a lack of understanding and support for the day-to-day circumstances that influence women's HIV risk contexts.

The key themes in this synthesis provide knowledge relevant to HIV prevention programming and policy, particularly in relation to the diverse populations and communities of women in Canada. The valuing of cultural identity and traditions, without making assumptions about the role that these traditions play in women's lives, requires being open and reflexive to the impact of, for example, language, culture, and ethnicity in our HIV prevention efforts. More specifically, HIV prevention for women requires enhancing public education about HIV, eliminating barriers to testing, improving the quality of HIV care, ensuring community-based governance of HIV prevention services (including develop-ment, implementation, delivery, and evaluation), developing culturally specific prevention programming, and partnering with local and existing services to create integrated health resources and to reduce HIV stigma. Additionally, HIV prevention services must provide support and safe spaces for women by ensur-ing health service providers understand the impact of the social determinants of health, such as culture, gender, and poverty, on women's HIV-related prevention needs. Women's experiential knowledge must be integrated into programming and policy to improve the fit, quality, and longevity of interventions. Existing HIV prevention programs and policies that apply biomedical approaches to HIV without exploring and addressing the root structural causes and social determin-ants of HIV need to be challenged and revised. The federal government should consistently require gender-based and sex-based analysis as mandatory in research and programming grants and provide adequate funding and support for gender-focused strategies. Lastly, Canadian women must continually be included in all stages of research investigating their HIV-related needs, from priority setting and planning to evaluation and dissemination in order to ensure that the research remains in line with their lived experiences and evolving needs.

FUTURE DIRECTIONS FOR RESEARCH ON HIV PREVENTION FOR WOMEN IN CANADA

Drawing parallels and identifying successes and challenges is necessary in order to move this important work forward with implications for HIV prevention policy, practice, and programming. The results of this synthesis suggest there are a number of significant gaps in need of further consideration in future research and program-ming efforts related to women and HIV prevention. The following section briefly outlines areas that may warrant further attention as specified by the authors of the literature. It should be noted that these issues may have been addressed in other re-search studies not included in this synthesis.

Cultural Rules

The cultural rules and expectations that serve to regulate and inform sexual behav-iours and practices of women require additional consideration. Research involving different populations of women, such as women living on reserves who are not HIV positive, may be necessary to further explore this question. For the women inter-viewed in the Mill (1997) study, it was critical to explore their life histories in order to develop a greater understanding of the factors that influenced their HIV infection.

Parenting

Links between HIV prevention, HIV/AIDS care, and reproductive health, including fertility options for people living with HIV, require additional attention by health care providers. The desire for parenthood among people living with HIV, access to fertility services, and coverage policies are important issues for future investigation and care initiatives. Parenting issues for women, both HIV-positive women wishing to become pregnant as well as those wishing to become pregnant where the serostatus of their partners may be unknown, requires additional attention. As well, parenting of infected and affected children within the same family and the differential approaches and consequent challenges this may cause is an important area that has been largely overlooked (Antle et al., 2001).

HIV Counselling and Testing

Despite the availability of HIV testing in Canada, barriers to testing differ in urban and rural areas (Bucharski et al., 1999). Obtaining both recipient and provider perspectives would provide a more complete understanding of how potentially differing views may influence the dynamics of care in HIV counselling and testing situations (Bucharski et al., 1999). Further, there are numerous Canadian studies that identify discrimination as a key barrier for Aboriginal women seeking health care services in general (Bucharski et al., 1999). These findings reinforce the need to address the issues of repeat negative testing in HIV test counselling practices. Further information on HIV counselling techniques that can allow for more effective approaches to addressing perceptions of safety associated with monogamy and HIV immunity may assist in reducing misinformation about risk (Ryder et al., 2005).

Although the national guidelines for HIV counselling and testing in Canada are being revised, focusing on HIV testing for women through prenatal care overlooks HIV testing for both heterosexual male partners and women who fall outside reproductive age. In addition, post-test counselling will continue to result in missed prevention opportunities if removed from the revised guidelines (Ryder et al., 2005). It is noteworthy that pre-test assessment of HIV risk behaviours was not seen as a significant barrier to testing and was rarely mentioned in the literature (Bucharski et al., 1999).

Stigma and Discrimination

To the extent that stigma and discrimination are significant components of the experience of Aboriginal people with HIV/AIDS, further community-based intervention research is needed to address these concerns (Clarke et al., 2005).

Health Protective Sexual Communication (HPSC)

Men and women may have different gender-based experiences and attitudes in relation to health protective sexual communication. Additional clarity on how one can engage in health protective sexual communication with a partner without sacrificing the relationship or one's sexual health may be warranted (Cleary et al., 2002).

Macro-Level Systemic Factors

It is clear from the data that further efforts are needed to address systemic inequities in HIV prevention education and stigma reduction at the macro-structural level (Flicker et al., 2008).

Determinants of HIV Risk

Future research may be needed to understand the particular social determinants of HIV risk of Aboriginal youth in diverse situations, including on-reserve youth and youth who migrate between cities and reserves (Larkin et al., 2007). Future research in treatment settings must take into account how addiction issues may be used as an important defence mechanism in buffering against the reality of HIV/AIDS (Nadeau et al., 2000).

Lesbian and Bisexual Women

Health care providers need to be aware of how lesbians' needs differ from those of heterosexual women in the area of reproductive health, including HIV prevention approaches. As well, acknowledging and addressing the barriers faced by lesbian/bisexual women in accessing basic services is crucial (Mathieson, Bailey, & Gurevich, 2002). Lesbians living with HIV remain a hidden and isolated population and as such are often unwilling to come forward as research participants. Further research with lesbian and bisexual populations, particularly from diverse youth populations, is required to attain a broader understanding of their needs (Travers & Paoletti, 1999). Further, understanding the regional differences in health care uptake patterns among lesbian and bisexual women may yield important HIV prevention interventions (Mathieson et al., 2002).

Treatment and Care

The decision as to when to begin HIV treatment may be problematic among certain populations who are more likely to be in care at a much later stage of illness. This may raise ethical issues regarding the basis of the knowledge that early treatment of HIV can prolong life. Further debate and discussion on this complex secondary prevention issue is necessary to ensure that treatment options that are congruent with individual- and community-level beliefs and values are both available and accessible (Mill, 2000).

Lived Experience of Women with HIV

Clearly there is a dire need to expand knowledge of the lived experiences of women affected by HIV—both in terms of primary and secondary prevention.

Black Women

The historical absence of Black women in the HIV prevention research and in terms of accessing prevention, treatment, support, and care initiatives is especially evident.

Although Black women and Aboriginal women make up a small proportion of the Canadian population, they are vastly overrepresented among those infected. Current HIV infection rates indicate an urgent need for further research with, by, and for populations of Black women to contextualize results obtained by statistical modelling and to better understand the psychosocial, cultural, and structural determinants of HIV risk (Tharao & Massaquoi, 2002).

Youth

HIV prevention for young women in Canada is characterized by significant barriers to HIV testing and access to treatments, and as such, this remains an area in need of further research (Travers & Paoletti, 1999).

Relationship with Health Professionals

The relationships women may have with health care professionals can serve as an important conduit to timely access to prevention interventions, HIV testing, and treatment. However, interacting with health care providers can be a significant source of anxiety, which has both policy and practice implications. Such anxiety is often related to service and social context issues, in addition to "anxious apprehension" about HIV test results. This is also the case with existing understandings of the power dynamic between clients and service providers, where the control exerted over the professional interaction by the client has been investigated only tangentially. More research is required in these areas (Worthington & Myers, 2003).

AIDS Widowhood

Those women who have lost their husbands or partners to AIDS remain a significant issue for future research. AIDS widowhood was described as "two in the one," which acknowledges the dual process of caring for a dying husband or partner while learning of and trying to adjust to their own diagnosis. This population appears to have several unique intrapsychic and support needs that have, until now, been largely overlooked. No reference to this particular finding was noted in the literature (Heath, 1999).

NEXT STEPS: THE WAY FORWARD

The results of this synthesis remind us of the need to reframe our collective understanding of the determinants of health that place women and men, and boys and girls in Canada at differential levels of risk for HIV infection. The shift away from focusing solely on individual-level factors and the recognition of the need to attend to the broader structural factors in HIV transmission resulted in a more complex analysis of the bio-psychosocial issues that, collectively, increase the likelihood of becoming HIV positive. This is particularly relevant to women as we regard gender as a key determinant of health and, more specifically, gender-related expectations regarding sexuality and how these gendered expectations impact both our primary and secondary HIV prevention efforts. The predominant message that emerged from the reviewed articles was the importance of women's day-to-day lived realities and the social and structural contexts that shape HIV risk.

Shifting the discourse away from a biomedical focus on individual HIV risk to "risk environments" or contexts acknowledges the historical interaction of social, political, and economic determinants of HIV risk. This in turn serves to create a more robust understanding of the intersecting and overlapping contexts of HIV risk, resulting in a more comprehensive approach to HIV prevention for women. We argue that such multi-sectoral approaches need to be widely adopted in prevention frameworks for government-led and community-based HIV programming and policy in Canada.

This synthesis recognizes the long history of HIV prevention efforts on the one hand while at the same time acknowledging the lack of integration and uptake of findings. This lack of integration has important implications for our future research-knowledge generation, as well as in terms of informing our policy responses and programming efforts. Clearly HIV research, policy, and programming responses for, by, and with diverse populations and communities of women require an augmented response across health, social, and legal sectors to ensure our efforts are meeting the unique primary and secondary HIV prevention needs of all women in Canada.

PROBLEM-BASED LEARNING CASE STUDY

Challenges in the development of novel prevention interventions are, in part, related to privileging particular approaches to research and the application of particular "ways of knowing." The utility of synthesizing our prevention knowledge is found in a greater understanding of what is working, what is not, and why. Despite this, different sectors working in HIV prevention—from community-based primary prevention to formal health care settings in secondary prevention—have distinct perspectives on what are seen as appropriate types of knowledge to inform their work. Consider each of the following sectors and how your approach to synthesizing knowledge would be regarded as useful, appropriate, and meaningful in developing prevention interventions for women in Canada:

- frontline service delivery
- policy analysis
- evaluation

CRITICAL THINKING QUESTIONS

1. How can our findings be better integrated into the next wave of both primary and secondary HIV prevention interventions for women while acknowledging the diverse populations of women?
2. How can we develop appropriate evaluation approaches of prevention interventions that take into consideration the lived experiences of women?

3. What are some alternative methodologies that would allow for a greater integration of approaches and yet include a gender-based analysis?
4. Based on your own disciplinary training, how would you bridge with other disciplines in the development of greater horizontality in our prevention efforts?

REFERENCES

Antle, B., Wells, L., Goldie, S., DeMatteo, D., & King, S. M. (2001). Challenges of parenting for families living with HIV/AIDS. *Social Work, 46*(2), 159–169.

Beazley, R. P., & Schmidt, K. M. (1996). Physicians as providers of reproductive health information to young women. *The Canadian Journal of Human Sexuality, 5*(1), 1–6.

Benoit, C., Carroll, D., & Chaudhry, M. (2003). In search of a Healing Place: Aboriginal women in Vancouver's Downtown Eastside. *Social Science and Medicine, 56*, 821–833.

Blueprint for Action on Women & Girls and HIV/AIDS. (2006). *Blueprint for action on women and girls and HIV/AIDS: Blueprint manifesto.* Retrieved from http://womensblueprint.org/userfiles/file/manifesto_e.pdf (site discontinued).

Bucharski, D., Brockman, L., & Lambert, D. (1999). Developing culturally appropriate prenatal care models for Aboriginal women. *The Canadian Journal of Human Sexuality, 8*(2), 48–54.

Bucharski, D., Reutter, L. I., & Ogilvie, L. D. (2006). You need to know where we're coming from: Canadian Aboriginal women's perspectives on culturally appropriate HIV counseling and testing. *Health Care Women International, 27*(8), 723–747.

Canadian HIV/AIDS Legal Network. (2005). *Aboriginal people and HIV/AIDS: Legal issues.* Retrieved from www.aidslaw.ca/publications/publicationsdocEN.php?ref=1

Clarke, J. N., Friedman, D. B., & Hoffman-Goetzb, L. (2005). Canadian Aboriginal people's experiences with HIV/AIDS as portrayed in select English language media. *Social Science and Medicine, 60*(10), 2169–2180.

Cleary, J., Barhman, R., MacCormack, T., & Herold, E. (2002). Discussing sexual health with a partner: A qualitative study with young women. *The Canadian Journal of Human Sexuality, 11*(3), 117–132.

DiCenso, A., Borthwick, V., Busca C., Creatura, C., Holmes, J. A., Kalagian, W. F., & Partington, B. M. (2001). Completing the picture: Adolescents talk about what's missing in sexual health. *Canadian Journal of Public Health, 91*(1), 35–38.

Dixon-Woods, M., Sutton, A., Shaw, R., Miller, T., Smith, J., Young, B., ... & Jones, D. (2007). Appraising qualitative research for inclusion in systematic reviews: A quantitative and qualitative comparison of three methods. *Journal of Health Services Research and Policy, 12*(1), 42–47.

Elliot, R. (1999). *After Cuerrier: Canadian criminal law and the non-disclosure of HIV-positive status.* Montreal, QC: Canadian HIV/AIDS Legal Network.

Elwood-Martin, R., Gold, F., Murphy, W., Remple, V., Berkowtiz, J., & Money, D. (2005). Drug use and risk of bloodborne infections: A survey of female prisoners in British Columbia. *Canadian Journal of Public Health, 96*(2), 97–101.

Flicker, S., Larkin, J., Smilie-Adjarkwa, C., Restoule, J-P., Barlow, K., Dagnini, M., & Mitchell, C.

(2008). "It's hard to change something when you don't know where to start": Unpacking HIV vulnerability with Aboriginal youth in Canada. *Pimatisiwin: A Journal of Aboriginal and Indigenous Community Health, 55*(2), 175–200.

Gardezi, F., Calzavara, L., Husbands, W., Tharao, W., Lawson, E., Myers, T., ... & Adebajo, S. (2008). Experiences of and responses to HIV among African and Caribbean communities in Toronto, Canada. *AIDS Care, 20*(6), 718–725.

Harvey, E., Strathdee, S. A., Patrick, D. M., Ofner, M., Archibald, C. P., Eades, G., & O'Shaughnessy, M. (1998). A qualitative investigation into an HIV outbreak among injection drug users in Vancouver, British Columbia. *AIDS Care, 10*(3), 313–321.

Health Canada. (1998). *Research on HIV/AIDS in Aboriginal people: A background paper.* Winnipeg, MB: Health Canada & the University of Manitoba.

Health Canada. (2003). *Gender-based analysis.* Ottawa, ON: Health Canada. Retrieved from www.hc-sc.gc.ca/hl-vs/pubs/women-femmes/gender-sexes-eng.php

Health Canada. (2009). *HIV/AIDS pandemic.* Ottawa, ON: Health Canada. Retrieved from www.hc-sc.gc.ca/ahc-asc/activit/strateg/int_aids-sida-eng.php

Heath, J. (1999). Psychosocial needs of women infected with HIV. *Social Work in Health Care, 29*(3), 43–57.

Hilton, B., Thompson, R., Moore-Dempsey, L., & Hutchinson, K. (2001). Urban outpost nursing: The nature of the nurses' work in the AIDS prevention street nurse program. *Public Health Nursing, 18*(4), 273–280.

Jackson, L., Bailey, D., Fraser, J., Johnson, J. K., Currie, A., & Babineau, D. D. (2002). Safer and unsafe injection drug use and sex practices among injection drug users. *Canadian Journal of Public Health, 93*(3), 219–222.

Kwong-Lai Poon, M., & Trung-Thu Ho, P. (2002). A qualitative analysis of cultural and social vulnerabilities to HIV infection among gay, lesbian, and bisexual Asian youth. *Journal of Gay and Lesbian Social Services, 14*(3), 43–78.

Larkin, J., Flicker, S., Koleszar-Green, R., Mintz, S., Dagnino, M., & Mitchell, C. (2007). HIV risk, systemic inequities, and Aboriginal youth: Widening the circle for HIV prevention programming. *Canadian Journal of Public Health, 98*(3), 179–183.

Mathieson, C., Bailey, N., & Gurevich, M. (2002). Health care services for lesbian and bisexual women: Some Canadian data. *Health Care for Women International, 23*, 185–196.

McKay-McNabb, K. (2006). Life experiences of Aboriginal women living with HIV/AIDS. *Canadian Journal of Aboriginal Community-Based HIV/AIDS Research, 1*, 5–16.

McKeown, I., Reid, S., & Orr, P. (2003). Experiences of sexual violence and relocation in the lives of HIV infected Canadian women. *Circumpolar Health, 63*, 399–404.

Metcalfe, K. A., Langstaff, J., Evans, S., Paterson, H. M., & Reid, J. L. (1998). Meeting the needs of women living with HIV. *Public Health Nursing, 15*(1), 30–34.

Mill, J. E. (1997). HIV risk behaviors become survival techniques for Aboriginal women. *Western Journal of Nursing Research, 19*(4), 466–489.

Mill, J. E. (2000). Describing an explanatory model of HIV illness among Aboriginal women. *Culture and Caring, 15*(1), 42–56.

Mill, J. E., Lambert, D. T., Larkin, K., Ward, K., & Harrowing, J. W. (2008). Challenging lifestyles: Aboriginal men and women living with HIV. *Pimatisiwin: A Journal of Aboriginal and Indigenous Community Health, 5*(2), 151–187.

Milton Keynes Primary Care Trust. (2002). *10 questions to help you make sense of qualitative research: Critical appraisal skills programme.* Retrieved from www.phru.nhs.uk/learning/casp_qualitative_tool.pdf

Mitra, D., Jacobsen, J. J., O'Connor, A., Pottie, K., & Tugwell, P. (2006). Assessment of the decision support needs of women from HIV endemic countries regarding voluntary HIV testing in Canada. *Patient Education & Counseling, 63*(3), 292–300.

Nadeau, L., Truchon, M., & Biron, C. (2000). High-risk sexual behaviors in a context of substance abuse: A focus group approach. *Journal of Substance Abuse Treatment, 19*(4), 319–328.

Newman, P., Williams, C., Massaquoi, N., Brown, M., & Logie, C. (2008). HIV prevention for Black women: Structural barriers and opportunities. *Journal of Health Care for the Poor and Underserved, 19*(3), 829–841.

Olivier, C., & Dykeman, M. (2003). Challenges to HIV service provision: The commonalities for nurses and social workers. *AIDS Care, 15*(5), 649–663.

Omorodion, F., Gbadebo, K., & Ishak, P. (2007). HIV vulnerability and sexual risk among African youth in Windsor, Canada. *Culture, Health and Sexuality, 64*(4), 429–437.

Public Health Agency of Canada. (n.d.). *Population health: What determines health?* Ottawa, ON: Centre for Health Promotion, Public Health Agency of Canada. Retrieved from www.phac-aspc.gc.ca/ph-sp/determinants/index-eng.php#What

Public Health Agency of Canada. (2004). *Federal initiative to address HIV/AIDS in Canada.* Ottawa, ON: Public Health Agency of Canada. Retrieved from www.phac-aspc.gc.ca/aids-sida/fi-if/index.html

Ryder, K., Haubrich, D. J., Calla, D., Myers, T., Burchell, A. N., & Calzavara, L. (2005). Psychosocial impact of repeat HIV-negative testing: A follow-up study. *AIDS and Behavior, 9*(4), 459–464.

Sandelowski, M., & Barroso, J. (2007). *Handbook for synthesizing qualitative research.* New York, NY: Springer Publishing.

Shannon, K., Kerr, T., Allinott, S., Chettair, J., Shoveller, J., & Tyndall, M. W. (2008). Social and structural violence and power relations in mitigating HIV risk of drug-using women in survival sex work. *Social Science and Medicine, 66*(4), 911–921.

Ship, S. J., & Norton, L. (2001). HIV/AIDS and Aboriginal women in Canada. *Canadian Woman Studies, 21*(2), 25–31.

Spittal, P. M., Small, W., Woods, E., Johnston, C., Charette, J., Laliberte, N., ... & Schechter, M. (2003). How otherwise dedicated AIDS prevention workers come to support state-sponsored shortage of clean syringes in Vancouver, Canada. *International Journal of Drug Policy, 15*, 36–45.

Strike, C., Challacombe, L., Myers, T., & Millson, M. (2002). Needle exchange programs: Delivery and access issues. *Canadian Journal of Public Health, 93*(5), 339–343.

Tharao, E., & Massaquoi, N. (2002). Black women and HIV/AIDS: Contextualizing their realities, their silence and proposing solutions. *Canadian Woman Studies/les cahiers de la femme, 21*(2), 72–82.

Travers, R., & Paoletti, D. (1999). Responding to the support needs of HIV-positive lesbian, gay and bisexual youth. *The Canadian Journal of Human Sexuality, 8*(4), 271–283.

Wardman, D., & Quarts, D. (2006). Harm reduction services for British Columbia's First Nation population: A qualitative inquiry into opportunities and barriers for injection drug users. *Harm Reduction Journal, 3*, 30.

Worthington, C., & Myers, T. (2003). Factors underlying anxiety in HIV testing: Risk perceptions, stigma, and the patient–provider power dynamic. *Qualitative Health Research, 13*(5), 636–655.

Chapter 4

WHEN WOMEN PICK UP THEIR BUNDLES: HIV PREVENTION AND RELATED SERVICE NEEDS OF ABORIGINAL WOMEN IN CANADA

Doris Peltier, Randy Jackson, Tracey Prentice, Renée Masching, LaVerne Monette, Monique Fong, Krista Shore, and the Canadian Aboriginal AIDS Network's Voices of Women (CAAN VOW) Standing Committee

INTRODUCTION

The members of the Canadian Aboriginal AIDS Network's (CAAN)[1] Voices of Women (VOW) Standing Committee prepared an Aboriginal[2] women's medicine bundle in the winter of 2010/2011. The preparation of a medicine bundle is a sacred process; each sacred item that is added to the bundle contributes to the healing potential of the bundle as a whole. The intent of this bundle is to help communities and community organizations in their efforts to contribute to healing for our peoples. This bundle was specifically prepared to support respectful and meaningful care, and treatment and support services—including prevention of HIV and AIDS—for Aboriginal women and their communities. This bundle has a life—it requires protection and nurturing and will be cared for by various organizations as the response to Aboriginal women's HIV-related needs is scaled up in different regions of Canada. The bundle began its journey with the Ontario Aboriginal HIV/AIDS Strategy (OAHAS), to support the work that is currently under way for Aboriginal women within this region, and to honour the vision of LaVerne Monette, who passed into the spirit world on December 1, 2010. When the bundle was presented to OAHAS, Grandmother Wanda Whitebird recalled the words of Elder Art Solomon: "When the women begin to pick up their [medicine] bundles, our nations will begin to heal." The intent of the CAAN VOW committee is to work in parallel to the bundle, seeing the scope of responsibility evolve to the community level and no longer rest with individuals.

This chapter is guided by a belief that health promotion and HIV prevention efforts for Aboriginal women and their communities must be led by Aboriginal women and "delivered in ways that are consistent with the norms and values of [their] cultures" (Unger, Soto, & Thomas, 2008, p. 125). In contrast to a mainstream public health discourse that privileges scientific evidence when addressing the needs of vulnerable populations, this chapter will highlight the importance of Aboriginal and decolonizing perspectives to explore the complex and unique healing and HIV-related service needs of Aboriginal women living with, at risk of, or affected by HIV infection. We will also describe some of the theoretical, methodological, and conceptual tensions that exist between Aboriginal and Western approaches to HIV prevention for this population. Drawing on examples from a broad-based community consultation aimed at defining strategic health goals for Aboriginal women both living with and affected by HIV and AIDS, this chapter highlights a culturally grounded community-based approach to HIV prevention for Aboriginal women. It also highlights a distinctively Aboriginal vision of Aboriginal women's HIV-related health, healing, and well-being—a vision that holistically includes women, men, children, families, and communities.

BACKGROUND

Almost three decades into the HIV epidemic, Aboriginal women continue to bear a disproportionate share of the burden of HIV infection. Between 1998 and 2008, females represented 48.8% of all HIV test reports among Aboriginal peoples compared to only 20.6% of the general population (Public Health Agency of Canada [PHAC], 2010). In studies of young people who use street drugs, researchers found that "Aboriginal women were three times more likely than men to be HIV positive" (Mehrabadi et al., 2008, p. 253) due to gendered experiences of trauma and sexual abuse. Root causes of poor health generally, and HIV infection specifically, are linked to determinants of health for everyone (Raphael, 2004); however, in the context of historical and continuing colonization, Aboriginal people's health and HIV infection is "widely understood to also be affected by a range of cultural factors, including racism, along with various Indigenous-specific factors, such as loss of language and connection to land, environmental deprivation, and spiritual, emotional, and mental disconnectedness" (King, Smith, & Gracey, 2009, p. 77; see also Loppie Reading & Wien, 2009). The ongoing and collective experiences of colonization, and historical and intergenerational trauma have left Aboriginal women particularly vulnerable to HIV infection (Pearce et al., 2008).

In response to the alarming rates of HIV among Aboriginal women, and in light of the need for more gender-appropriate and culturally relevant HIV prevention and related services for Aboriginal women (Prentice, 2004), in 2008 the Canadian Aboriginal AIDS Network implemented a nationwide consultation with more than 300 Positive Aboriginal Women (PAW), Aboriginal women "at risk" of or affected by

HIV infection, and their service providers. In 11 cities across the country, Aboriginal women participated in a series of focus groups aimed at identifying the most pressing HIV-related service needs for Aboriginal women and how best to address these needs. Building on Aboriginal women's strengths, with attention to overcoming structural barriers and consideration of structural oppression, effective HIV-related services will recognize and embed a range of cultural assets (e.g., connection to family, community, spirituality, and traditional healing practices) within program design (Walters & Simoni, 2002; Walters, Simoni, & Evans-Campbell, 2002; Gone, 2007). Specifically, the consultation highlighted the need to strengthen and increase the network of support for PAW, increase availability and accessibility of culturally relevant HIV-related services across all regions, address the structural barriers that impede health and well-being, increase the number of prevention programs, and address gaps or make research related to Aboriginal women more accessible (Peltier, 2010). Women participating in these sessions were made aware that this community-driven, by-women-for-women consultation was being conducted by the Canadian Aboriginal AIDS Network to inform the development of a five-year strategic action plan to address HIV and AIDS among Aboriginal women in Canada.

Prior to the release of this strategy, a new identity grounded in an assets-based model for Aboriginal women living with HIV was widely adopted by the Canadian Aboriginal AIDS Network's Voices of Women Standing Committee. The new acronym PAW was introduced by VOW co-chair Kecia Larkin and refers to HIV-Positive Aboriginal Women. Adopting this new identity is important because it is self-chosen and gives a dual and culturally relevant meaning to being "positive." For many Aboriginal women, the mother bear and bear paws are powerful cultural symbols of women-centred strength. When consulted, an elder highlighted the following qualities of the female bear: she is family-oriented, aware of her surroundings, and knowledgeable about the healing properties of nature. These are qualities that PAW strive to realize in their own lives.

The national Aboriginal women's strategy was released in December 2010 and is known as *EONS*, or *Environments of Nurturing Safety: Aboriginal Women in Canada, Five Year Strategy on HIV and AIDS* (see Peltier, 2010). Rather than a review of the consultation results, this chapter will offer a critique of the ways in which Western scientific evidence (Public Health Agency of Canada [PHAC], 2005) has particular implications for Aboriginal women and HIV prevention in Canada. Evidence-based practice often means that the HIV-related programs used by Aboriginal peoples living with and affected by HIV are shaped by Western perspectives (Hodge, Limb, & Cross, 2009). A review of HIV/AIDS scholarship highlights how current approaches are dominated by a Western biomedical perspective (McKay-McNabb, 2006; Lavallee & Clearsky, 2006); overwhelmingly emphasize perceived socio-behavioural deficits of Aboriginal peoples without meaningful appreciation for women and community cultural strengths (Valaskakis, Dion Stout, & Guimond, 2009; Bond, 2006; Adelson,

2008); have a tendency to homogenize program responses at the expense of cultural diversity (Kirmayer, Tait, & Simpson, 2009); emphasize primary care versus secondary care approaches; and lean toward favouring the "model client" as a gay male while ignoring cultural and gender diversity within Aboriginal experiences.

A handful of HIV scholars, particularly those that adopt decolonizing or other critical lens approaches, have recognized the damaging effects of colonialism and residential school experiences on the health of Aboriginal peoples in Canada (Mehrabadi et al., 2008; Mill, 1997; Pearce et al., 2008). Far fewer HIV studies in Canada, however, have considered the equally valid positioning that Indigenous knowledge can inform research processes that in turn contribute findings that "indigenously" ground approaches to HIV prevention, care, support, and treatment (Duran & Walters, 2004) for Aboriginal women. Amid struggles to assert the need for cultural continuity and community development grounded in Aboriginal knowledge, Aboriginal women must "reconcile the numerous disconnects between their holistic world view and the Western view that is so often atomistic, mechanistic, and antagonistic" (Valaskakis, Dion Stout, & Guimond, 2009, p. 1), to say nothing about its reductionist leanings. These challenges were reflected on by Duran and Walters (2004), who acknowledge the value in the tensions between Indigenous and post-colonial approaches and Western science to the research, design, and delivery of HIV prevention programs.

CONCEPTUAL TENSIONS: RESPONDING TO ABORIGINAL WOMEN'S HIV-RELATED SERVICE NEEDS

In thinking about and discussing the national Aboriginal women's consultation, as described above, we have come to understand how Aboriginal HIV and AIDS "health inequalities arise from general socioeconomic factors in combination with culturally and historically specific factors particular to the people affected" (King, Smith, & Gracey, 2009, p. 76). The community consultation highlighted community assets and a range of cultural factors that must be considered when designing HIV prevention and related services for Aboriginal women living with and affected by HIV (see Peltier, 2010). Using Western approaches to HIV prevention as a point of contrast, we turn our attention now to the conceptual challenges in designing and delivering those services.

Western Knowledge versus Indigenous Knowledge

What is Indigenous knowledge? How is this knowledge applied in the context of HIV prevention and other health services? In what ways is Indigenous knowledge creating a needed conceptual tension with Western-defined notions of health and responses to these health challenges? The answers to these questions are exceedingly difficult to provide, but to paraphrase Finlay (2000) anyone who has had the opportunity to work with Aboriginal peoples knows the tremendous wealth of wisdom that Aboriginal peoples can offer. Yet the space that separates Western knowledge as the dominant construct informing public health approaches and HIV prevention and related policies, programs, and services from the holistic quality of Indigenous knowledge is real and not easily resolved—even though health education strategies have attempted to approach health in increasingly holistic and patient-centred ways (Gilbert, 2005). Nonetheless, strategies that promote complementary approaches that support a person's well-being, alongside delivery of mainstream health services, appear to be making headway (LaValley & Verhoef, 1995). Cultural synthesis—that of foregrounding the culturally embedded worldviews of one's patient or client—incorporates skills such as reflection of one's own cultural position, respect for the needs of others, empathy, and communication strategies (Darlington, 2011).

As advocates and allies push the Western medical model away from a focus on homogeneity and toward support for diversity, an awareness of Indigenous knowledge when providing care to Aboriginal peoples is critical. Indigenous knowledge related to health is far from uniform; it is localized, and thus spread across space and geography (Battiste & Youngblood Henderson, 2000). Equally important is the consideration of the richly layered knowledge that is found against the backdrop of gender, age, and sexuality (Ladson-Billing & Donnor, 2008). For example, Loppie Reading and Wien (2009) provide an Aboriginal perspective on the social determinants of health, which takes into account a range of intersecting factors (see also Raphael, 2004, for an interesting discussion on Aboriginality as a social determinant of health). Given the "tremendous diversity of peoples, languages, cultures, traditions, beliefs, and values" (Battiste, 2008, p. 499), writing about a singular Indigenous concept of health is an exceedingly complicated and challenging, if not inappropriate, task. Given this diversity, as authors of this chapter we acknowledge that universal definitions of health compromise the validity of localized and multiple Indigenous knowledge systems. Nonetheless, and drawing on the Ojibway cultural tradition of two of the chapter's authors, Indigenous concepts of health emphasize "the importance of balance. All four elements of life, the physical, emotional, mental, and spiritual, are represented in the four directions of the medicine wheel. These four elements are intricately woven together and interact to support a strong and healthy person" (King et al., 2009, p. 76) through active and meaningful engagement that extends beyond the individual to include family, community, spirit worlds, and the environment. While biological processes also remain an important core focus, this must also be extended to include other aspects of self (i.e., mental, emotional, and spiritual).

Indigenous knowledge therefore pushes against assumptions made by "the medical model of categorization, pathologization and treatment" (Lavallee & Poole, 2010, p. 271) to a position that favours Indigenous experiential knowledge as equally valuable. Knowledge in Indigenous systems is felt to be subjective and is conveyed through congruence of mind, heart, and spirit to outward experience. As Brant Castellano states, "Knowledge of the physical world, which forms an essential part of praxis of inner and outward learning, does not flow exclusively or primarily through the intellect … [but rather, there is] the need to walk on the land in order to know it" (2000, p. 29). This prerequisite presents an additional challenge for both Aboriginal people working cross-culturally with other Aboriginal groups and for allied non-Aboriginal health care professionals. Health workers must consider and be willing to move beyond text, printed material, or even brief clinical encounters. As Battiste reminds us, "to acquire Indigenous knowledge [and then use it effectively in the context of health] … one must come to know through extended conversation and experiences with elders, peoples, and places of Canada" (2008, p. 502). This is not meant to suggest that involvement is impossible; rather, what many Aboriginal scholars, community leaders, and Aboriginal women living with HIV insist upon is long-term engagement and involvement in Aboriginal communities, and a willingness to listen and learn, to be humble, and to respect principles of self-determination.

The national consultation with Aboriginal women living with or affected by HIV revealed that their voices are often relegated to the periphery, where they are offered little to no involvement or control over the design and delivery of HIV prevention and care services. As a result, Aboriginal women are often left feeling powerless, unsafe, or made more vulnerable in ways that potentially impact how, when, or if they access these services. As articulated by participants, the inclusion of women-specific ceremonies, for example, is important in that they can potentially reverse this sense of exclusion and contribute to healing and well-being (Peltier, 2010). Positive health outcomes for Aboriginal women will only be viable in so far as they resonate with the localized, culturally defined, age-appropriate, and gendered experiences of Aboriginal women. In other words, despite what appear to be similarities in experience for Aboriginal women vis-à-vis other cultural groups experiencing HIV, health programs that are designed to be malleable will more positively attend to and ground responses in specific and differing meaning attached to localized contexts through attention to traditions, customs, and local conditions specific to each person, family, and community (Peltier, 2010). In addition, in regards to honouring cultural assets, Aboriginal women call upon all children, men, community leaders, and Elders in their communities to also be involved in formulating, responding to, and delivering HIV programs. Healing from this perspective attends to the notion of relational connection and invites and cultivates a mutually supportive environment in which health and well-being are fostered and maintained. In other words, Aboriginal women cannot heal in isolation. An effective response to HIV risk for Aboriginal women is a community response in which men, women, children, families, and community members are all working towards the common goal of HIV prevention via greater health and well-being (Peltier, 2010). Unlike Western knowledge, Indigenous scholars tell us that Indigenous knowledge is "revealed and contextualized through relationships [and becomes] … validated not through the notion of 'truth value' but rather through connection" (Holmes, 2000, pp. 40–42; see also Battiste, 2008).

Homogenization versus Population Diversity

Aboriginal peoples in Canada are enormously diverse. They speak more than 55 languages in 11 major language groups (Norris, 2007), include 615 formal First Nations bands, 2,284 reserves, 52 Inuit communities (Kirmayer et al., 2009), and countless Métis settlements. Just over half of all people who self-identify as Aboriginal are female (Statistics Canada, 2009). Recognition of the diversity among Aboriginal women is foundational to *Environments of Nurturing Safety (EONS)* (Peltier, 2010). However, the limited HIV prevention literature for women in general, and Aboriginal women in particular, tends to treat women as a homogenous group, both conceptually and methodologically (Gahagan & Ricci, 2011), ignoring and erasing differences in culture, geography, age, sex and gender, religion, health status, and so on. For example, most, if not all, HIV prevention studies for Aboriginal women are based on mixed samples of Aboriginal women and do not provide separate analyses for First Nations, Métis, or Inuit women, geographic representation, age, or sexual orientation. This may be appropriate in some cases due to small sample sizes; however, the lack of specificity within these studies can also lead to a lack of specificity within HIV prevention programs, policies, and services. This is a situation that does not serve Aboriginal women well, as the voices of those most marginalized within the population are not heard, and therefore their HIV prevention needs are not met. Métis and Inuit women are particularly marginalized within this context, as are First Nations women living on-reserve or in rural areas.

Current literature and prevention initiatives also ignore non-normative contexts, such as HIV prevention for two-spirit women, or women who have both male and female sexual partners. The focus instead is on "normative" contexts, such as reducing mother-to-child transmission (Bucharski, 1999) or "high-risk" contexts, such as street involvement, involvement in the sex trade, or injection drug use (Shannon et al., 2008; Pearce et al., 2008). In other words, prevention literature and initiatives tend to address contexts of "risk behaviours," while ignoring the prevention needs and the socio-cultural contexts of those women who do not fall neatly into these categories. The same can be said for age as a key determinant of health and Aboriginal women's HIV prevention. HIV prevention literature and initiatives ignore and erase differences in age, implicitly assuming that the prevention needs of all ages of Aboriginal women are the same, whether they be 18 or 58 years old. However, an increasing number of positive Aboriginal women are long-term survivors, and aging with HIV is becoming a more common situation. New research is beginning to address these issues in the general population; however, targeted HIV prevention research, policy, and programs that address the unique needs of older Aboriginal women are lacking.

The Gendered Impacts of Colonization

Aboriginal and allied scholars agree that gender roles in Aboriginal communities experienced a dramatic shift as a result of the imposition of Eurocentric governance systems and social values (Weaver, 2009; Healey, 2008; Kubik, Bourassa, & Hampton, 2009). Prior to colonization, gender roles were typically balanced and egalitarian with complementary roles for males and females. Some Aboriginal scholars, with consideration given to the diversity among Aboriginal traditions, have compared the traditional relationship between men and women to the eagle who flies to tremendous heights on the strength of one male and one female wing (Monture-Angus, 1995; Valaskakis et al., 2009). If either of these wings is weaker or stronger than the other, the eagle is out of balance and cannot fly. Such were the traditional roles of males and females in Aboriginal communities: if the powers of one were stronger or weaker than the other, the community could not function effectively. Historically, while men were the hunters and protectors of their communities, Aboriginal women carried "major responsibility for transmitting their cultures and assuring the well-being of their communities" (Weaver, 2009, p. 1552; see also Healey, 2008). Considered to be the heart of their nations (Brant Castellano, 2009), women were teachers, healers, and givers of life (Wolski, 2009). Thus, "women were seen as sacred human beings and were protected by the men of their communities" (Hawkins, Reading, & Barlow, 2009, p. 13).

In order for Aboriginal communities and Aboriginal women's health to move forward, the negative impact of colonization and its effect on the way Aboriginal men and women, and Aboriginal and non-Aboriginal peoples, relate to each other must be understood (Gracey & King, 2009; King et al., 2009). This will require a hard look back at the gendered impacts of colonization and then a conscious move into the future by Aboriginal communities to redress the historical hurts, particularly those that shaped male and female relations. As Elder Lyle Longclaws once said, "Before the healing can happen the poison has to be exposed" (D. Peltier, personal communication, September 27, 2010).

Effective HIV prevention and related services for Aboriginal women will recognize this central need and, where appropriate, invite families, men, and children into the circle of healing. In addition, they will employ culturally attuned staff who recognize the needs of a diverse Aboriginal women population, and work towards embedding core Aboriginal worldviews in their HIV prevention and related programs (Benoit, Carroll, & Chaudry, 2003). This is so even in urban areas, where sex work involvement and/or drug and alcohol use does not end the core connection many Aboriginal women feel toward their cultural identity. HIV prevention and related services, even in urban settings, should remain tied to Aboriginal ontological beliefs that are centred on the importance of balancing physical, spiritual, mental, and emotional aspects of self (Majumdar, Guenter, & Browne, 2010).

Strength (or Asset)-Based Approaches versus Deficit-Model Approaches

The predominance of a disease-oriented paradigm in research about Aboriginal people living with HIV and AIDS has created an overall picture of suffering, disease, and dysfunction among Aboriginal peoples and communities that is an incomplete and disempowering representation of the Aboriginal HIV and AIDS experience (Bond, 2006; Reading & Nowgesic, 2002). As O'Neil, Reading, and Leader (1998), for example, point out:

> Portraits of Aboriginal sickness and misery act as powerful social instruments for the construction of Aboriginal identity. Epidemiological knowledge constructs an understanding of Aboriginal society that reinforces unequal power relationships; in other words, an image of sick and disorganized communities can be used to justify patterns of paternalism and dependency. (p. 230)

In the case of Aboriginal HIV and AIDS issues, particularly among women, researchers have shown great interest in the negative health outcomes associated with physical and sexual abuse (Varcoe & Dick, 2008; Pearce et al., 2008), substance use including injection drugs (Pearce et al., 2008), engagement in sex work (Shannon et al., 2008), barriers to health care (CAAN, 2005; Benoit et al., 2003), and colonialism and historical trauma (Varcoe & Dick, 2008; Pearce et al., 2008). This approach has done much to advance our understanding of the inequitable burden of HIV and AIDS on Aboriginal women and has undeniably been useful in developing public policy to address the health outcomes associated with these adversities. One might argue, however, that researchers have been so focused on understanding the determinants of Aboriginal ill health that few attempts have been made to model "thriving" health, (Richmond, Ross, & Egeland, 2007) including wellness, for Aboriginal women living with or affected by HIV and AIDS.

As recognized by the Aboriginal women who participated in the nationwide consultation, additional research is needed that identifies and elaborates on protective or resiliency factors (Andersson et al., 2008) for Aboriginal women and the strengths and assets of individuals and communities (Dion Stout, Kipling, & Stout, 2001) that promote and maintain health and well-being (Walters & Simoni, 2002; Walters et al., 2002). This health-focused research is increasingly recognized as essential to reorienting health services and (re)building healthy communities (Kretzman & McKnight, 2007). The community consultation outlined above emphasized a culturally attuned, strengths-based approach that potentially informs the continuum of care from prevention to support, care, and treatment. It points to a community-defined desire to reorient the perception of Aboriginal women living with HIV and AIDS away from negative associations of illness and vulnerability and toward strengths and assets focused on relational connections (Peltier, 2010). Attempts to circumvent deficit models of constructing Aboriginal women's realities in the context of HIV and AIDS are, however, often related to narrowly defined notions of resiliency that are focused on individual agency and are rooted in and reflect a "Eurocentric perspective ... [that embodies] the notion that 'if only you would take responsibility for your health and healing" (Lavallee & Clearsky, 2006, p. 4). While we acknowledge the importance of these individually focused resiliency studies in moving the discussion beyond a focus on gaps and deficits, we encourage care and attention to the often Eurocentric and victim-blaming assumptions that underpin some resiliency approaches. By contrast, we encourage the use of resiliency models that consider Aboriginal perspectives and that take collective, cultural, and relational factors into account (Kirmayer et al., 2011; Fleming & Ledogar, 2008). Similarly, approaches that adopt culturally competent service delivery models without attention to shifting services toward embedding cultural values and perspectives do not go far enough (Barlow et al., 2008). Rather, as articulated by women participating in the national consultation, a first step in reorienting services is to honour the essence of Aboriginal women's communities, challenge negative socio-structural aspects of women's gendered experience of HIV and AIDS as grounded in colonial processes, and support more culturally based values and perspectives (Peltier, 2010).

"Prevention Is For Everybody": Positive Aboriginal Women (PAW) as Leaders in HIV Prevention

Biomedical approaches to HIV prevention have historically categorized prevention interventions as primary or secondary (Gordon, Stall, & Cheever, 2004). These labels and categories reflect the focus of the prevention effort on remaining HIV-negative, on living well with HIV, and on minimizing the health effects of symptomatic HIV respectively. These categories are not without dispute: some feel that this division of prevention interventions into "primary" and "secondary" "implies a hierarchy of importance when it comes to targeting people for prevention programmes" (NAM aidsmap, 2010), while others feel that it emphasizes individual responsibility over "risk environments" or structural determinants of health (Gordon, Stall, & Cheever, 2004). Nonetheless, it represents the dominant approach to HIV prevention generally, and the dominant approach to HIV prevention for Aboriginal women (Gahagan & Ricci, 2011). We suggest, however, that HIV prevention for Aboriginal women must move beyond these targeted Western categories that divide the world by HIV status, and embrace a culturally appropriate, holistic perspective that bridges the divide between primary and secondary HIV prevention. As highlighted in *EONS* (Peltier, 2010), culturally appropriate HIV prevention interventions for Aboriginal women will ideally be holistic, contribute to community as well as individual healing, and be inclusive of all Aboriginal women, whether they are living with, affected by, or "at risk" of HIV. This is not to say that targeted HIV prevention is inappropriate; rather, that it must be seen in the context of a broader whole that has the healing of communities as its end goal. Refocusing on structural environments or "environments of risk" is one way of bridging this divide rather than simply reinforcing individual behavioural aspects of HIV prevention.

Another way of ensuring that HIV prevention for Aboriginal women is holistic and culturally appropriate is to involve PAW in the design and development of prevention programs, policies, or services. Several decades of advocacy around the GIPA (Greater Involvement of People Living with HIV/AIDS) principle have raised awareness of the importance of involving people living with HIV/AIDS in policies, programs, and services that affect them. More recently, the Canadian Aboriginal AIDS Network has advocated for the Meaningful Involvement of Aboriginal People Living with HIV/AIDS strategy (Stratton, Jackson, & Barlow, 2006). These philosophical positions and their practical applications have received widespread support from governments (Public Health Agency of Canada [PHAC], 2007), yet PAW continue to be invisible or marginalized in Aboriginal women's HIV prevention and research. We suggest a "by and for approach," with Aboriginal women at the forefront of HIV prevention, guiding and shaping the response to meet their communities' needs. In the following section, we provide three such examples.

MEETING THE HIV-RELATED SERVICE NEEDS OF ABORIGINAL WOMEN

The community consultation, although critical of the lack of Aboriginal women-centred approaches and services across Canada (Peltier, 2010), revealed several unpublished Aboriginal women-specific prevention and treatment programs that attempt to circumvent the tensions described above. Characteristic of these approaches are attempts to understand HIV and AIDS from Aboriginal women's perspectives. Shared here in the following first-person descriptions are the important principles that guide these approaches. They include views that conceptualize Aboriginal women as firmly connected to cultural strengths and to community, and as voicing and acting on the concerns they themselves have identified and defined, as well as the active positioning of Indigenous knowledge as valid and integral to the development and delivery of HIV and AIDS prevention, care and support, and treatment programs.

Ontario Aboriginal HIV/AIDS Strategy[3]

LaVerne Monette

In 2005, we were reviewing recommendations contained in our new strategic plan. We were concerned about the focus on Aboriginal women in Ontario. We knew that the epidemiological data indicated that Aboriginal women were quickly approaching 50% of the total Aboriginal HIV epidemic. However, we were not seeing many positive Aboriginal women in our work. If they were not coming to see us, where were they going? The greatest concern we had, of course, is that they were not seeing anyone and not receiving appropriate care, treatment, and support. We decided that we had to get out there and find out what Aboriginal women were hearing about HIV, given that Aboriginal women were at such high risk.

We decided to do a series of two-day women-only workshops and to go to various urban centres in Ontario and talk to Aboriginal women who are HIV positive or at risk of HIV and AIDS, and their service providers. In order to create a safe space for all, participants were asked to say only their names and where they were from. Workshop topics included historical reasons Aboriginal women are at high risk for HIV, the nuts and bolts of HIV, and issues such as stigma and discrimination and the slippery slope of non-disclosure of HIV status in relationships. Abbott Virology generously sponsored a doctor to provide a workshop on HIV and women from infancy to menopause. Included as part of this was a powerful session given by a Positive Aboriginal Woman (PAW) about finding her voice. We also talked about healthy sexuality and women's sexual and reproductive rights.

Although our work here is far from complete, so far we have held nine of these sessions across the province and plan to do a few more. We hope to learn from women across the province and plan to conduct an impact study on what has happened for Aboriginal women participants since our workshop series.

Healing Our Nations[4]
Monique Fong

Over the last 14 years, there has been a shift in the number of Aboriginal people becoming infected with HIV and AIDS. The number of Aboriginal women who are testing positive is increasing with each passing year. As a mother and stepmother of three girls, I wondered how these numbers would affect them. Were other parents thinking the same thing? What about our communities? How could we assist our families, and Aboriginal women?

At Healing Our Nations, we discussed the issue and proposed an idea to our funders. We obtained funding to do some focus groups with women and to develop training from what we learned when meeting with the women. This initiative came to be known as "The Empowering Aboriginal Women Project." What we learned from the project is that women still needed basic HIV information and they also wanted to learn how to make healthy sexual decisions. The three themes that came up consistently were self-esteem, boundaries, and healthy relationships. For example, we discussed how low self-esteem places Aboriginal women at risk for HIV and AIDS, and ways of building up self-esteem so they can negotiate safer sex. "The Empowering Aboriginal Women Project" is an ongoing piece of work, and the response has been amazing. Women are stating that they are learning techniques that they can pass on to their daughters, nieces, and other female family members.

All Nations Hope AIDS Network[5]
Krista Shore

My vision is to develop a Positive Aboriginal Women's (PAW) traditional talking/healing circle in my region. This vision was inspired by a gathering I had the opportunity to attend in Toronto in 2010, where I attended a similar healing circle. This was a profound moment for me because it solidified my own vision of healing circles for positive Aboriginal women in my region. The Elder who conducted the talking/healing circle is a well-known woman in her region, an Anishinabe sister whom I had the opportunity and privilege to meet on my journey. We were educated on the meaning, purpose, and symbolism of the talking/healing circle, and although it was an emotional experience, I feel we were given an important teaching that would help us go ahead in our communities to help our people in this way.

As I was sitting there, I thought—as an Aboriginal First Nations woman—that we need to take our power back and make initiatives to integrate our cultural teachings in our process of healing, growth, leadership, and mentorship, and bring this into each and every one of our communities. From my point of view, this is a necessity, not only for the benefit of healing, growth, and support, but when Aboriginal women flourish, as well as their children, family, and community, then the whole world gains. Furthermore, there is a need for more activism and advocacy to improve our determinants of health, and we will be able to bring forth changes in policy that exists here in Canada.

I have gained significantly by meeting other Aboriginal women who live their truth within our movement, and they have generously shared their knowledge and mentored me. They shared with me the importance of the need to address the lack of support for Aboriginal women who are feeling the impacts of this epidemic. The mentorship has had the effect where I believe that I can see myself grow, and if I can grow, my community will also grow and the world grows, too. I carry with me a teaching from my Elder who told me that a healthy me plus healthy children will result in a healthy world. My vision is that when we come together as PAW within our healing circle, each of the women will also go forth and start another healing circle in their community. This way, the vision will grow!

DISCUSSION AND CONCLUSION

In thinking about the results of the consultation, and particularly the theoretical and conceptual tensions inherent in designing and delivering HIV-related health services for Aboriginal women, several dominant themes have emerged. First, despite increasing rates of HIV infection among Aboriginal women, the majority of HIV prevention and related services are designed for men (e.g., gendered aspects of HIV are not considered) or other dominant cultural groups (e.g., Aboriginal notions of health and well-being are not included). Second, Aboriginal women tend to be excluded from the design and delivery of programs and services that target Aboriginal women. Consequently, Aboriginal women can be left feeling further marginalized in ways that impact their use of HIV-related services. Third, constrained by funding considerations, services are often based on pan-Aboriginal approaches and, as a result, tend to ignore cultural diversity among Aboriginal groups in Canada. While concepts of resiliency have been explored, they have often focused on individual agency and risk, emphasizing individual responsibility and ignoring a sense of connection to the broader environment, including family, community, men, and children. Guided by a relational ethic, a position of strength, Aboriginal approaches on the other hand promote a mutually supportive environment in which health and well-being are maintained. Lastly, in recent years, the literature examining Aboriginal HIV is moving away from a strict focus on "HIV risk behaviour" to include consideration of a range of structural inequalities, including a focus on the negative effects of colonization. Particularly, we are concerned about the lack of HIV prevention, care, and support, and treatment literature that is grounded in Aboriginal women's culture and traditional heritage. A systematic review of Aboriginal health literature across the social sciences, for example, revealed a lack of studies focusing on traditional approaches to healing and/or access to traditional healers/medicines (Wilson & Young, 2008). Although fruitful in terms of shifting blame away from individuals to broader structural and community concerns, much of this research unfortunately continues to further marginalize Aboriginal women living with and affected by HIV and AIDS.

In many ways, this chapter has been about "walking backwards to the future" (Valaskakis et al., 2009, p. 4). It is about recognizing that the inner individual and community strength necessary to mount effective resistance, to reclaim, and to act in the present is wholly contingent on the past (Grande, 2004). It is recognition and validation that "even though [W]estern culture does not encourage us to work with our ancestors (especially dead ones), that doesn't (necessarily) mean they don't have anything to offer!" (Anderson, 2000, p. 30). In couching our thinking about the consultation in the past while walking forward, this chapter highlights the need for historically and culturally grounded HIV and AIDS prevention and social services to effectively confront the HIV epidemic among Aboriginal women living with and at risk of HIV and AIDS. As noted at the outset of this chapter, Aboriginal women are beginning to "pick up their bundles," to heal themselves, their families, and the communities to which they belong. This is an invitation to Aboriginal leadership, community activists, health and social professionals, and Canadian political leadership at all levels to join them in a firm commitment to redress the structural factors that give rise to environments of risk that lead to and shape experiences of living with HIV infection for Aboriginal women.

PROBLEM-BASED LEARNING CASE STUDY

There are two HIV-positive Aboriginal women living at home in their First Nations community. Jeannie is a 44-year-old recovering drug addict who has left her addiction behind. She is dealing with her issues and trying to come to terms with her experiences with childhood sexual abuse through weekly counselling sessions. The counselling also helps her to come to terms with her recent HIV diagnosis, and she finds her greatest strength is coming from reconnecting to her spiritual beliefs and to the Creator. Linda is the other HIV-positive woman. She is a 24-year old woman who continues her problematic use of drugs and alcohol. She is not dealing well with her HIV diagnosis. Neither Jeannie nor Linda has knowledge of each other's HIV status, but some people in the community have knowledge of both women's HIV status, as is usually the case in a small community where everyone knows your business.

One day, Jeannie receives a call from a childhood friend of hers in the community to tell her about Linda, and that she is worried that Linda might be spreading HIV around the community. She tells Jeannie, "Everyone knows Linda is HIV positive and yet she is still out there partying away, and I think she is spreading HIV and someone has to stop her!" Her friend goes on to say she has heard that Linda has been at some parties in the community and on a couple of occasions she has woken up naked on the couch. Jeannie's friend is concerned that Linda is infecting other people. It is obvious that Linda is still having sex and she wants Jeannie to do something. She suggests that perhaps Jeannie can talk to Linda to tell her to stop partying and having unprotected sex.

CRITICAL THINKING QUESTIONS

1. This chapter suggests a community-driven approach to HIV prevention for Aboriginal women that embeds cultural assets in the program design. What might a community-driven approach to the above scenario look like?
2. How can a community-driven approach to HIV prevention for Aboriginal women, such as the examples included in this chapter, be adapted to address this situation?
3. One of the tensions highlighted in this chapter is the tendency to homogenize the HIV prevention and related needs of Aboriginal women. How might a community-driven HIV prevention initiative designed to address the above situation be different if Linda were 13 years old? 27 years old? 56 years old?
4. What would you need to consider if Linda were Métis? Inuit? Living in an urban centre?

ACKNOWLEDGEMENTS

The authors of this chapter honour the diversity of Aboriginal women who connected with their inner strengths and, through this, shared their voices in a national consultation process.

DEDICATION

We dedicate this chapter and the work to come to LaVerne Monette, a strong warrior woman who left us for the spirit world on December 1, 2010; we honour and acknowledge her many years of dedicated work within the Aboriginal HIV/AIDS movement. In one of her keynote addresses, she challenged us all to take action by stating the obvious: "If our Aboriginal women and youth are being impacted by HIV and AIDS at such high rates, where is our future?"

NOTES

1 The Canadian Aboriginal AIDS Network is a not-for-profit national coalition of individuals and organizations that provides leadership, support, and advocacy for Aboriginal people living with and affected by HIV/AIDS, regardless of where they reside.

2 The Canadian Aboriginal AIDS Network uses the term "Aboriginal" to refer to First Nations (both Status and non-Status), Métis, and Inuit. This signifies the solidarity and mutual good-will among these groups, but in no way denies or erases the differences between them.

3 The Ontario Aboriginal HIV/AIDS Strategy's goal is to provide culturally respectful and sensitive programs and strategies to respond to the growing HIV/AIDS epidemic among Aboriginal women in Ontario through promotion, prevention, long-term care, and treatment and support initiatives consistent with harm-reduction principles.

4 Healing Our Nations' mandate is to teach and support our people in a manner that is respectful of our Native ways of life.

5 All Nations Hope AIDS Network's mission is to holistically, traditionally, and spiritually support and assist First Nations, Métis, and Inuit, and all other people and their families living with HIV/AIDS and hepatitis C to live meaningful lives, and to provide professional training and awareness of HIV/AIDS and hepatitis C to the community.

REFERENCES

Adelson, N. (2008). Discourses of stress, social inequalities, and the everyday worlds of First Nations women in a remote northern Canadian community. *Ethos, 36*(3), 316–333.

Anderson, K. (2000). *A recognition of being: Reconstructing Native womanhood.* Toronto, ON: Canadian Scholars' Press.

Andersson, N., Shea, B., Archibald, C., Wong, T., Barlow, B., & Sioui, G. (2008). Building on the resilience of Aboriginal people in risk reduction initiatives targeting sexually transmitted infections and bloodborne viruses: The Aboriginal community resilience to AIDS (ACRA). *Pimatisiwin: A Journal of Aboriginal and Indigenous Community Health, 6*(2), 89–110.

Barlow, K., Loppie, C., Jackson, R., Akan, M., MacLean, L., & Reimer, G. (2008). Culturally competent service provision issues experienced by Aboriginal people living with HIV/AIDS. *Pimatisiwin: A Journal of Aboriginal and Indigenous Community Health, 6*(2), 155–180.

Battiste, M. (2008). Research ethics for protecting Indigenous knowledge and heritage: Institutional and researcher responsibilities. In N. Denzin, Y. Lincoln, & L. Smith (Eds.), *Handbook of Critical and Indigenous Methodologies* (pp. 497–509). Thousand Oaks, CA: Sage Publications, Inc.

Battiste, M., & Youngblood Henderson, J. (2000). *Protecting Indigenous knowledge and heritage: A global challenge.* Saskatoon, SK: Purich Publishing Ltd.

Benoit, C., Carroll, D., & Chaudhry, M. (2003). In search of a healing place: Aboriginal women in Vancouver's Downtown Eastside. *Social Science & Medicine, 56,* 821–833.

Bond, C. (2005). A culture of ill health: Public health or aboriginality? *Medical Journal of Australia, 183*(1), 39–41.

Brant Castellano, M. (2000). Updating Aboriginal traditions of knowledge. In G. Sefa Dei, B. Hall,

& D. Goldin Rosenburg (Eds.), *Indigenous knowledges in global contexts: Multiple readings of our world* (2nd ed., pp. 21–36). Toronto, ON: University of Toronto Press.

Brant Castellano, M. (2009). Heart of the nations: Women's contributions to community healing. In G. Valaskakis, M. Dion Stout, & E. Guimond (Eds.), *Restoring the balance: First Nations women, community, and culture* (pp. 203–235). Winnipeg, MB: University of Manitoba Press.

Bucharski, D. (1999). Developing culturally appropriate prenatal care models for Aboriginal women. *The Canadian Journal of Human Sexuality, 9*(2), 151–154.

Canadian Aboriginal AIDS Network. (2005). *Aboriginal women living with HIV/AIDS: Care, treatment and support issues.* Vancouver, BC: Canadian Aboriginal AIDS Network.

Darlington, A. (2011). Raising a critical consciousness for the reformation of health care culture. *Canadian Journal of Respiratory Therapy, 47*(3), 6–12.

Dion Stout, M., Kipling, G., & Stout, R. (2001). *Aboriginal women's health research synthesis project: Final report.* Winnipeg, MB: Prairie Women's Health Centre of Excellence.

Duran, B., & Walters, K. (2004). HIV/AIDS prevention in "Indian Country": Current practice, Indigenist etiology models, and postcolonial approaches to change. *AIDS Education and Prevention, 16*(3), 187–201.

Finlay, L. (2000). Foreword. In M. Battiste (Ed.), *Reclaiming Indigenous voice and vision* (pp. ix–xiii). Vancouver, BC: UBC Press.

Fleming, J., & Ledogar, R. (2008). Resilience, an evolving concept: A review of literature relevant to Aboriginal research. *Pimatisiwin: A Journal of Aboriginal and Indigenous Community Health, 6*(2), 7–23.

Gahagan, J., & Ricci, C. (2011). *HIV/AIDS prevention for women in Canada: A meta-ethnographic synthesis.* Halifax, NS: Dalhousie University.

Gilbert, J. (2005). Interprofessional education for collaborative, patient-centred practice. *Canadian Journal of Nursing Leadership, 18*(2), 32–38.

Gone, J. (2007). "We never was happy living like a whiteman": Mental health disparities and postcolonial predicament in American Indian communities. *American Journal of Community Psychology, 40*(3/4), 290–300.

Gordon, C., Stall, R., & Cheever, L. (2004). Prevention interventions with persons living with HIV/AIDS: Challenges, progress, and research priorities. *Journal of Acquired Immune Deficiency, 37*(Suppl. 2), S53–S57.

Gracey, M., & King, M. (2009). Indigenous health part 1: Determinants and disease patterns. *The Lancet, 374*(9683), 65–75.

Grande, S. (2004). *Red pedagogy: Native American social and political thought.* Lanham, MD: Rowman & Littlefield, Inc.

Hawkins, K., Reading, C., & Barlow, K. (2009). *Our search for safe spaces: A qualitative study of the role of sexual violence in the lives of Aboriginal women living with HIV/AIDS.* Ottawa, ON: Canadian Aboriginal AIDS Network.

Healey, G. (2008). Tradition and culture: An important determinant of Inuit women's health. *Journal of Aboriginal Health, 4*(1), 25–33.

Hodge, D., Limb, G., & Cross, T. (2009). Moving from colonization toward balance and harmony:

A Native American perspective on wellness. *Social Work, 54*(3), 211–219.

Holmes, L. (2000). Heart knowledge, blood learning and the voice of the land: Implications of research among Hawaiian elders. In G. J. Sefa Dei, B. L. Hall, & D. Goldin Rosenberg (Eds.), *Indigenous knowledges in global contexts: Multiple readings in our world* (pp. 54–69). Toronto, ON: University of Toronto Press.

King, M., Smith, A., & Gracey, M. (2009). Indigenous health part 2: The underlying causes of the health gap. *The Lancet, 374*(9683), 76–85.

Kirmayer, L., Dandenau, S., Marshall, E., Phillips, M., & Williamson, K. (2011). Rethinking resilience from Indigenous perspectives. *Canadian Journal of Psychiatry, 56*(2), 84–91.

Kirmayer, L., Tait, C., & Simpson, C. (2009). The mental health of Aboriginal peoples in Canada: Transformations of identity and community. In L. Kirmayer & G. Valaskakis (Eds.), *Health traditions: The mental health of Aboriginal peoples in Canada* (pp. 3–35). Vancouver, BC: UBC Press.

Kretzman, J., & McKnight, J. (2007). *Building communities from the inside out: A path towards finding and mobilizing a community's assets.* Skokie, IL: ACTA Publications.

Kubik, W., Bourassa, C., & Hampton, M. (2009). Stolen sisters, second class citizens, poor health: The legacy of colonization in Canada. *Humanity & Society, 33*(February/March), 18–34.

Ladson-Billing, G., & Donnor, J. (2008). Waiting for the call: The moral activist role of critical race theory scholarship. In N. Denzin, Y. Lincoln, & L. Smith (Eds.), *Handbook of critical & Indigenous methodologies* (pp. 61–83). Thousand Oaks, CA: Sage Publications.

Lavallee, B., & Clearsky, L. (2006). "From woundedness to resilience": A critical review from an Aboriginal perspective. *Journal of Aboriginal Health, 3*(1), 4–6.

Lavallee, L., & Poole, J. (2010). Beyond recovery: Colonization, health and healing for Indigenous people in Canada. *International Journal of Mental Health, 8*(2), 271–281.

LaValley, W., & Verhoef, M. (1995). Integrated complementary medicine and health care services into practice. *Canadian Medical Association Journal, 153*(1), 45–49.

Loppie Reading, C., & Wien, F. (2009). *Health inequalities and social determinants of Aboriginal peoples' health.* Victoria, BC, and Halifax, NS: National Collaborating Centre for Aboriginal Health.

Majumdar, B., Guenter, D., & Browne, G. (2010). HIV prevention in an Aboriginal community in Canada. *Journal of the Association of Nurses in AIDS Care, 21*(5), 449–454.

McKay-McNabb, K. (2006). Life experiences of Aboriginal women living with HIV/AIDS. *Canadian Journal of Aboriginal Community-Based HIV/AIDS Research, 1,* 5–16.

Mehrabadi, A., Craib, K., Paterson, K., Adam, W., Moniruzzaman, A., Ward-Burkitt, B., … & the Cedar Project Partnership. (2008). The Cedar Project: A comparison of HIV-related vulnerabilities amongst young Aboriginal women surviving drug use and sex work in two Canadian cities. *International Journal of Drug Policy, 19*(2), 159–168.

Mehrabadi, A., Paterson, K., Pearce, M., Patel, S., Craib, K., Moniruzzaman, A., … & the Cedar Project Partnership. (2008). Gender differences in HIV and hepatitis C related vulnerabilities among Aboriginal people who use street drugs in two Canadian cities. *Women & Health, 48*(3), 235–260.

Mill, J. (1997). HIV risk behaviors become survival techniques for Aboriginal women. *Western Journal of Nursing Research, 19*(4), 466–489.

Monture-Angus, P. (1995). *Thunder in my soul: A Mohawk woman speaks.* Halifax, NS: Fernwood Publishing.

NAM aidsmap. (2010). *Differing philosophies of HIV prevention.* Retrieved from http://aidsmap.com/Differing-philosophies-of-HIV-prevention/page/1061505/

Norris, M. J. (2007, May). *Aboriginal languages in Canada: Emerging trends and perspectives on second language acquisition.* Retrieved from www.statcan.gc.ca/pub/11-008-x/2007001/9628-eng.htm

O'Neil, J., Reading, J., & Leader, A. (1998). Changing the relations of surveillance: The development of a discourse on resistance in Aboriginal epidemiology. *Human Organization, 57*(2), 230–237.

Pearce, M., Christian, W., Patterson, K., Norris, K., Moniruzzaman, A., Craib, K., ... & the Cedar Project Partnership. (2008). The Cedar Project: Historical trauma, sexual abuse and HIV risk among young Aboriginal people who use injection and non-injection drugs in two Canadian cities. *Social Science & Medicine, 66*(11), 2185–2194.

Peltier, D. (2010). *Environments of Nurturing Safety (EONS): Aboriginal women in Canada, five year strategy on HIV and AIDS.* Vancouver, BC: Canadian Aboriginal AIDS Network.

Prentice, T. (2004). *HIV/AIDS and Aboriginal women, children, and families: A position statement.* Ottawa, ON: Canadian Aboriginal AIDS Network.

Public Health Agency of Canada. (2005). *Leading together: Canada takes action on HIV/AIDS (2005–2010).* Ottawa, ON: Public Health Agency of Canada.

Public Health Agency of Canada. (2007). *Statement of meaningful engagement of Aboriginal people.* Ottawa, ON: Public Health Agency of Canada. Retrieved from www.phac-aspc.gc.ca/aids-sida/fi-if/aboriginal/state-eng.php

Public Health Agency of Canada. (2010). *HIV/AIDS Epi Updates, July 2010.* Ottawa, ON: Public Health Agency of Canada. Retrieved from www.phac-aspc.gc.ca/aids-sida/publication/epi/2010/index-eng.php

Raphael, D. (Ed.). (2004). *Social determinants of health: Canadian perspectives.* Toronto, ON: Canadian Scholars' Press.

Reading, J., & Nowgesic, E. (2002). Improving the health of future generations: The Canadian Institutes of Health Research Institute of Aboriginal Peoples' Health. *American Journal of Public Health, 92*(9), 1396–1400.

Richmond, C., Ross, N., & Egeland, G. (2007). Social support and thriving health: A new approach to understanding the health of Indigenous Canadians. *American Journal of Public Health, 97*(9), 1827–1833.

Shannon, K., Kerr, T., Allinott, S., Chettiar, J., Shoveller, J., & Tyndall, M. (2008). Social and structural violence and power relations in mitigating HIV risk of drug-using women in survival sex work. *Social Science & Medicine, 66*(4), 911–921.

Statistics Canada. (2009). *Aboriginal identity (8), sex (3) and age groups (12) for the population of Canada, provinces, territories, census metropolitan areas and census agglomerations, 2006 census -*

20% sample data. Catalogue no. 97-558-XCB2006007. Ottawa, ON: Statistics Canada.

Stratton, T., Jackson, R., & Barlow, K. (2006). *Making it our way: A community mobilization toolkit*. Ottawa, ON: Canadian Aboriginal AIDS Network.

Unger, J., Soto, C., & Thomas, N. (2008). Translation of health programs for American Indians in the United States. *Evaluation & the Health Professions, 31*(2), 124–144.

Valaskakis, G., Dion Stout, M., & Guimond, E. (2009). Introduction. In G. Valaskakis, M. Dion Stout, & E. Guimond (Eds.), *Restoring the balance: First Nations women, community, and culture* (pp. 1–9). Winnipeg, MB: University of Manitoba Press.

Varcoe, C., & Dick, S. (2008). The intersecting risks of violence and HIV for rural Aboriginal women in a neo-colonial Canadian context. *Journal of Aboriginal Health, 4*(1), 42–52.

Walters, K., & Simoni, J. (2002). Reconceptualizing Native women's health: An "Indigenist" stress-coping model. *American Journal of Public Health, 92*(4), 520–524.

Walters, K., Simoni, J., & Evans-Campbell, T. (2002). Substance use among American Indians and Alaska Natives: Incorporating culture in an "Indigenist" stress-coping paradigm. *Public Health Reports, 117*(Suppl. 1), S104–S117.

Weaver, H. N. (2009). The colonial context of violence: Reflections on violence in the lives of Native American women. *Journal of Interpersonal Violence, 24*(9), 1552–1563.

Wilson, K., & Young, K. (2008). An overview of Aboriginal health research in the social sciences: Current trends and future directions. *International Journal of Circumpolar Health, 67*(2/3), 179–189.

Wolski, E. (2009). The role of culturally relevant gender-based analysis in reconciliation. In G. Younging, J. Dewar, & M. DeGagne (Eds.), *Response, responsibility, and renewal: Canada's reconciliation journey* (pp. 271–279). Ottawa, ON: Aboriginal Healing Foundation.

Chapter 5

AN EVIDENCE-BASED INTERVENTION TO SUPPORT AFRICAN, CARIBBEAN, AND BLACK WOMEN IN CANADA TO DISCLOSE THEIR HIV-POSITIVE STATUS

Wangari Tharao, Marvelous Muchenje, and Mira Mehes

INTRODUCTION

African, Caribbean, and Black (ACB) communities are disproportionately affected by HIV/AIDS, with women bearing the greatest burden of the disease. Despite representing 2.2% of the total national population, approximately 16% of new infections occur within the ACB demographic subset (Public Health Agency of Canada [PHAC], 2009). In recent years, public health interventions and awareness campaigns have sought to decrease the rate of HIV infection. However, Black Canadians continue to experience an increased incidence of transmission. Over the past two decades, the rate of HIV infection has doubled within the ACB population, from 7.3% to 14.5%, between 1988 and 2008 (PHAC, 2009). Epidemiological data also indicates a steady increase in positive diagnoses among Canadian women, with the most recent reports placing the national rate of infection at 26% (PHAC, 2009). ACB women are particularly impacted by HIV and AIDS, accounting for more than 70% of new infections among all Canadian women. Within the HIV-endemic subcategory, women represent more than 50% of new infections and just over 40% of AIDS cases (PHAC, 2007).

While it is recognized that women are more physiologically susceptible to contracting HIV than men, ACB women often face the additional challenges of institutional discrimination, gender imbalances, cultural and social stigmatization, migration issues, and economic disparities. These compounding factors may contribute to a higher incidence and risk of HIV among Black women. Additionally, social determinants such as poverty, gender, and structural discrimination play a role in the disempowerment and marginalization experienced by women of colour (PHAC, 2005; Newman, Williams, Massaquoi, Brown, & Logie, 2008). Although social stigma surrounding HIV is often linked to behavioural or lifestyle assumptions, most women contract HIV through heterosexual contact. Nevertheless, HIV stigmatization in Canada continues to contribute to discriminatory experiences, emotional distress, and a fear of disclosure among HIV-positive women (Black & Miles, 2002; PHAC, 2007).

The present situation faced by ACB women illustrates the importance of developing and supporting effective HIV prevention interventions designed with consideration for the multiple intersecting factors that contribute to each woman's unique experience. Adaptable and appropriate HIV prevention interventions should move beyond individual women's behavioural choices (Webber, 2007) to the broader factors that reduce their ability to exercise individual agency and free will when faced with situations where HIV transmission is possible (Gardezi et al., 2008; Gray et al., 2008; Tharao, Massaquoi, & Teclom, 2006; UNAIDS, 2005).

Factors that influence a woman's situation include: (1) a lack of knowledge and skills required to protect oneself and others; (2) factors pertaining to the quality and coverage of services (e.g., inaccessibility of service due to distance, cost, or other factors); and (3) systemic or structural factors such as migration, immigration and settlement, human rights violations, and existing socio-cultural norms (Gardezi et al., 2008; Gray et al., 2008; Tharao et al., 2006; UNAIDS, 2005). For HIV-positive women from the ACB community, these factors are often compounded by intersecting dimensions of stigma and discrimination, ranging from those that are HIV and gender-related to racism and homophobia. The impact of these experiences encompasses an important consideration that must be incorporated into HIV transmission interventions that are adapted to meet the needs of women of colour.

The experience of HIV-positive women has recently been complicated by the increasing criminalization of HIV non-disclosure. Failure to disclose one's serostatus when engaging in activities that pose a significant risk of transmitting HIV can result in criminal prosecution and public exposure (Mykhalovskiy, Betteridge, & Mclay, 2010). Criminalization of HIV non-disclosure has become a highly racialized issue, with Black men representing more than half of heterosexual men prosecuted between 2004 and 2009 (Mykhalovskiy et al., 2010). Racialization is the process by which groups are designated as different and singled out for unequal treatment on the basis of race, ethnicity, language, religion, or culture (Larcher & Symington, 2010). The media portrayal of HIV-infected people as irresponsible, dishonest, and criminally dangerous has aggravated HIV-related stigma and fear (Mykhalovskiy et al., 2010), particularly within the ACB community (Larcher & Symington, 2010).

The process of disclosure is viewed as an important public health strategy for reducing HIV transmission. Effective disclosure has been linked to reductions in HIV transmission (Kalichman, Rompa, & Cage, 2005), adherence to medical regimens (Stirratt et al., 2006; Peretti-Watel, Spire, Pierret, Lert, & Obadia, 2003), access to support services (Abdool et al., 2008), improved mental health status (Emlet, 2007), and effective adaptation to living with HIV. On the other hand, ineffective disclosure can lead to strained relationships, loss of employment, discrimination, and even violence (Greeff et al., 2008; World Health Organization [WHO], 2004).

Disclosure of HIV-positive serostatus is an ongoing process that is intimately personal but has a considerable effect on families and communities, and impacts access to information and services intended to help people deal effectively with HIV/AIDS. To support HIV-positive women throughout the experience of disclosing their HIV status, it is imperative to understand the intricacies of the process, the unique pathways and strategies that individuals will use to disclose their status, and the factors that influence their decisions. This information should be used to inform any disclosure intervention developed to support women. At present there is a paucity of support materials and interventions available to ACB women and their providers. When considering the complex interplay of factors that influence disclosure and the unparalleled experience of Black women and women of colour, it becomes apparent that there is a pressing need to establish tools and resources for disclosure that are tailored to the needs of this group.

Women's Health in Women's Hands (WHIWH) Community Health Centre, in partnership with Toronto People with AIDS Foundation (PWA), The Black Coalition for AIDS Prevention (Black CAP), Africans in Partnership Against AIDS (APAA), The Teresa Group, and CASEY House Hospice, recently introduced an HIV disclosure intervention that has been designed with consideration for the unique needs and circumstances faced by HIV-positive women from the ACB community. WHIWH, a community health centre based in Toronto, is uniquely positioned to lead the development of this intervention as an ally to the ACB community, providing primary health care services and psychosocial support for Black women and women of colour within an anti-racism and anti-oppression framework.

The intervention was collaboratively developed by researchers, service providers, and HIV-positive women from the community who explored disclosure barriers, facilitators, and opportunities. The group also explored the literature to identify existing interventions and strategies designed to meet the needs of similar populations. Although there were no interventions established specifically for the needs of ACB women, existing strategies served to inform the development of the intervention. Once a general framework was established, the group conducted a series of focus groups and in-depth interviews with HIV-positive women and with support workers working in the community. The purpose of these sessions was to gain a better understanding of the multiple factors influencing the experience of ACB women in Canada who were navigating disclosure or contemplating initiating the process. Participants provided feedback and recommendations that were integrated into the intervention design. Following the development of the initial model, a pilot project was conducted in collaboration with local service providers, trained peers, support workers, and women who were actively engaged in working through the disclosure process. The outcomes of this pilot study were used to develop a preliminary evidence-based HIV disclosure intervention tailored to the needs of women from the ACB community.

The resulting intervention is designed to serve as a resource for women undergoing or contemplating HIV disclosure to their heterosexual sexual partners, children, and family members. It is also intended as a resource for service providers assisting women throughout this complex journey, who often must draw from multiple disparate resources, adapting materials to meet the needs of their clients. The complete HIV disclosure intervention package contains a disclosure handbook that outlines various disclosure scenarios and processes, resources for referral, and a training package to build the capacity of HIV-positive peers who can be partnered with women seeking support throughout their disclosure experiences.

This chapter highlights the process that was used to develop a culturally and socially adapted HIV disclosure intervention for HIV-positive women. The evidence-based model that we present is intended to work as a starting point and complementary guide for ACB women living with HIV/AIDS as they navigate through processes of voluntary and involuntary disclosure.

We present a review of the current literature, drawing from examples that provide models and strategies for disclosure of HIV status. Next, we offer an overview of the main themes and messages emerging from focus groups and in-depth interviews that were conducted with ACB women living with HIV/AIDS, as well as service providers working in the community through AIDS Service Organizations (ASOs), cultural groups, and other support organizations. The findings from these sessions were used to inform the content and structure of the intervention. Finally, we discuss the intervention pilot-testing experience and suggest recommendations for broader rollout of a socio-culturally based intervention.

INTERVENTION DEVELOPMENT PROCESS

The disclosure study took place in three stages. The first stage involved a broad-scope literature review that explored existing data on disclosure and more specifically on the disclosure experiences of women from ACB communities. The second stage of the study involved a series of focus groups and in-depth interviews to gain insight into the experiences and perceptions of women from the ACB community and staff from various social and health care systems. Finally a pilot-testing phase introduced the intervention to HIV-positive women and service providers as they worked through the disclosure process.

Limitations

While this study seeks to understand factors influencing the perceptions and the experiences of ACB women engaging in the process of disclosure or contemplating disclosure, it is important to recognize the limitations of this study. African,

Caribbean, and Black women are often grouped into the same category; however, individual disclosure processes will be different. When reflecting on the literature, it is evident that studies often do not consider the distinct cultural, historical, faith-based, and social differences experienced by Black women and women of colour. For instance, women from the Caribbean diaspora were particularly under-represented in the literature, with only one study focusing specifically on their disclosure experiences and needs (Anderson et al., 2009). This is concerning in light of the particular culture of silence and the stigma associated with HIV that has been anecdotally observed within this community. Given the specific challenges of creating a "one-size-fits-all" disclosure process, the proposed model will reflect a pragmatic framework that can be adapted to the specific cultural and psychosocial needs of each woman.

Literature Review

We conducted an extensive literature review exploring factors that influence disclosure. For the most part, studies about HIV serostatus disclosure have largely overlooked the experiences of women from African, Caribbean, and Black communities. To address this discrepancy, we wanted to examine how the experiences of this group are distinct from those of other people living with HIV and AIDS. While the social location of a woman has implications for her well-being, we also searched the literature for factors influencing disclosure in HIV-positive men and women of different backgrounds to see if themes, patterns, or models could be adapted to the experiences of ACB women in Canada.

This review explored the challenges that emerge at various stages of disclosure and the role of support systems. We also identified interventions that have been developed and tested with similar populations that may be promising, relevant, and feasible. Identified interventions were critically appraised to capture the elements of each intervention, the duration and frequency of intervention, the geographic location of each intervention, and the outcomes measured, and to assess whether participant perceptions or evaluations were conducted.

Through the literature search we identified a number of promising interventions and models; however, none of the available studies examined the specific experience of ACB women. For the most part, we identified disclosure theories and models that were designed to meet the requirements of broader demographic subsets, including people categorized according to risk exposure group (Bairan et al., 2007), gender (Derlega, Winstead, Greene, Serovich, & Elwood, 2002; Kalichman, DiMarco, Austin, Luke, & DiFonzo, 2003; Serovich & McDowell, 2008), and sexual orientation (Driskell, Salomon, Mayer, Capistrant, & Safren, 2008). While one study provided a model for disclosure of African-American women to intimate sexual partners (Hudson, 2008), it is important to note that the experience of this demographic group is largely distinct from that of Canada's ACB diaspora.

Some studies focused on the role of social support systems (Kalichman et al., 2003;

Simoni, Demas, Mason, Drossman, & Davis, 2000), as well as the effects of stigma and discrimination on an individual's ability and agency to disclose (Abdool et al., 2008). Additionally, a number of studies were divided according to the disclosure category, including family (Fekete et al., 2009; Serovich, Craft, & Yoon, 2007), children (Delaney, Serovich, & Lim, 2009), and sexual partners. Although one intervention provided a valuable context for disclosure to children, the scope of this resource did not encompass the cultural, social, and economic factors faced by ACB women when contemplating disclosure to HIV-positive and HIV-negative children (Nelms & Zeigler, 2008).

Among the studies that examined the experience of women, a number of challenges and consequences to disclosure were identified, including violence and rejection (Carlson Gielen et al., 2000), privacy and self-blame (Derlega, Winstead, Greene, Serovich, & Elwood, 2004), and stigma and discrimination (Abdool et al., 2008). These considerations were incorporated into the development of our disclosure intervention framework. Finally, two additional studies provided a strong theoretical and conceptual basis for developing an adaptable HIV disclosure intervention (Kimberly & Serovich, 1996; Medley, Garcia-Moreno, McGill, & Maman, 2004).

Focus Groups

Following the completion of the literature review, we conducted four focus groups. Two of the focus groups included 18 HIV-positive women from the ACB community: one group included women who had publicly disclosed their status and the other group was for women who had not yet revealed their status but who were considering disclosure to a partner, a child, or a family member. Two additional focus groups were conducted with 12 service providers who work with women from the ACB community within the capacity of psychosocial and biomedical support systems. More than half of the service providers were women from the ACB community. Some of the service providers participating in the interviews were also HIV positive.

Key Informant Interviews

Following the completion of focus groups, we identified four women from the ACB community to serve as key informants to the study. Interviews were open-ended. Questions were based on information gathered from the literature review and throughout the focus groups. Both focus groups and interviews were recorded and transcribed. The transcripts were then coded and analyzed thematically using a grounded approach informed by transnational and feminist and critical race theories.

Pilot-Testing Phase

A modified draft intervention was reviewed by providers and pilot tested with HIV-positive women who had indicated to their service providers that they were contemplating disclosure. Pilot testing was supported by trained HIV-positive peers. We then refined the draft intervention based on pilot-testing findings and discussions from a disclosure "think tank" meeting that we organized to bring together experts from the field, including researchers, service providers, policy-makers, HIV-positive women, and community members, to inform the development of the intervention.

FACTORS INFLUENCING THE DISCLOSURE PROCESS

For any intervention to be effective, it has to incorporate needs and issues that are relevant to the population or group to which the intervention is targeted. Review of literature revealed that experiences of the disclosure process are incredibly diverse and vary across race and ethnicity (Arnold, Rice, Flannery, & Rotheram-Borus, 2008; Elford, Ibrahim, Bukutu, & Anderson, 2008), sexual identity (Korner, 2007), nationality (Miller & Rubin, 2007; Pulerwitz, Michaelis, Lippman, Chinaglia, & Diaz, 2008), age (Emlet, 2008), and gender, geographic location, and culture (Rasera, Vieira, & Japur, 2004; Liu et al., 2006). Disclosure is also influenced by knowing one's partners' HIV status, fear of abandonment, and history of abuse (King et al., 2008), concern for others (Emlet, 2007) and one's community, the need to break the silence and end the secrecy of one's HIV-positive status, the need to be understood and supported practically or spiritually (Greeff et al., 2008), and the fear of others knowing one's status.

Narratives of ACB women and providers who participated in focus groups and key informant interviews also indicated that the intersection of race, gender, culture, and other dimensions of difference created unique experiences of HIV that impacted on the disclosure process directly or indirectly. What follows is a discussion of factors identified as being important by ACB women and their providers.

A Process of Self-Acceptance and Empowerment

ACB women discussed disclosure in terms of a process involving self-awareness and acceptance of who one has become as a person living with HIV. Most depicted a process involving ongoing counselling and education around HIV-related issues. Once a certain level of comfort and understanding has been achieved, women feel better equipped and more empowered to undertake the journey of disclosure. Feelings of anger, shame, regret, sadness and other emotional and psychological issues become easier to deal with.

> They got counselling ... lots of education about HIV and AIDS. And, hey, now they have reached that stage where they can say, "Okay, this is me. I have to live with this, and it's not a problem for me to tell someone." (African woman)

Raising Awareness, Education, and Promoting Testing

A number of women also viewed disclosure as an opportunity to promote general awareness about HIV/AIDS, and to challenge pervasive stereotypes by demystifying misconceptions about what it means to live with HIV. Some women described how they found the courage to share their own stories with friends or family members who were hesitant to have an HIV test or who were contemplating disclosure. In this sense, the women were encouraging access to treatment and giving others hope for the future. Others used this opportunity to prepare their families before they disclosed their HIV status to them. The strategy allowed women to assess reactions and beliefs, to challenge misconceptions, and sometimes even to shift negative perceptions about HIV and AIDS.

> We were talking at a church group once and I got up there and asked, "Do you know of anyone who is HIV positive in the room?" They looked around and said, "No, everyone looks healthy." That's when I told them that I'm HIV positive ... People think HIV is in the face, not in the blood. I disclose to educate people. (Caribbean HIV-positive woman)

Ability to Deal with Multiple Facets of Stigma and Discrimination

The experience of stigma is complex and multi-faceted. HIV-positive women from the ACB diaspora are exposed to prejudice across multiple overlapping spheres, encompassing the broader societal stereotypes attributed to women of colour and people living with HIV/AIDS, the discrimination that exists within socio-cultural communities, and the biases that are experienced within intimate support networks (Emlet, 2007; Gardezi et al., 2008; Tharao et al., 2006; Newman et al., 2008). Narratives emerging from our study highlighted that women's conceptualization of HIV was based on the pervasive views of HIV within their families and communities and contributed to feelings of shame and fear, with their secrecy leading to self-stigmatization and marginalization. Gender inequalities, views of women as "carriers" of HIV/AIDS, links to race, culture, and ethnicity, or association of HIV with homosexuality, prostitution, drug use, poverty, and so forth, contributed to women's decisions to disclose or not to disclose. In all cases, the way HIV/AIDS is perceived within the Canadian context contributes to feelings of fear and shame, leading to marginalization.

Self-stigmatization

> I stigmatize myself even before I give other people the chance to stigmatize me ... I don't want my kids to share my soap. In my mind I feel I'm dirty ... Even with the baby, when I put his soother in my mouth, my husband says: "You are giving my child HIV." We are the ones stigmatizing ourselves against our kids ... That's corrupting and I feel guilty. (African HIV-positive woman)

Gender-based stigma

> I told my partner that if between us, if one of us should die, they would think right away that it was me. For people who do not know me, even though he was positive when we met, those who don't know that will blame me. If everything is going well in the home, it's the man. If anything goes wrong, it's the women. If a man gets sick with HIV, it's the woman. (African HIV-positive woman)

Racial discrimination

> Only Black people get HIV—the colour of your skin stands out … When a Black person infects someone else, they will show the faces, the images. There is more respect for white people, not showing their images as much. (Caribbean HIV-positive woman)

Association of HIV with other marginalized groups

> If you have HIV and AIDS, you're either a prostitute or a drug user. Or you're gay if you're a man. But they don't say lesbians, because apparently lesbians don't get HIV. People associate you with HIV—birds of the same feather fly together. They think if you have HIV, your friends have HIV. Certain people don't want to interact with my kids. They associate HIV with them. (Caribbean HIV-positive woman)

The Need to Relieve the Burden of Silence and Secrecy

Non-disclosure can represent an incredible burden in the lives of ACB women. The stigma attached to HIV, and the consequent need to conceal a positive status, operates to isolate an HIV-positive person even from their own community. That silence is permeated by fear (Korner, 2007), and the associated despair, hopelessness, and desolation have serious implications for any and all provision of health and social support services (Worth, Reid, Ackroyd, & Tamarite-Bowden, 2001). Many ACB women described how the secrecy attributed to concealing a positive status created barriers to accessing support and services. After disclosing, one woman said: "I feel better about myself. It's like lifting a house off my shoulders. I feel lightness and relief" (Caribbean HIV-positive woman).

> I believe that when we are sick, we should not keep this secret to ourselves; otherwise, you will begin to deteriorate. You can always find people to support you, to keep your secret and to get advice … But if

you keep the secret to yourself, I don't think it's good. Even when you begin taking medications, if you don't have anyone to talk to, they won't have the same impact. (African HIV-positive woman)

Access to Treatment, Care, and Support

Visible symptoms of disease progression were a strong determinant of disclosure as an enabler of access to medical care and treatment. Reasons given for disclosure at this time included gaining access to better medical care and treatments while receiving support from friends or family members, and having an emergency contact person who could provide medical history and treatment information to health care providers in the event that critical medical episodes arose. While support was often accessed from existing organizations and support networks, many women also discussed the role of peer support and the importance of having a confidant who understands what it means to live with a positive diagnosis and who had moved forward to live a positive life.

> To my daughter I only say: "If I'm ever sick, this is where my medication is." And I have one friend who knows about my status … Yeah, some people, they disclose because of the pressure. Let's say, maybe you are very sick … You feel that pressure to disclose, not because you want to, but just because you are very sick. Maybe you think you are dying, that you need to disclose it. (Caribbean HIV-positive woman)

> If you live with your family and you're taking medications, you may be prone to disclose. It's a relief to be able to come home and bring materials and leave them on the table. I can say, "I'm going to one of THOSE meetings!" I can live freely. You don't have to hide anything. My mother looked at every bottle … none of them say HIV. So she asked: "Who gave you all these bottles? The doctor gave you all these vitamins?" … She was looking for it, but I wasn't ready to tell her. (Caribbean HIV-positive woman)

Having partners and family members living in countries of origin was particularly challenging since women were worried about the impacts of disclosure to family members abroad without being close by to support them or for them to see that they were okay. Women made plans to disclose during in-person visits when everyone could see that they were healthy and thriving.

Gender-Based Violence: Safety and Security

The threat or possibility of physical, psychological, or verbal abuse or violence by a partner was a critical factor influencing a woman's ability to disclose. It remains at the forefront of many women's minds for their own safety and well-being and that of their children. ACB women participating in this project discussed why and how disclosure might lead to partner abuse, threats of being separated from their children, and deportation in cases where a woman had no legal status to stay in Canada. Psychological abuse, which was very prevalent throughout women's narratives, had an impact on women's self-worth and confidence and influenced, in many ways, decisions to disclose their status or access to support. Additionally, both women and service providers described experiences of targeted physical violence and psychological aggression from within the community, occurring anonymously and overtly.

Threats from HIV-negative partners

> Most of the time what I see for example is that, ah, women who are HIV positive and their partners are not HIV positive, there is that conflict … It's almost like a weapon whereby I am going to say that you are HIV positive, and then you're going to lose your children to CAS, because I'm going to tell them that … you're not capable of taking care of these children because you're sick most of the time. (African HIV-positive woman)

Immigration status

> Many women are sponsored. They are on the sponsorship of the husbands. The children are also on the sponsorship of the husbands. So any kind of, ah, disclosure that can affect, or break, or separate that husband/wife relationship … immediately impacts the immigration status of the woman. So I think sponsorship is a huge issue … Immigration is a huge issue that really will play an important role in whether … the woman will disclose or not. (Service provider)

Legal Issues: Criminalization of HIV Non-Disclosure

Criminalization of HIV non-disclosure can be both a facilitator and an inhibitor of disclosure of HIV status. The prospect of criminalization linked to non-disclosure resulted in several animated discussions among women and service providers. Many women explained that they had no choice but to disclose their status to potential or current partners, as required by the law. For the most part, fear was the primary driving factor. The women described the fear of being taken to court for not disclosing, resulting in public disclosure: "The entire court house and media will know." Subsequently, for most women, the fear of such a consequence motivated them to reveal their status to partners.

At the same time, many women felt that if they took necessary precautions, like using a condom during consensual sex, they were protecting themselves and their partner. Hence, they felt that they should not be prosecuted in the absence of disclosure. The possible rejection, anger, or aggression on the part of both casual and long-term partners was among the reasons given for foregoing disclosure. Others worried that if they disclosed to their partner and, later, the relationship broke down, they could be accused of not disclosing their status even when they had. The law does not protect them against these accusations.

> And the other thing they also fear is the legal system. If they leave, and their partner is also HIV positive, then the partner will say, "She gave me HIV. I was not HIV. She's the one who brought it to me." So we need to educate ... It's a hard thing, because if you don't disclose you can get into trouble. This person can criminalize you; they can take you to court even if you use a condom. Because that's what they're saying, is, you know, it's in the law, they say that if you, even if you use a condom, and then the person finds out after, they can still criminalize you because they can say, "What if this condom had broken?" And things happen; you didn't say that you are. So for me, if you're going to have sex with somebody, or you're going to go into a relationship with somebody, it's best you tell them, okay this is who I am, so they know what they are getting into. I disclosed because there is no choice in Canada. (African HIV-positive woman)

Financial Support and Security

Financial security is critical to accessing appropriate housing, ensuring food security, and providing for individual and family needs. In many cases the ability to obtain and maintain gainful employment or economic support represents an important consideration when ACB women consider disclosure (Tharao et al., 2006). Women's narratives covered a wide scope of issues, ranging from workplace discrimination, institutional barriers to employment, PHA-specific jobs (PHA refers to a person or people living with HIV/AIDS), and financial support accessed through ASOs to alleviate poverty. These narratives also reflected the reality that many women from the Canadian ACB diaspora send a portion of their income back home to support extended family members.

> I know by my disclosing or not disclosing at my workplace, or at the hospital, or wherever it is, medical coverage or work, am I qualified enough for work? Will my qualifications get me a job? If I get the job, and there's some level of disclosure there, where will my medical coverage be from? You know? So I think that is the second thing that ... hugely plays a role on whether women disclose or not. (Service provider)

Culture and Community

Cultural influences play an important role in the way a woman perceives disclosure, and a number of women expressed apprehension about revealing their status in relation to culture and community. Others were advised by counsellors and service providers that they should be cautious about disclosing within their own communities. Lack of understanding, myths about HIV within communities, experiences of HIV in country of origin, and cultural differences were cited as some of the factors that discourage disclosure.

Lack of understanding about HIV

> Some cultures do not understand HIV. If you have HIV, you are a bad person; you are going to die tomorrow. (African HIV-positive woman)

Conflicting ways of dealing with HIV between country of origin and that of destination

> I started to go to support groups and wanted to disclose but support workers and outreach workers told me that you don't have to disclose, you shouldn't disclose. And I thought, why are you teaching me to lie? But even though you might think you're in a safe space and you disclose, they go out in the community and talk about your business. (African HIV-positive woman)

Myths about HIV

> In my country, there is a belief that if HIV comes into a house, it's the wife who has bewitched the husband to get all the money ... His parents used to come to my house when my husband was sick. I would cook food, and they wouldn't eat. When my husband died in the house, the family made the arrangements and then disappeared. Normally, you would stay in the house ... My mother-in-law said: "My foot will never step in this house again. Those two kids are yours. We don't want to see them again." And I never saw them again ... Somehow I ended up believing that I killed him. Those next two years were very difficult. I felt guilty. I was going to the witch doctor to see what I did wrong. (African HIV-positive woman)

Different approaches to dealing with HIV between African and Caribbean women

> My values as an African woman and maybe someone else from a Caribbean background are totally different ... from an African and

Caribbean context … Women from each of these different communities live totally different kinds of lives. We can't address a problem without looking at the socio-cultural context, for sure. (Service provider)

Religion/Faith-Based Groups

Faith organizations offer hope while at the same time many stigmatize based on their beliefs and stereotypes about HIV and groups that are affected. The fear of being ostracized from one's faith community and the spiritual support groups offered by these institutions prevented many women from disclosing to anyone from their church, including their pastors. The benefits received from religion-based groups, for example, prayers, outweighed their desire to access support for challenges related to HIV.

> The only person I wanted to tell was my pastor. I said: "I want to talk to you about something after church." But then during the service he started talking about AIDS, saying, if you don't live right, if you jump from one partner to another, you don't have to wait long, it will come out in HIV and AIDS … so I didn't disclose to him … They have many prayers for the sick, so the church does pray for me then. But I have not disclosed my status. (African HIV-positive woman)

In summary, facilitators and inhibitors of disclosure for ACB women are varied and complex, and range from individual-based, to familial and communal, to systemic, as highlighted above. The journey starts with the acceptance of one's HIV status facilitated through support, education, and resiliency building. To raise awareness in oneself and others through education and to strengthen one's support system while eliminating stigma and discrimination are also important steps in the journey. The social environments within which women are living, within family, community, and where they access services, also have major impacts on their ability to disclose. Any intervention developed to support ACB women go through this process needs to take all these issues into consideration.

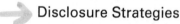

Disclosure Strategies

Distinct disclosure processes have been identified in particular communities (Ontario HIV Treatment Network, 2009). Participants identified several disclosure strategies, ranging from point-blank disclosure to subtle hints such as a discussion of treatment options, or support groups one is participating in, or other indices that might be an indication of HIV-positive status. Others used partial or incremental disclosure where they would reveal a little information at a time. Involuntary disclosure also happened, particularly within social contexts and situations, ranging from rumours within the community to breach of confidentiality by service providers or peers. Sometimes disclosure happened accidentally through family members, friends, or children. All these factors illustrated the struggles women go through in their efforts to tell others about their HIV status. This highlights the importance of developing systematic and culturally appropriate ways to support disclosure of HIV status.

INTERVENTION FRAMEWORK

ACB HIV-positive women experience systemic inequality in relation to gender, race, class, and sexuality that intersects with HIV status. Their role in Canadian society is socially and culturally limited and is navigated within legal, financial, religious, and economic systems that discriminate against them (Gardezi et al., 2008; Tharao et al., 2006). To support women's disclosure of HIV status effectively and safely within these contexts, we have placed the proposed intervention within a feminist and critical race theoretical framework that emphasizes justice, fairness, and rights (Brown, Macintyre, & Trujillo, 2003; Thompson, 2003; Walters, 2005) and links research to action (Bennett, 2008). It helps to shed light on the organizational and structural nature of intersecting oppressions (gender oppression, racism, homophobia, etc.) and the interdependent and mutually constitutive relationship between social identities and social inequities (Derlega et al., 2002; Medley et al., 2004; Salter-Goldie et al., 2007). It helps to connect research to resistance with emancipatory aims to challenge oppression and promote social justice. Locating the intervention within this framework will place HIV disclosure within the broader context in which ACB HIV-positive women live their lives and where HIV is just one of the many issues with which they are struggling.

We have also utilized a transnational theoretical framework that best describes the multiple and hybrid identities of ACB people living in Canada. This framework takes into consideration the multiple locations of the social life of ACB women as migrant populations or "people on the move." It recognizes that the social life of migrants is not confined to the boundaries of the nation-state of destination (Levitt & Glick Schiller, 2004; Wagner, 2002). They maintain ties between societies of origin and of settlement, taking part in the social life of both societies, rendering the nation-state boundaries invisible. They simultaneously live aspects of their lives in their country/culture of origin while they are incorporated into the countries of destination (Levitt, 2001; Levitt & Glick Schiller, 2004). This framework will help us to understand better identity politics, space contestations, and discourses around HIV and their impacts on HIV disclosure among ACB women in Canada. This framework goes beyond the exploration of the individual into the multi-layered and multi-sited networks and connections that influence their sense of self, their actions, and the impact of these actions on their loved ones across boundaries.

INTERVENTION STRUCTURE AND ELEMENTS

Our findings indicate that disclosure is a multi-faceted and multi-layered process that involves a number of incremental stages to move a woman from a diagnosis of HIV and acceptance of this diagnosis, all the way to increased ability and comfort to tell someone else about this diagnosis. Every woman experiences disclosure differently. However, most women will undergo similar stages of disclosure each time the disclosure process is initiated. Understanding the primary phases of disclosure can help prepare a woman for the process of discussing her serostatus, whether she is coming to terms with her own diagnosis or guiding a partner, child, or family member through the process.

Figure 5.1: The Disclosure Process

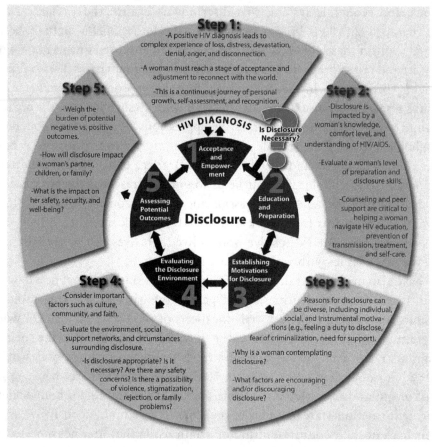

STAGES OF DISCLOSURE

Step 1: Acceptance and Empowerment

Acceptance and adjustment to an HIV-positive diagnosis

An HIV diagnosis involves great distress, experiences of loss, and such feelings as being victimized, regret, sadness, loss of future dreams, hopelessness, and fear. The isolation and depression that often accompany a diagnosis of HIV may result in suicidal thoughts, anger, anxiety, and grieving. To be prepared for disclosure, a woman needs support to deal with all these feelings, to come to terms with her diagnosis, and to adjust to being a person living with HIV. Some studies have drawn links between identity development and HIV disclosure, documenting the steps of adapting to living with HIV and their corresponding place on the approach to disclosure (Arnold et al., 2008; Baumgartner, 2007). This stage represents a continuous process of personal growth, self-assessment, recognition, and acceptance of the new self one has become. Self-acceptance is a sign that one is ready to move to the second step of the disclosure journey.

Step 2: Education and Preparation
Evaluation of a woman's level of preparation and disclosure skills
A woman's level of understanding of different aspects of HIV and her comfort with discussing HIV/AIDS-related topics can facilitate disclosure and the disclosure experience. Throughout the process, and even beforehand, it is beneficial for a woman to evaluate her own level of preparation. This can involve determining her level of knowledge about HIV and related issues, recognizing potential outcomes, benefits and challenges of disclosing, and accessing support services and care as she continues to deal with HIV and its impacts on her life. This stage is increasingly associated with involvement with the HIV community (Miller & Rubin, 2007; Serovich, Oliver, Smith, & Mason, 2005) in an effort to access information and services for support, care, and/or treatment. This stage may involve counselling and peer support to provide guidance and the support required to navigate the process of disclosure, training in the basics of HIV 101, becoming comfortable discussing HIV, and answering questions about transmission, prevention, treatment, support, and care. This stage ensures that a woman is prepared not only to deal with her own status but also to provide basic information, education, and support to the person being disclosed to.

Step 3: Establishing Motivations for Disclosure
Instrumental, individual, and social motivations for disclosure
At this stage a woman identifies and explores her reasons for wanting to disclose her HIV-positive status. As highlighted earlier, disclosure motivations may range from a need or desire to access resources, services, additional social supports, to meeting legal (criminalization of HIV non-disclosure) and public health requirements (e.g., partner notification, educating others to reduce stigma and discrimination, and encouraging HIV testing). This stage helps a woman undertake a self-assessment to determine why she wants to disclose, if it's even necessary, and the legal considerations that might need to be taken into account, particularly if there are issues of unprotected sex prior to disclosure.

Step 4: Evaluating the Disclosure Environment
Assessing whether the setting and circumstances are appropriate for disclosure
This step involves an evaluation of the social environment to determine what

support is needed, what is available, and what needs to be put in place to facilitate an effective disclosure. There is recognition that culture, community, faith, and social supports will impact the disclosure setting. In particular, the role and impact of multiple facets of stigma and discrimination are determined, and a plan is made to mitigate them to ensure that disclosure does not threaten the safety and well-being of a woman and her family. The following questions need be answered at this stage: Is there a possibility of violence, blame, stigmatization, rejection, or family problems? If so, what is the plan to resolve them? Are disclosure circumstances favourable? Does the woman have appropriate resources and supports in place? What will disclosure look like? Answers to these questions facilitate movement to the next stage or lead to further planning if it is determined that a woman is not ready to move forward.

Step 5: Assessing Potential Outcomes

Assessing the potential outcomes of disclosure

Prior to deciding to reveal a positive serostatus, it is important to determine potential reactions, weighing positive outcomes against potentially detrimental repercussions (a cost–benefit analysis). What are the potential reactions to disclosure? Is safety and well-being accounted for? How will disclosure affect a woman's future? How will it affect her health and well-being? How might it impact her family? Ultimately, this stage helps to ensure a woman's safety and well-being throughout the disclosure process. Ideally, the benefits resulting from disclosure should outweigh the risks associated with revealing an HIV-positive status.

If a woman is ready to move forward, preparations for the actual disclosure event are made. This requires making decisions as to the location where the event will take place, the other person(s) who will be present for support if needed, and the protocols that will be followed to ensure that the person being disclosed to is supported effectively. Plans are also made to protect the well-being of a woman and her family, in case of negative repercussions.

Regardless of whether a woman has reached a stage where she is prepared to disclose her status, ongoing support should be provided on a continual basis, even after a point of disclosure has been reached. Each woman will likely require ongoing counselling and follow-up, both for herself and for the person to whom she has disclosed her status. The guidance of a counsellor, support worker, or service provider will be critical to helping both parties navigate through the repercussions and outcomes of disclosure. To encompass the non-linearity of the disclosure experience, the proposed model is circular, allowing for the woman and her service provider to move back and forth between various phases of preparation. In instances where non-disclosure does not present the risk of HIV transmission, the model can help to relieve undue pressure to disclose until the woman and her partner, children, or family members have been adequately prepared.

DISCUSSION

HIV disclosure is a process that needs to be located within the individual and broader contexts within which Canadian ACB women live and experience their identity. This environment is often defined by a woman's relationships with intimate partners, family members, community, and society at large. As such, the experience and influence of stigma and discrimination within these relationships can determine if, when, where, how, and to whom a woman discloses her HIV status (Brown et al., 2003; Mahajan et al., 2008; UNAIDS, 2005). Moreover, news travels very quickly within ACB social networks. Many experiences reveal that once a woman divulges her status to a member of her community, information about her serostatus will often be disseminated throughout her entire network, including immediate and extended family, community members, and friends. In some instances, the news will even reach family members and friends living in her country of origin (Larcher & Symington, 2010). Beyond concern over public disclosure, a number of women are fearful that their positive status may be attributed to promiscuous or sinful behaviour, resulting in rejection and alienation from family and community (Gardezi et al., 2008; Tharao et al., 2006).

A number of myths distort how HIV is perceived within the ACB community, including assumptions that heterosexuals are not at risk for infection; that HIV/AIDS is associated with promiscuity, extramarital sex, and sex work; that the virus comes from "outsiders"; or that HIV infection only happens to those who transgress their culture or religion. The deep-seated stigma associated with HIV in the ACB community can create barriers that prevent women from accessing counselling and resources to help them navigate their experience with HIV/AIDS. Oftentimes, these mistaken beliefs will dissuade ACB women from seeking support and guidance from ethnocultural organizations that deliver linguistic and culturally appropriate services, or from family members, friends, and communities who traditionally form the social support system to rely on in times of need (Larcher & Symington, 2010). HIV-related stigma also intersects with other dimensions of stigma and discrimination including racism, gender discrimination, and homophobia, further complicating the ability to disclose HIV-positive status (Gardezi et al., 2008; Tharao et al., 2006). Adopting a culturally appropriate intervention can help positive women and their support workers to move beyond looking at stigma through a single lens, opting instead for a perspective that encapsulates the multi-layered dimensions and experiences of ACB women within the institutions of family, community, and institutional organizations (Collins, 2000; Crenshaw, 1989; Hancock, 2007). Developing a clear understanding of the complexity of stigma experienced by ACB women also helps to inform the development and implementation of stigma-reduction interventions to support women in their disclosure efforts.

Disclosure for ACB women is further complicated by criminalization of HIV non-disclosure and debates that have emerged in response to recent allegations.

Non-disclosure of HIV status has been declared a criminal offence, invalidating consent and transforming otherwise consensual sex into sexual assault (Larcher & Symington, 2010; Mykhalovskiy et al., 2010). Efforts to reduce HIV transmission through other methods, such as consistently using condoms and diligently complying with treatment regimens to reduce transmissibility of HIV through reduced viral load, are underappreciated, thereby limiting approaches to HIV prevention and sexual intimacy that characterize real-life sexual encounters and failing to recognize the differing social contexts that empower or disempower individuals in sexual interaction (Larcher & Symington, 2010) based on race, gender, sexual orientation, economics, and other dimensions of difference.

Violence emerges as an additional issue of concern, limiting ACB women's ability and agency to disclose their HIV status. Numerous studies from around the world indicate that violence against women is one of the major risk factors for acquiring or transmitting HIV. Violence and the threat of violence dramatically increases the vulnerability of women by making it difficult or impossible to negotiate safe behaviours to prevent HIV transmission (Dworkin & Ehrhardt, 2007; Maman et al., 2002; Wingood & DiClemente, 1997; WHO, 2000). Inability to negotiate safer sexual practices within communities that condone multiple sexual partnerships, are patriarchal in nature, and in which discussions of sex and sexual relationships are taboo increases the risk of ACB women acquiring or transmitting HIV (Gardezi et al., 2008; Tharao et al., 2006). This makes it difficult for women to disclose their HIV status and access essential HIV prevention care and treatment services (UNAIDS, 2009). Women often learn of their HIV-positive status before their sexual partners, since they are more likely to access health services, particularly when seeking prenatal care. As a result, women may be blamed for bringing HIV into their home (UNAIDS & UNDP, 2007). Fear of violence, abandonment, or other negative consequences such as legal ones resulting from the criminalization of HIV non-disclosure are highlighted in our chapter as being of concern to many ACB women. The proposed intervention brings up these issues for discussion and ensures that they are addressed as part of supporting women through the process of disclosure.

ACB women also live their lives amid abject poverty, with high rates of unemployment or underemployment making it difficult to make ends meet financially (Tharao et al., 2006). Studies have linked food security (Weiser et al., 2007), poverty (Gardezi et al., 2008; Kalichman et al., 2006; Tharao et al., 2006), and women's decreased access to means of production and credit, and inadequate guarantees of the right to inherit and own property as factors that increase the risk of acquiring or transmitting HIV (Hankins, 2008; UNAIDS/PCB, 2007). Economic dependence on male partners can result in women staying in risky relationships to ensure their own financial well-being and that of their children (Tharao et al., 2006). HIV-positive women are fearful of disclosing their HIV status for fear of rejection or abandonment by their partners, thereby jeopardizing their economic safety net. Our disclosure intervention takes this into consideration.

Migration has resulted in movements of large numbers of the ACB population from their countries of origin in search of safety or better opportunities for themselves and their families (Interagency Coalition on AIDS and Development, 2004; European Conference Report, 2007). Settling in a new country takes first priority, leaving access to HIV prevention and care services for later, if ever, even for those living with HIV. Factors contributing to this include unstable legal status; language and cultural differences; lack of information, education, and work; poor access to prevention, harm reduction, and health care services; social exclusion; and gender-related factors (European Conference Report, 2007; PHAC, 2009; Tharao et al., 2006). All of these factors are further exacerbated by stigma and discrimination. Travel restrictions, deportation, and policies that make it illegal for migrants to stay in a country may also threaten their lives and well-being, as well as violate their human rights (European Conference Report, 2007). ACB HIV-positive women are usually uncertain about immigration law and policy regarding HIV and whether HIV-positive people are accepted as legal residents in Canada, leading to avoidance of health care, social assistance benefits, or regular employment (Gardezi et al., 2008) to avoid disclosure. Avoidance of services limits awareness of individual legal rights, leaving women at the mercy of husbands or long-term partners who threaten them with withdrawal of immigration sponsorship or threaten to report to public health or police that they did not disclose their HIV status to them.

CONCLUSION

HIV counselling and disclosure are viewed as positive public health interventions for preventing further transmission of HIV/AIDS. As highlighted in this chapter, ACB women face many challenges unique to their situation and experience. For many women from this community, disclosure represents a journey that will be influenced by multiple cross-cutting factors. Recognizing that the experiences of HIV-positive Black women and women of colour will often be framed within the contexts of experienced and perceived stigma and discrimination, historic experiences of marginalization or exclusion, physical and emotional violence, and socio-political injustice, these are critical considerations when guiding and counselling a woman from the community. Additional obstacles that ACB women face include criminal prosecution, loss of financial sustainability, rejection from community, family, and faith-based networks, fear of deportation, and lack of knowledge surrounding migration laws.

We developed an evidence-based HIV intervention, incorporating literature review findings, and feedback from ACB women living with HIV and service providers working in the community. Following the development of the proposed disclosure model, we pilot tested the intervention with a group of women from the ACB community, with the support of trained peers and service providers who had an ongoing relationship with the women. Drawing from participant feedback and think tank recommendations, we adapted the model to better fit the gaps and needs identified within the ACB community. This study provides an example of the development of an evidence-based HIV disclosure intervention that can be used by service providers and by women contemplating HIV disclosure to their partners, children, or family members. As the HIV/AIDS epidemic enters its fourth decade of prevalence in Canada, there is an increasing need for adaptable and effective HIV prevention interventions that are respectful and inclusive of ethnicity, gender, sexual orientation, faith, and other socio-cultural characteristics.

PROBLEM-BASED LEARNING CASE STUDY

Disclosure is a multi-layered process that can take place in many different contexts and rarely takes place in a single step. A woman may use a variety of approaches or strategies when revealing her serostatus, including point-blank disclosure, subtle hints, partial disclosure, and incremental disclosure. In most cases, disclosure takes place over time and involves various degrees of revelation. Preparation and education are important first steps, both for the woman and for the people to whom she is disclosing. It is a significant life experience and a nuanced procedure that calls for counselling, support, and access to appropriate resources that ensure a woman's psychosocial and physical well-being.

Gloria is a woman from the ACB community who has lived in Canada without any legal immigration status for seven years. She has been accessing health care services at a community health centre for women in Toronto. The centre encouraged her to apply for legal status, and with their help, she filed a refugee claim two years ago. As required by Citizenship and Immigration Canada, her immigration medical included an HIV test. She tested positive for HIV and was referred to the medical care of an HIV specialist. Thanks to an effective antiretroviral regimen, she has managed to maintain an undetectable viral load. Gloria disclosed her HIV status to the social worker at the community health centre and has continued to receive counselling, psychosocial support, and educational resources and referrals to AIDS Service Organizations for further support. These tools have helped her to gain greater understanding and acceptance of her HIV-positive status.

Partner notification was originally dealt with by Public Health when she tested positive. After that time, Gloria met a new partner and engaged in protected sex but did not disclose her HIV status to him. She wanted to disclose but was fearful of the repercussions, although she indicated that her partner was caring and supportive.

With support, Gloria worked through the stages of the disclosure intervention and felt much more confident in her ability to disclose to her partner. She also identified educational materials, resources, and service agencies that could provide additional support for her and her partner following the initial disclosure. Feeling empowered, Gloria initiated a conversation about HIV/AIDS with her partner and revealed that she is HIV positive. Surprised, confused, and shocked, her partner went directly to his doctor's office for an HIV test, which came back negative. His family practitioner strongly encouraged the man to file a police report and to press charges against Gloria. The same day the man's doctor contacted the police, and Gloria was placed under house arrest, unable to access additional support to help her cope with the repercussions of her disclosure.

Meanwhile, the man began to read through some of the resources Gloria provided him with when she first spoke to him about HIV/AIDS. He discovered that he could access support from an AIDS Service Organization that works specifically with the ACB community. In search of support, he began to access counselling and educational services from this organization, which helped him to better understand Gloria's experience with HIV and disclosure decisions. Based on this more informed understanding, Gloria and her partner have reconciled. They have begun accessing counselling for serodiscordant couples. Although Gloria is no longer under house arrest, she still faces a court date that may result in serious charges for HIV nondisclosure. Her partner would like to have her charges dropped but in Canada it is not possible to repeal such a charge.

CRITICAL THINKING QUESTIONS

1. What is the basis for Gloria's fears about disclosure? What would help alleviate these fears?
2. What are the legal, privacy, and confidentiality issues highlighted by this case, and how can they be resolved?
3. How can you ensure that a woman's security, well-being, and livelihood will be protected after she discloses her HIV status?
4. What opportunities for further HIV education and awareness can you identify in this scenario?
5. What is and should be the role of Gloria's partner in ensuring his own well-being and protection from acquiring HIV?
6. Based on current science and use of condoms, mount a legal defence for Gloria's case.

GLOSSARY

ACB: African, Caribbean, and Black

AIDS Service Organization (ASO): A centre that provides community-based services as well as support for people living with HIV/AIDS, including psychosocial support, peer programming, capacity and skills building, HIV testing, wellness initiatives, and referral services. ASOs will often extend their services to family members, intimate partners, and friends. Additional initiatives include prevention, research, and advocacy for people living with HIV/AIDS.

AIDS endemic: The Public Health Agency of Canada uses the term *HIV-endemic* to describe a country with an adult prevalence of HIV that exceeds 1% and that meets one of the following criteria: (1) heterosexual transmission represents more than

50% of all HIV infections; (2) women account for more than 33% of all infections; or (3) an HIV prevalence that exceeds 2% among women seeking antenatal care.

Ally: A member of a dominant social group who works in partnership with populations that have experienced marginalization and disempowerment. Ally organizations work within a framework of anti-oppression and anti-racism, questioning and challenging power imbalances. AIDS Service Organizations that are allies to the ACB community can provide ethno-specific and culturally appropriate support to their clients, recognizing the unique societal factors, political pressures, and cultural norms that influence their clients' identity and experience.

Anti-racism/anti-oppression framework (AR/AO): Power and privilege are inherent to all relationships. The AR/AO framework recognizes and seeks to overcome existing power imbalances based on gender, age, culture, social and geographic location, physical ability, and sexual orientation. An organization working within an AR/AO framework identifies areas of systemic racism and oppression, and challenges these power imbalances through advocacy, policy reform, and socially equitable practices.

Community health centre: A community health care centre works within an integrated model of care, providing primary health care, and a complement of health promotion programs and community development services.

Criminalization of non-HIV disclosure: Criminalization is the process by which a person is held criminally accountable for engaging in activities that pose a *significant risk* of transmitting HIV without disclosing his or her HIV serostatus or taking reasonable precautions to prevent transmission. In Canada, people living with HIV have a legal duty to disclose their status to their partners before engaging in sexual activity.

Discrimination: This term signifies an unjust or unfavourable treatment of a person or group on the basis of prejudice, often associated with aspects of social location, including race, gender, ethnicity, sexual orientation, or socio-economic status. HIV-related discrimination is described by the Joint United Nations Programme on HIV/AIDS (UNAIDS) as "any measure entailing any arbitrary distinction among persons depending on their confirmed or suspected HIV serostatus or state of health" (UNAIDS, 2005).

Racialization: The process by which groups are designated as different and singled out for unequal treatment on the basis of race, ethnicity, language, religion, or culture.

Stigma: HIV-related stigma includes prejudicial behaviours, attitudes, and practices that are directed toward an individual based on the knowledge or belief that the person is living with HIV/AIDS.

Serodiscordant couple: This term describes a couple that includes one partner who is HIV positive and another who is HIV negative. Serodiscordant couples will often face unique challenges, including prevention of HIV transmission, emotional and psychological stressors, family planning decisions, and caregiving concerns. Many ASOs provide counselling services and support groups for serodiscordant partners.

REFERENCES

Abdool, K. Q., Meyer-Weitz, A., Mboyi, L., Carrara, H., Mahlase, G., Frohlich, J. A., & Abdool, K. S. (2008). The influence of AIDS stigma and discrimination and social cohesion on HIV testing and willingness to disclose HIV in rural KwaZulu-Natal, South Africa. *Global Public Health*, 3(4), 351–365.

Anderson, M., Elam, G., Solarin, I., Gerver, S., Fenton, K., & Easterbrook, P. (2009). Coping with HIV: Caribbean people in the United Kingdom. *Qualitative Health Research*, 19(8), 1060–1075.

Arnold, E. M., Rice, E., Flannery, D., & Rotheram-Borus, M. J. (2008). HIV disclosure among adults living with HIV. *AIDS Care—Psychological and Socio-Medical Aspects of AIDS/HIV*, 20(1), 80–92.

Bairan, A., Taylor, G. A., Blake, B. J., Akers, T., Sowell, R., & Mendiola, R. (2007). A model of HIV disclosure: Disclosure and types of social relationships. *Journal of the American Academy of Nurse Practitioners*, 19(5), 242–250.

Baumgartner, L. M. (2007). The incorporation of the HIV/AIDS identity into the self over time. *Qualitative Health Research*, 17(7), 919–931.

Bennett, J. (2008). Researching for life: Paradigms and power. *Feminist Africa*, 11, 1–12.

Black, B. P., & Miles, M. S. (2002). Calculating the risks and benefits of disclosure in African American women who have HIV. *Journal of Obstetric, Gynecologic, and Neonatal Nursing*, 31, 688–697.

Brown, L., Macintyre, K., & Trujillo, L. (2003). Interventions to reduce HIV/AIDS stigma: What have we learned? *AIDS Education and Prevention*, 15(1), 49–69.

Carlson Gielen, A., Fogarty, L., O'Campo, P., Anderson, J., Keller, J., & Faden, R. (2000). Women living with HIV: Disclosure, violence, and social support. *Journal of Urban Health*, 77(3), 480–491.

Collins, P. H. (2000). Gender, Black feminism, and Black political economy. *Annals of the American Academy of Political and Social Science*, 568, 41–53.

Crenshaw, K. W. (1989). Demarginalizing the intersection of race and sex: A Black feminist critique of antidiscrimination doctrine, feminist theory and antiracist politics. In J. James & T. D. Sharpley-Whiting (Eds.), *The Black feminist reader* (pp. 208–238). Malden, MA: Wiley Blackwell.

Delaney, R., Serovich, J., & Lim, J-Y. (2009). Psychological differences between HIV-positive mothers who disclose to all, some, or none of their biological children. *Journal of Marital and Family Therapy*, 35(2), 175–180.

Derlega, V. J., Winstead, B. A, Greene, K., Serovich, J., & Elwood, W. (2002). Perceived HIV-related stigma and HIV disclosure to relationship partners after finding out about the seropositive diagnosis. *Journal of Health Psychology*, 7(4), 415–432.

Derlega, V. J., Winstead, B. A., Greene, K., Serovich, J., & Elwood, W. N. (2004). Reasons for HIV disclosure/nondisclosure in close relationships: Testing a model of HIV-disclosure decision making. *Journal of Social and Clinical Psychology*, 23(6), 747–767.

Driskell, J., Salomon, E., Mayer, K., Capistrant, B., & Safren, S. (2008). Barriers and facilitators of HIV disclosure: Perspectives from HIV-infected men who have sex with men. *Journal of HIV/ AIDS & Social Services*, 7(2), 135–156.

Dworkin, L. S, & Ehrhardt, A. A. (2007). Going beyond "ABC" to include "GEM": Critical reflections on progress in the HIV/AIDS epidemic. *American Journal of Public Health, 97*(1), 13–18.

Elford, J., Ibrahim, F., Bukutu, C., & Anderson, J. (2008). Disclosure of HIV status: The role of ethnicity among people living with HIV in London. *Journal of Acquired Immune Deficiency Syndromes, 47*(4), 514–521.

Emlet, C. A. (2007). Experiences of stigma in older adults living with HIV/AIDS: A mixed-methods analysis. *AIDS Patient Care and STDs, 21*(10), 740–752.

Emlet, C. A. (2008). Truth and consequences: A qualitative exploration of HIV disclosure in older adults. *AIDS Care—Psychological and Socio-Medical Aspects of AIDS/HIV, 20*(6), 710–717.

European Conference Report. (2007, June). *Migration and HIV/AIDS: Community recommendations based on the European conference.* The Right to HIV/AIDS Prevention, Treatment, Care and Support for Migrants and Ethnic Minorities in Europe: The Community Perspective, Lisbon, Portugal.

Fekete, E. M., Antoni, M. H., Durán, R., Stoelb, B. L., Kumar, M., & Schneiderman, N. (2009). Disclosing HIV serostatus to family members: Effects on psychological and physiological health in minority women living with HIV. *International Journal of Behavioral Medicine, 16*(4), 367–376.

Gardezi, F., Calzavara, L., Husbands, W., Tharao, W., Lawson, E., Myers, T., … & Adebajo, S. (2008). Experiences of and responses to HIV among African and Caribbean communities in Toronto, Canada. *AIDS Care, 20*(6), 718–725.

Gray, K., Calzavara, L., Tharao, W., Johns, A., Burchell, A., Remis, R., … & Chalin, C. (2008). *The East African health study in Toronto (EAST): Results from a survey of HIV and health-related behaviour, beliefs, attitudes, and knowledge.* HIV Social, Behavioural, and Epidemiological Studies Unit, Dalla Lana School of Public Health, University of Toronto, Toronto.

Greeff, M., Phetlhu, R., Makoae, L. N., Dlamini, P. S., Holzemer, W. L., Naidoo, J. R., … & Chirwa, M. L. (2008). Disclosure of HIV status: Experiences and perceptions of persons living with HIV/AIDS and nurses involved in their care in Africa. *Qualitative Health Research, 18*(3), 311–324.

Hancock, A. M. (2007). When multiplication doesn't equal quick addition: Examining intersectionality as a research paradigm. *Perspectives on Politics, 5*(1), 63–79.

Hankins, C. (2008). Gender, sex, and HIV: How well are we addressing the imbalance? *Current Opinion in HIV and AIDS, 3*, 514–520.

Hudson, R. (2008, February). *When shame-proneness hinders HIV disclosure: New evidence-based practice approaches to a chronic and enduring problem.* Paper presented at the National Association for Christian Social Workers (NACSW) Convention, Orlando, Florida.

Interagency Coalition on AIDS and Development. (2004). *International migration and HIV/AIDS* [Fact sheet]. Ottawa, ON: Interagency Coalition on AIDS and Development.

Kalichman, S. C., DiMarco, M., Austin, J., Luke, W., & DiFonzo, K. (2003). Stress, social support, and HIV-status disclosure to family and friends among HIV-positive men and women. *Journal of Behavioural Medicine, 26*(4), 315–332.

Kalichman, S. C., Rompa, D., & Cage, M. (2005). Group intervention to reduce HIV transmission risk behavior among persons living with HIV/AIDS. *Behavior Modification, 29*(2), 256–285.

Kalichman, S. C., Simbayi, L. C., Kagee, A., Toefy, Y., Jooste, S., Cain, D., & Cherry, C. (2006). Associations of poverty, substance use, and HIV transmission: Risk behaviors in three South African communities. *Social Science & Medicine, 62*(7), 1641–1649.

Kimberly, J. A., & Serovich, J. M. (1996). Perceived social support among persons living with HIV/AIDS. *American Journal of Family Therapy, 24,* 41–53.

King, R., Katuntu, D., Lifshay, J., Packel, L., Batamwita, R., Nakayiwa, S., ... & Johansson, E. (2008). Processes and outcomes of HIV serostatus disclosure to sexual partners among people living with HIV in Uganda. *AIDS and Behavior, 12*(2), 232–243.

Korner, H. (2007). Negotiating cultures: Disclosure of HIV-positive status among people from minority ethnic communities in Sydney. *Culture, Health and Sexuality, 9*(2), 137–152.

Larcher A. A., & Symington, A. (2010). *Criminals and victims? The impact of the criminalization of HIV non-disclosure on African, Caribbean and Black communities in Ontario.* Toronto, ON: The African and Caribbean Council on HIV/AIDS in Ontario.

Levitt, P. (2001). *The transnational villagers.* Berkeley and Los Angeles: University of California Press.

Levitt, P., & Glick Schiller, N. (2004). Transnational perspectives on migration: Conceptualizing simultaneity. *International Migration Review, 38*(3), 1002–1039.

Liu, H., Hu, Z., Li, X., Stanton, B., Naar-King, S., & Yang, H. (2006). Understanding interrelationships among HIV-related stigma, concern about HIV infection, and intent to disclose HIV serostatus: A pretest-posttest study in a rural area of eastern China. *AIDS Patient Care and STDs, 20*(2), 133–142.

Mahajan, A. P., Sayles, J. N., Patel, V. A., Remien, R. H., Sawires, S. R., Ortiz, D. J., ... & Coates, T. J. (2008). Stigma in the HIV/AIDS epidemic: A review of the literature and recommendations for the way forward. *AIDS, 22*(Suppl. 2), S67–S79.

Maman, S., Mbwambo, K. J., Hogan, M. N., Kilonzo, P. G., Campbell, C. J., Weiss, E., & Sweat, D. M. (2002). HIV-positive women report more lifetime partner violence: Findings from a voluntary counseling and testing clinic in Dar es Salaam, Tanzania. *American Journal of Public Health, 92*(8), 1331–1337.

Medley, A., Garcia-Moreno, C., McGill, S., & Maman, S. (2004). HIV status disclosure to sexual partners: Rates, barriers and outcomes. *Bulletin of the World Health Organization, 82*(4), 299–307.

Miller, A. N., & Rubin, D. L. (2007). Factors leading to self-disclosure of a positive HIV diagnosis in Nairobi, Kenya: People living with HIV/AIDS in the Sub-Sahara. *Qualitative Health Research, 17*(5), 586–598.

Mykhalovskiy, E., Betteridge, G., & Mclay, D. (2010). *HIV non-disclosure and the criminal law: Establishing policy options for Ontario.* Toronto, ON: Ontario HIV Treatment Network.

Nelms, T. P., & Zeigler, V. L. (2008). A study to develop a disclosure to children intervention for HIV-infected women. *JANAC, 19*(6), 461–469.

Newman, P. A., Williams, C. C., Massaquoi, N., Brown, M., & Logie, C. (2008). HIV prevention for Black women: Structural barriers and opportunities. *The Journal of Health Care for the Poor and Underserved, 19*(3), 829–841.

Ontario HIV Treatment Network. (2009). *HIV disclosure: Rapid review response.* Toronto, ON: Ontario HIV Treatment Network, Rapid Response Service.

Peretti-Watel, P., Spire, B., Pierret, J., Lert, F., & Obadia, Y. (2003). Management of HIV-related stigma and adherence to HAART: Evidence from a large representative sample of outpatients attending French hospitals. *AIDS Care—Psychological and Socio-Medical Aspects of AIDS/HIV, 18*(3), 254–261.

Public Health Agency of Canada. (2005). *HIV/AIDS Epi Updates*. Ottawa, ON: Centre for Infectious Disease Prevention and Control, Public Health Agency of Canada.

Public Health Agency of Canada. (2007). *HIV/AIDS Epi Updates*. Ottawa, ON: Surveillance and Risk Assessment Division, Public Health Agency of Canada.

Public Health Agency of Canada. (2009). *Population-specific HIV/AIDS status report: People from countries where HIV is endemic—Black people of African and Caribbean descent living in Canada.* Ottawa, ON: Public Health Agency of Canada. Retrieved from www.phac-aspc.gc.ca/aids-sida/publication/ps-pd/africacaribbe/index-eng.php

Pulerwitz, J., Michaelis, A. P., Lippman, S. A., Chinaglia, M., & Diaz, J. (2008). HIV-related stigma, service utilization, and status disclosure among truck drivers crossing the Southern borders in Brazil. *AIDS Care—Psychological and Socio-Medical Aspects of AIDS/HIV, 20*(7), 764–770.

Rasera, E. F., Vieira, E. M., & Japur, M. (2004). Influence of gender and sexuality on the construction of being HIV positive: As experienced in a support group in Brazil. *Families, Systems and Health, 22*(3), 340–351.

Salter-Goldie, R., King, S. M., Smith, M. L., Bitnun, A., Brophy, J., Fernandes-Penney, A., ... & Read, S. E. (2007). Disclosing HIV diagnosis to infected children: A health care team's approach. *Vulnerable Children and Youth Studies, 2*(1), 12–16.

Serovich, J. M., Craft, S. M., & Yoon, H. J. (2007). Women's HIV disclosure to immediate family. *AIDS Patient Care and STDs, 21*(12), 970–980.

Serovich, J. M., & McDowell, T. (2008). Women's report of regret of HIV disclosure to family, friends and sex partners. *AIDS and Behavior, 12*(2), 227–231.

Serovich, J. M., Oliver, D. G., Smith, S. A., & Mason., T. L. (2005). Methods of HIV disclosure by men who have sex with men to casual sexual partners. *AIDS Patient Care and STDs, 19*(12), 823–832.

Simoni, J. M., Demas, P., Mason, H., Drossman, J. A., & Davis, M. L. (2000). HIV disclosure among women of African descent: Associations with coping, social support, and psychological adaptation. *AIDS and Behavior, 4*(2), 147–158.

Stirratt, M. J., Remien, R. H., Smith, A., Copeland, O. Q., Dolezal, C., & Krieger, D. (2006). The role of HIV serostatus disclosure in antiretroviral medication adherence. *AIDS and Behavior, 10*(5), 483–493.

Tharao, E., Massaquoi, N., & Teclom, S. (2006). *Silent voices of the AIDS epidemic: African and Caribbean women, their understanding of the various dimensions of HIV/AIDS and factors that contribute to their silence.* Toronto, ON: Women's Health in Women's Hands Community Health Centre.

Thompson, N. (2003). *Promoting equality: Challenging discrimination and oppression.* Basingstoke, UK: Palgrave Macmillan.

UNAIDS. (2005). *HIV-related stigma, discrimination and human rights violations: Case studies of successful programmes.* Geneva: UNAIDS.

UNAIDS. (2009, November 10). *Violence against women and HIV.* Feature story. Retrieved from www.unaids.org/en/resources/presscentre/featurestories/2009/november/20091110vaw/

UNAIDS/PCB. (2007, April). *Presentation of policy guidance to address gender issues.* Provisional agenda item 4.2 at the 20th meeting of the UNAIDS Programme Coordinating Board, Geneva, Switzerland.

UNAIDS/UNDP (2007, October–November). *Summary of main issues and conclusions.* Report on the International Consultation on the Criminalization of HIV Transmission, Geneva, Switzerland.

Wagner, S. (2002). *Putting a face on transnationalism: Migration, identity, and membership in the transnational city of Johannesburg.* Paper presented at a graduate seminar, Department of Anthropology, Harvard University, Cambridge, Massachusetts.

Walters, M. (2005). *Feminism: A very short introduction.* New York: Oxford University Press.

Webber, G. C. (2007). Chinese health care providers' attitudes about HIV: A review. *AIDS Care, 19*(5), 685–691.

Weiser, S. D., Leiter, K., Bangsberg, D. R., Butler, L. M., Percy-de Korte, F., Hlanze, Z., ... & Heisler, M. (2007). Food insufficiency is associated with high-risk sexual behavior among women in Botswana and Swaziland. *Public Library of Science Medicine, 4*(10), 1589–1597.

Wingood, G. M, & DiClemente, R. J. (1997). The effects of an abusive primary partner on the condom use and sexual negotiation practices of African-American women. *American Journal of Public Health, 87*, 1016–1018.

World Health Organization. (2000, October). *Violence against women and HIV/AIDS: Setting the research agenda.* Meeting report. Retrieved from www.who.int/gender/violence/vawandhiv/en/index1.html

World Health Organization. (2004). *Gender dimensions of HIV status disclosure to sexual partners: Rates, barriers and outcomes.* Review paper. Retrieved from www.who.int/gender/documents/en/genderdimensions.pdf

Worth, H., Reid, A., Ackroyd, J., & Tamarite-Bowden, E. (2001). *Silence and secrecy: HIV positive refugees in New Zealand.* Auckland, NZ: Institute for Research on Gender, University of Auckland.

Chapter 6
HOUSING AS HIV PREVENTION AND SUPPORT OF AND FOR HIV-POSITIVE MOTHERS IN CANADA: THE WAY FORWARD

Saara Greene, Lori Chambers, Khatundi Masinde,
and Chantal Mukandoli

INTRODUCTION

Our approach to understanding the needs and experiences of HIV-positive mothers "emphasizes the relationship between social marginalization and marginalized ways of knowing, focusing on the relevance of epistemological values for social work practice, education, and research" (Tangenberg, 2000, p. 31). This has enabled us to examine gender and other societal inequalities, such as poverty, racism, and immigration status, in relation to women's health and to capture the social world and housing situations in which HIV-positive mothers live. Hence, our understanding of these women's experiences challenges current thinking about traditional definitions of mothering and, in particular, mothering with HIV, which goes beyond white, middle-class experiences. Moreover, our theoretical and methodological framework has been based on an understanding and belief that the health, housing, and social care policies and practices that will be most effective in meeting the housing needs of HIV-positive mothers will include forms of knowledge that reflect their intersecting social positionings and the diversity of their daily lived experiences and needs. This has resulted in our decision to ground our research in a "social determinants of women's health" (Bent-Goodley, 2007; Wuest, Meritt-Gray, Berman, & Ford-Gilboe, 2002) framework as it applies to the housing experiences of HIV-positive African and Caribbean mothers living in Toronto, Ontario.

A social determinants of women's health framework recognizes the importance of differences between women, men, and other gender groups, as well as differences between and within groups of women based on social factors, identity statuses, geographical locations, and access to key material and ideological resources. It also recognizes that although women play multiple roles in our society, including mothering, they continue to have unequal access to power. This suggests that a social determinants of women's health framework is necessary when engaging in applied research aimed at developing more effective practice and policy-based outcomes. This is because, as Benoit and Shumka (2007) argue, "a health determinants approach that incorporates gender [should] allow us to first, investigate variations in how women experience and recount different aspects of their health and then, secondly, link these accounts to socio-structural forces and within particular sociocultural contexts" (p. 16). Yet, even with our commitment to creating space for marginalized voices to be heard and responded to, our reflections on this process have raised questions about our theoretical framework and methodology and how we can respond to these tensions as we contemplate the way forward for research on and about HIV-positive mothers.

This chapter will begin with an overview of some of the critical findings regarding the unique housing needs and experiences of HIV-positive parents, as well as a presentation of our own findings from our research on the housing needs and experiences of HIV-positive mothers from African and Caribbean communities in Toronto. This will be followed by our reflections on how these findings correspond with the assertion that "housing is prevention" (Aidala, Cross, Stall, Harre, & Sumartojo, 2005). This chapter will also highlight the key conceptual, theoretical, and methodological tensions we experienced when engaging in a community-based research study that was grounded in a social determinants of health framework and consider the ways that researchers can respond to these multiple tensions as they work with communities to develop appropriate and meaningful prevention strategies in the housing sector. Finally, in light of both our research findings and a critique of the theoretical and methodological framework underpinning our findings, we will also highlight some of the key issues to consider for the way forward in developing future housing research with and for HIV-positive mothers that will lead to the prevention of the key concerns presented by HIV-positive mothers. This will be achieved by

1. Presenting an overview of the findings from secondary research on the housing needs and experiences of HIV-positive mothers and our own findings from the Families, HIV, and Housing study
2. Presenting a social determinants of women's health framework that acknowledges the intersecting identities and diverse spaces of marginality that impact on the housing experiences of, and thus preventative strategies for, HIV-positive mothers
3. Highlighting the implications this has on the development of housing policies and practices that reflect the prevention needs of HIV-positive mothers in Canada
4. Providing concrete suggestions for housing prevention research, practice, and policy for HIV-positive mothers in Canada

BACKGROUND

This chapter is based on our reflections of the conceptual, theoretical, and methodological tensions and deliberations related to the future development of preventative approaches to establishing appropriate housing policies and practices for HIV-positive women and their children in Canada. These considerations initially emerged out of qualitative findings on the housing experiences and needs of HIV-positive mothers from the Positive Spaces Healthy Places (PSHP) community-based research study (Greene et al., 2010), and have further evolved through the Families, HIV, and Housing study (FHH), a qualitative community-based research project that explored the impact of unstable housing on HIV-positive mothers and their children. Data from both studies highlighted a number of themes related to the gendered experience of housing for HIV-positive mothers, in particular the need to situate these experiences within a social determinants of women's health framework that acknowledges and can respond to the multiple social positionings experienced by HIV-positive mothers.

WOMEN, HIV, AND HOUSING

Recent studies have shown that women are particularly at risk for poor health outcomes as a result of being at the centre of two converging epidemiological trends: HIV transmission and homelessness (Kilbourne, Herndon, Andersen, Wenzel, & Gelberg, 2002). Canadian HIV prevalence estimates indicate that the number of women in Canada living with HIV continues to grow. By the end of 2002, an estimated 7,700 women were living with HIV, accounting for about 14% of the national total, an increase of 13% from the estimate of 6,800 at the end of 1999 (Geduld, Gatali, Remis, & Archibald, 2003). Statistics indicate that about 3,895 of these women live in Ontario, 344 of which were diagnosed in 2006 alone (Remis, Swantee, Schiedel, & Liu, 2008).

Studies in both Canada and the U.S. show that homeless women are particularly vulnerable to HIV/AIDS (Culhane, Gollub, Kuhn, & Shpaner, 2001; Weinreb, Goldberg, Lessard, Perloff, & Bassuk, 1999) and that HIV has been found to be among the leading causes of death of homeless women between the ages of 18 and 44 (Cheung & Hwang, 2004). This highlights the importance of understanding the role that housing plays in the increase in HIV/AIDS among women, particularly as it relates to the risk factors associated with contracting HIV, such as drug use, sex trade work, mental health, domestic violence, and sexual abuse (Kilbourne et al., 2002; Song, 2003; Wenzel, Tucker, Elliot, & Hambarsoomian, 2007). Women who are prone to living in unstable housing situations are at a disproportionate risk of contracting HIV/AIDS, regardless of their lifestyle (Zierler & Krieger, 2000). This is because housing instability, homelessness, and transience compromise access to adequate health care (Parish, Burry, & Pabst, 2003) and create barriers to accessing appropriate and effective social supports (Fisher, Hovell, Hofstetter, & Hough, 1995). Homeless mothers, in particular, have been found to subordinate their own health care needs for the needs of their children (Song, 2003), which leads to competing subsistence needs and caregiver roles that have been found to adversely influence health care access for women living with HIV/AIDS (Shelton, 1993). As such, HIV-infected parents, mothers in particular, may have unique housing needs that are related to both their physical and mental health. This suggests that there is a need to develop a deeper understanding of how HIV and housing instability are implicated within their overall parenting experience.

HIV-POSITIVE PARENTS AND HOUSING INSTABILITY

Little is known about the impact of homelessness and housing instability on Canadian families. The information that is available is found mainly in government reports or research that is based on very small population samples that often fail to reflect the "spectrum of homeless families" in Canada (Waegemakers Schiff, 2007). Families who experience homelessness live on the streets, in cars or abandoned buildings, in temporary or emergency shelters, in shelters for those fleeing domestic violence, in temporary or transitional housing, with family or friends, or in motel rooms rented on a monthly basis. Just as in the general population of people experiencing homelessness, some families may have only one homeless incident while other families may experience multiple episodes of homelessness. Many families also experience housing instability or the threat of homelessness due to the imminent risk of losing their housing (Waegemakers Schiff, 2007).

Included in the spectrum of homeless families are families with children who are affected by HIV. These families share many of the same experiences as homeless families in addition to unique challenges related to the impact that HIV has on the entire family system. Most of what we currently know about the experiences of HIV-positive parents and their children is based on research conducted in the U.S. These families are characterized by chronic poverty, homelessness, multiple losses, substance use, and racialization. Racialized women living on a low income have been particularly affected by HIV, and it is mainly these women who tend to be the sole or primary caregivers in families affected by HIV (Pequegnat & Bray, 1997). More recently, studies have shown that HIV-positive parents continue to cope with discrimination, stigma, poverty, secrets about HIV status, and planning for the possibility of sickness or death, as well as the everyday issues of life and parenting (Antle, Wells, Salter Goldie, Matteo, & King, 2001). These unique experiences, concerns, and challenges negatively impact their physical and mental health and quality of life (DeMatteo, Wells, Salter Goldie, & King, 2002). These issues are often exacerbated for HIV-positive mothers who are living in overcrowded housing or who remain in violent relationships in order to have a place to live (Kappel Ramji Consulting Group, 2002). Other concerns include unwanted family separation and/or the involvement of social service agencies that have a mandate for the welfare of children, and the longer term intergenerational impact of both HIV/AIDS and housing instability, particularly in cases where children take on roles beyond those of their peers in terms of caregiving and providing emotional support (Kappel Ramji Consulting Group, 2002). Hence, it has been argued that while interventions that support parents around challenges such as disclosure to children, planning for illness, helping children adjust to new caregivers, and goals in the event of parental death are important, unless basic survival and security needs (food, shelter, employment, heath care) are met first, these interventions are unlikely to succeed (Rotheram-Borus, Weiss, Alber, & Lester, 2005).

More recently, findings from the Positive Spaces Healthy Places study highlight the complex and unique needs of HIV-positive mothers who live with and care for their children in Ontario, and the central role that housing plays in their lives (Greene et al., 2010). This study found that HIV-positive mothers experience a number of interconnected barriers to living in appropriate and stable housing for both themselves and their children, including concerns related to the safety of the neighbourhood and/or the building in which they live; the stability of their housing situation as it relates to their physical and emotional safety; the potential for experiencing HIV-related stigma and discrimination; and the impact on their mental health. Perhaps the most salient issue that emerged from this study is the multiple day-to-day and future concerns that HIV-positive mothers live with regarding stigma, in particular as it relates to their social positioning as HIV-positive mothers who live in poverty and, subsequently, in unsafe and unstable housing situations. The losses associated with this stigma and discrimination are most often reflected in relation to their children. This is due to both the reality and/or the perceived potential of losing their children to the child welfare system as a direct result of their housing situation (Greene et al., 2010).

Anxiety, stress, and depression are also associated with housing conditions, housing costs, and neighbourhood safety. Most parents had to make accommodations that resulted in choosing between an appropriate number of bedrooms for themselves and their children and/or living in unsafe neighbourhoods or in shelters. The research conducted by Greene and colleagues resulted in the impetus to do further research that would highlight the complexity of housing in the lives of HIV-positive mothers from ethnoracial communities. What follows is a discussion of the themes that emerged from in-depth interviews with HIV-positive mothers from African and Caribbean communities about their housing experiences, in addition to the implications their experiences have for the future development of prevention-focused housing policies and practices.

THE FAMILIES, HIV, AND HOUSING STUDY: EXPERIENCES OF HIV-POSITIVE MOTHERS FROM AFRICA AND THE CARIBBEAN
Methodology
This study was funded by an Ontario HIV Treatment Network (OHTN) Community Scholar Award. The award supported the researcher and Fife House, Toronto's largest HIV/AIDS supportive housing organization, to develop a community-based research partnership and project that sought to address the housing needs of HIV-positive parents in Toronto. From its inception, the Families, HIV and Housing (FHH) study

was grounded in a community-based research (CBR) framework that was community driven and controlled. The community-based researcher was chosen by the agency and, from the very beginning of the research process, Fife House partnered with external community stakeholders, including people living with HIV (PHAs) and organizations that provided health, housing, and other related services and programs to women, families, parents, or children affected by HIV/AIDS. In line with our community-based and social determinants of women's health framework, English- and French-speaking community members were hired and trained as research assistants on the study. The research assistants were involved in developing research questions, conducting in-depth interviews, completing qualitative analysis, and disseminating findings.

The findings that follow are based on our sub-analysis of in-depth qualitative interviews with 17 HIV-positive mothers from Africa or the Caribbean. These participants represented a diverse sample of families including refugees, immigrant newcomers, and first-generation Canadian citizens; families with one or two or multiple heads of households; a range of dependents; and racial and linguistic diversity. The interview questions focused on the unique needs of parents living with HIV and their experiences of caregiving, specifically with accessing resources, barriers and facilitators to accessing health and social services in connection to their housing situation, experiences of discrimination regarding housing, and experiences related to housing transitions. Interviews were conducted in local community-based agencies and were conducted in both English and French. Interviews were taped and transcribed verbatim, and were approximately 1 to 1.5 hours in length. The interviews underwent thematic analysis, peer debriefing, and investigator triangulation. Names and places were changed and pseudonyms were used to protect the identity of the participants.

OVERVIEW OF KEY FINDINGS
Ethnocentrism
The overarching theme that touched the lives of the mothers in the FHH study was their experience of ethnocentrism and how ethnocentric policies and practices impacted their daily lives. Many of the African and Caribbean mothers interviewed discussed their exclusion as newcomers from the housing system in Toronto because of their lack of knowledge and experience with the health and social service system and, in particular, supportive housing services and programs.

> You know, in Africa, when the white people come and visit us, the tourist, everything is laid down. They just go to this information thing and they are told everything. They even hold their hand and take them. They don't say, "Here is the address." We take them there and we speak and say, "Okay, here, meet sir, sir, sir," [Yeah, yes] meet the mzungu and treat them well and for sure, because I've taken

> there to say, "Please take care of this man, show him everything that
> they need to know." ... But I come here, I'm taken to a place where
> they're supposed to tell me all the information but they never tell me
> everything. They tell me bits and pieces. That's why I'm saying I don't
> know whether that's how it's designed ... so that I don't make it, so
> that I have to suffer a little bit? (Abida)

Abida echoes the experience of the majority of the women who participated in this study, many of whom were new immigrants. For them, housing systems in Canada were difficult to navigate, assumed prior knowledge of housing policies and processes, and assumed cultural understandings of such practices as locating housing, finding support services, or using public transit, practices that are learned over time through living in a new country.

It is not surprising then that this ethnocentric view of appropriate housing was even more apparent to mothers who were in the midst of the reunification process. These participants found that immigration and social service policies conflicted with housing policies. Where housing policies did not allow a single resident to apply for more than a single bedroom, family service policies required parents to have a separate room for their children. For immigrant parents, where reunification with their children is a common experience, this created problems in trying to find appropriate housing for their children.

> The challenge with Immigration, too, was that I needed to come up
> with five thousand dollars in my account for me to apply, to prove to
> the government that I am able to take care of my son when he gets
> here ... So as I was applying for this two-bedroom house, the chal-
> lenge was housing was not going to provide it until the kid was here
> ... It was, it was out of question. So it's like the two messages were
> conflicting on their own, you know, coming from the local govern-
> ment, you know, but I just had to do what I had to do. (Betty)

Betty's narrative resonates with the experience of immigrant mothers more generally, given that it is common for immigrants to migrate in a "stepwise" fashion. Through this process, the head of the household will migrate prior to the migration of their children, which can often be complicated by structural hurdles such as immigration laws and laws governing children and family (Suarez-Orozco, Todorova, & Louie, 2002). In order to gain the proper housing for their children, many of these parents felt that they had to adapt to such policies as obtaining appropriate housing at market rents they could not afford, because the current policies did not accommodate their needs as newcomers with children living abroad. This suggests that the narratives that follow must be viewed through a social and political lens that seeks to understand and acknowledges how HIV-positive mothers confront ethnocentrism within the context of inequitable gender and economic relations, and how this underpins the housing experiences of HIV-positive mothers from Africa and the Caribbean.

When a House Becomes a Home

> I want a house, even if it's a townhouse, even if it's in an apartment building. I'm fine with that. I just want a, I want a home—not a "house" but a HOME where there are other homes. That's how I look at it. I don't just want a house. I want a home. (Esther)

Home Is ... Family

Many of the African and Caribbean women interviewed continued to have strong ties with their family back home; in some cases, the mothers still had children remaining "back home" that they wished to sponsor in immigrating to Canada. The separation from their family was a profoundly isolating experience that highlighted their need to have an appropriate home in Canada. Dinah, an African woman who came from a large, close family, found living alone, as a single parent without her family, a difficult experience.

> Emotionally it's very challenging. It's difficult to be alone ... When you look at that picture [takes a breath] ... I was born in a family of so many people. Look, look at that picture ... it's difficult to be [alone]. (Dinah)

Moreover, in situations where the participants cared for a larger family, barriers to finding appropriate housing were constantly preventing them from being housed.

> We come from environments where we have large families and then we get confined into apartments and it's challenging. (Esther)

Hence, the mothers in this study also shared specific challenges that were related to finding housing and social supports that accommodated the size of their family. The ability to care for their children was often challenged by rigid policies that did not accommodate the definition of family used by these mothers.

> I needed help, I needed to get out of that neighbourhood, and they couldn't help me. They told me that, oh, mostly they help small families like single parent, not big family. (Hazel)

Current housing policies (i.e., with a rigid view of family shaped by the Canadian norm that are challenged with accommodating the diverse, fluid view of family) were also experienced as barriers to being housed.

> [M]y dream for the future, if there's going to be projects, will you consider especially larger families. I mean, like, I don't know how many units or how many rooms the units may ... have, but, um, I mean, like just this one woman who has, what? Six kids or eight kids? How do you accommodate such a person? (Betty)

Previous studies of housing and immigrant experience have suggested that immigrants often experience discrimination when accessing housing, particularly those immigrants who are racialized (Li, 2003a). Interestingly, when some African and Caribbean mothers were asked directly if they experience discrimination in relation to housing, they discussed discriminatory experiences in relation to their HIV status rather than in relation to their ethnoracial status. Yet, many of these mothers discussed housing and social supports as being non-accommodating to their lived experiences as an immigrant, as a newcomer, and as an African or Caribbean mother, all of which meet the definition of ethnocentrism, another form of ethnoracial prejudice. The experiences of ethnocentrism reflect the immigration discourse where, despite the multicultural tenet often espoused in Canadian policies and practices, immigrants are expected to "integrate" and "adapt" to a monolithic Canadian culture that remains intolerant to cultural experience outside of the mainstream (Li, 2003b). In these narratives, African and Caribbean women were treated as the social "other." It was "assumed" that they understood Canadian culture even as newcomers, they were expected to adapt to meet the requirements of housing policies, and their cultural understandings of home, and of family, were typically not reflected in the Canadian context. Ethnocentrism within housing was a predominant theme in the narrative of African and Caribbean mothers, where their ideals of housing, home, community, support, and family were often not reflected in the housing services and supports they received in Ontario.

Home Is ... Community

> Stigma and discrimination is still out there. Most of us are hesitant to move in because that's the "HIV building." You know? Right. So when you have kids you want your kids to, you know, grow up in a happy environment and not, not have that feeling of, "Oh, you live in the HIV building?" (Betty)

Many African and Caribbean mothers such as Betty described HIV designated housing as "marked" housing and discussed its potential for HIV-related stigma. An added concern was the potential impact living in a HIV designated building would have on their children: they might expose their children to stigma and discrimination if they chose to live in "marked" housing. Many of the African and Caribbean mothers interviewed, especially newcomers to Canada, had not disclosed their status to their children to protect them from HIV-related stigma and discrimination. Yet if these women are put in a position where they must choose HIV designated housing in order to secure housing for their families, they may have to disclose their status to their child.

HIV-related stigma also emphasized for the participants the important link between home and living in a place that was in a "community" or a place where other families with children resided.

> Well, you know, I'm faced with this and I'm trying to … look for a new home, but I'm looking for a home in a community 'cause I have a young child so I want to move into a community that has children. And they say, you know, "Maybe you should talk to ABC because we can't help you. You know, we deal with single, single people or we deal with couples or we deal with abused, um, abused women, or—" you know, or something like that, right? Because I don't want to call somebody and say, "Hey, this is my name, so on and so on, I'm looking for this," and they say, after they take all your information, they say, "Well, you know, maybe you should talk to this person." (Winnie)

In this case, having to disclose one's HIV-positive status in order to access housing is in opposition to mothering work activities, such as information work— "Where and what kind of housing is in the best interest of my children?"—and surveillance and safety work—"Will disclosing my HIV status expose my children to HIV-related stigma?" (Sandelowski & Barroso, 2003). This is particularly stressful given the fears that HIV-positive mothers have with regard to the relationship between their HIV status, housing situation, and Children's Aid Society (CAS) involvement (Greene et al., 2010). Even in situations where these African and Caribbean women are comfortable with disclosing their status and willing as PHAs to live in HIV designated housing, this completely shifts for them as mothers who are considering the housing needs of their children.

Finding a home within a "community" often meant having to disclose one's HIV status, a decision that was at times stressful and demeaning and, as Sandelowski and Barroso (2003) suggest, calls into question the work that HIV-positive mothers do in order to reflect their identities as "good mothers."

> With me, I'm okay with my status. I feel like now, right now, living in [HIV designated housing] I feel like I'm safe. But will they [my children] be safe, too? That's the big question I have. Will they feel okay with that … it's, it's marked—I don't want to say "it's marked" but somehow

> somewhere they might know that this house belongs to HIV, something
> like that. So I'm like, how are they going to respond? (Sophie)

Sophie notes the tensions between the individual experience versus the collective for HIV-affected families who contemplate living in HIV designated housing. For her, HIV designated housing signifies "safe" housing that provides her with an opportunity to be free about her status and also with a sense of belonging to a community of people who share her HIV seropositive status. She may feel safe living in HIV designated housing, but she questions if her children will feel as safe living in this type of housing. For her children, HIV designed housing signifies "marked" housing: a place where the HIV designation may be known to others, and with that disclosure comes the potential for HIV-related stigma. Hence, in a housing situation where they are offered HIV designated housing because of their status, or either asked to disclose in order to receive housing or feel they need to disclose in the hope that it will get them housing, many African and Caribbean mothers are put in a catch-22 situation. They have to consider how they will protect their children: through the provision of safe, secure housing or from HIV-related stigma. Forcing these mothers to choose how they will protect their children can increase the stigma they experience as HIV-positive mothers, as racialized women, and as marginalized members of Canadian society, and can erect additional barriers to housing these African and Caribbean HIV-affected families safely.

Home Is ... Safety

> He uses this, this HIV thing. He uses it as if, as if he can hurt me with
> it, and, you know, it—it's a kind of a psychological torment. (Winnie)

Another theme that emerged from the participants' narratives were experiences of violence in relationships that impacted their housing stability. As HIV-positive mothers, relationship violence often put these women in precarious housing situations where they had to consider what was best for them and for their children. Many of these women were also survivors of violence. Not only had they experienced forms of violence that were typically associated with intimate partner violence, such as physical or verbal abuse, but they had also been exposed to psychological abuse, where their HIV status had been used as a weapon against them, including the threat of status disclosure if they chose to leave with their child. Many of the mothers told their stories about violence within their relationship, especially of psychological abuse where the threat of disclosure was used as a means of controlling them. While these women could see the threat of disclosure as a "psychological torment" and as an unsafe place for them, it was harder for these women to understand that this form of violence was also unsafe for their children, especially in situations where the woman considered a two-parent "home" as a form of housing security or as a cultural expectation.

> What it boils down to is, at the end of the day, if this has to get nasty it will end up in family court, and all these things and at the—and what it is that they—it's the interests of the child. We have one child. He knows we have one home and that his mom is in one room and his dad is in one room and that we are always there. That's all he knows. (Winnie)

Other HIV-positive African and Caribbean women's experience of violence provided a means for them to secure safe, secure housing. After leaving her abusive partner, Sela was able to secure safe housing. She recognizes not only the barriers that exist in housing services to obtaining secure housing for HIV-positive mothers in an abusive relationship, but also that her status as a survivor of violence rather than her need for safe housing as a HIV-positive mother was the predominant factor that secured her housing.

> I would say that the situation that I went through with my ex was a sad situation, but at the same time, and even though it was a sad situation, it is because of that situation that I was able to get housing, so when you look at it that way, it is really sad. So it means that, does a woman need to be abused or does she need to be sick … so that you can have housing? (Sela)

Housing insecurity within a violent relationship was compounded by fragmentation in the housing system. The fragmentation of social services results in these women not knowing how to access services or in their being passed on to multiple agencies with no guarantees of service. This can be a real barrier both for women who are trying to leave an abusive relationship and for those who are trying to find appropriate housing for their children. This barrier is especially burdensome for women who don't understand the social systems that can support their housing outcomes. The complexity of service navigation, such as the fragmentation of service, can place a woman in a dilemma where she is asking herself, "Should I stay or should I go?" Should she leave her abusive partner, only to navigate a housing system that might be just as psychologically or emotionally draining? These women may feel they lack the resources, the know-how, or the energy to navigate a fragmented or complex system, and this becomes a secondary form of violence.

DISCUSSION

The study findings suggest that in order to address the housing experiences and needs of HIV-positive mothers from newcomer, African, and Caribbean communities in Toronto, two main factors must be considered. First, HIV-positive mothers have intersecting identities that result in multiple sites of marginalization and oppression, which can have a detrimental impact on their housing experiences. Second, to effectively address housing issues within this context, the development of housing models that not only view housing as a social determinant of health, but that integrate and coordinate housing, health, and social issues into models of care is essential in addressing the social care needs of HIV-positive parents from ethnoracial communities. This has been made particularly apparent through the mothers' narratives of "home" and what this means to them when considered in the context of their family, their community, and their experience or fear for the safety of both themselves and their children.

Another important narrative that emerged from the interviews was that women make "choices" about whether or not to live in what could be constituted as "risky" housing situations that are unstable, undesirable, or unsafe. This is because of the lack of options available to them and the fear of what this could mean in situations where having "any kind of housing" will, at the very least, allow them to remain with their children. It is also interesting that different "identities" figure more prominently for the participants depending on the immediate issues they are confronted with at any given time, including HIV-related stigma, sexism, racism, and the impact of ethno-centrism. For example, experiences of navigating an unfamiliar housing system result in the prominence of racism and ethnocentrism, whereas in situations where violence becomes the most urgent concern, gender-based oppression and the subsequent experience of powerlessness and marginalization become the most pressing issue.

In reviewing both the secondary and primary research, it is clear that HIV-related stigma continues to be an overarching concern and one that has both short- and long-term effects on HIV-positive mothers and their children. Moreover, concerns about HIV-related stigma appears to exacerbate the housing needs, concerns, and experiences for HIV-positive mothers. These multiple and fluid experiences of oppression highlight the need to reconceptualize the social determinants of health framework, in particular the social determinants of women's health that will address the complex and unique positioning of HIV-positive mothers. Suggestions for how this is to be achieved include conceptualizing the housing experiences of HIV-positive mothers within a notion of intersectionality, particularly as we consider a way forward in the development of policies and programs that are aimed at preventing housing instability among HIV-positive mothers from diverse communities.

HOUSING AS PREVENTION I: CONCEPTUAL, THEORETICAL, AND METHODOLOGICAL TENSIONS WHEN DOING HOUSING RESEARCH ON AND WITH HIV-POSITIVE MOTHERS

Our experience researching the lives of HIV-positive mothers has brought into question the conceptual framework that underpins our work, and the subsequent theoretical and methodological tensions that ultimately emerge. What follows is a discussion of both the theoretical and methodological tensions we experienced as we engaged in this area of research, and the implications this will have on the way forward in doing prevention research on the housing needs of HIV-positive mothers.

Intersectionality and Ethnocentrism

Our findings from the FHH study suggest that the notion of intersectionality should be at the core of any conceptual framework that seeks to understand the multiple issues and concerns that face HIV-positive women in Canada. This is because the notion of intersectionality moves beyond the assumption that health outcomes may be caused by a number of contributing causes, by asserting that numerous factors are always at play and that "intersectionality examines gender, race, class and nation as systems that 'mutually construct one another'" (Collins, 1998, p. 63). Moreover, intersectionality encourages a contextual analysis that probes beneath single identities, experiences, and social locations to consider a range of axes of difference to better understand any situation of disadvantage (Yuval-David, 2006). In the context of the lives of HIV-positive women, Crenshaw's (2001) illustration of the experience of intersectionality is particularly powerful:

> [I]ntersectionality is what occurs when a woman from a minority group … tries to navigate the main crossing in the city … the main highway is "racism road." One cross street can be Colonialism, then Patriarchy street … [S]he has to deal not only with one form of oppression but with all forms, those named as road signs, which link together to make a double, a triple, multiple, a many layered blanket of oppression.

It is important, however, for researchers who are committed to social justice and working toward creating change in health and social care prevention policies to view intersectionality as more than merely a concept; it is a term that can be enacted to address social inequalities. This is echoed by Phoenix and Pattynama (2006), who argue that "intersectionality can inspire political action and policy development … by understanding how individual stories are politically embedded and have political consequences" (p. 189).

Intersectionality and the Social Determinants of Health

Health differences among Canadians result primarily from experiences of qualitatively different environments associated with the social determinants of health. These social determinants include ethnicity, Aboriginal status, early life education, employment and working conditions, food security, health care services, housing, income and its distribution, and social safety net and support (Raphael, 2006). They also include issues of gender, race, culture, and HIV stigma and discrimination, all of which have been found to contribute to HIV infection and to disease progression (Ontario Advisory Committee on HIV/AIDS, 2002). Nevertheless, Raphael has argued that "one of the shortcomings in the work on social determinants of health is the failure to consider 'a master conceptual scheme' that illuminates the political, economic, and social processes by which the quality of social determinants of health is shaped" (Raphael, 2006, p. 654). We argue that a master conceptual scheme is an illusive notion, given the complexity and fluidity of people's lives and the ways in which the political, economic, and social process impact women's lives differently from men's, as well as from each other.

Taking these ideas further, it is perhaps more productive for women's health researchers to consider one of the key conclusions of the Canadian Women's Health Surveillance project, which highlights the "need for coherent theoretical frameworks that help to explain the dynamic interrelationships among the social and biological determinants of health, including processes of human resilience and vulnerabilities, causal pathways and cumulative effects of circumstances and risks over the life cycle" (Tudiver, Kantiebo, Kammermayer, & Mayrak, 2004). Of particular relevance to this research are the social determinants of women's health, which urged us to incorporate a gender analysis into the social determinants of health framework. This incorporation provided us with a critical lens from which to consider the way forward in developing practice and policy-based knowledge and interventions that address the housing needs of Canada's diverse population of HIV-positive mothers. This echoes Wuest et al.'s (2002) assertion that

> [t]his shift in emphasis toward social determination of health also draws attention to and legitimizes women's health research that moves beyond traditional science and epidemiology to questioning previously unquestioned societal norms and structures that influence women's health ... Without such research, our knowledge of how social factors that underpin women's health interact will be faceless and will not address the interplay of health and social policy within women's lives. (p. 795)

This view aligns well with the notion of intersectionality in that it acknowledges the notion that health and wellness are multi-dimensional and cut across biology, society, and culture. Hence, it continues to be important for us to integrate intersectionality as both a concept and an action, because it challenges the dominant analyses of health determinants by "revealing how to better conceptualize the cumulative, interlocking dynamics that affect human experiences, including human health" (Hankivsky & Christofferson, 2008, p. 276). Further, Hankivsky and Christofferson urge Canadian health researchers to recognize the indispensability of an intersectional approach for challenging and transforming dominant approaches to health determinants to embrace and respond to a whole range of social inequalities, including inequality in health and housing systems and policies. It is with this notion in mind that we consider the implications this will have on the development of "housing as prevention" strategies in the Canadian social policy and practice arenas.

HOUSING AS PREVENTION II: IMPLICATIONS FOR HOUSING PRACTICE AND POLICY

The research presented in this chapter highlights some of the key issues that require further attention in the development of housing policies and practices that will prevent HIV-positive women and their children from living in unstable and unsafe housing situations. Furthermore, preventing housing instability will prevent HIV-positive mothers from experiencing a whole range of emotional and mental health concerns that are primarily related to the impact of HIV stigma and discrimination. Our research shows that the negative effects of housing instability are exacerbated for HIV-positive mothers as a result of their HIV-positive status, combined with the intersecting issues of poverty, racism, sexism, and HIV-related stigma and discrimination. Echoing Robertson (2007), who argues that "notions of home are ordered by gender and culture expectations and these are anchored to individual biographies, to dynamic relationships among people and between places" (p. 529), housing solutions for women must address the context of their lives and the places and spaces that they traverse at any given time.

Our research also highlights the need to critically inquire into what we mean by "stable" housing, since staying in once place does not necessarily mean HIV-positive mothers are living in appropriate or safe housing situations. It is particularly important that prevention efforts do not reflect a one-size-fits-all approach to housing and housing support; this will not work for HIV-positive mothers, given the diversity of this population and how intersecting identities relate to gender, HIV stigma, race, poverty, and motherhood. Rather, understanding the housing needs and experiences of HIV-positive mothers, particularly those from ethnoracial and otherwise marginalized communities, will require a critical evaluation of current housing policies and programs that act as facilitators and/or barriers to a whole range of health and social services.

One issue that requires further attention as we consider developing housing as a prevention strategy for HIV-positive mothers (and women) is in the area of intimate partner violence (IPV). According to a recent study of housing and homelessness among female-headed households living in a shelter, housing instability was a common experience among the participants surveyed, with many of the women interviewed living at an average of four places including a shelter at the time of the interview (Paradis, Novac, Sarty, & Hulchanski, 2009). The most common reason for these women leaving their last stable place of residence was relationship violence, with nearly one-third of participants leaving because of abuse. Women of colour who are HIV positive may be more at risk of mental and physical impacts of IPV due to systemic barriers such as racism, ethnocentrism, immigration status, and poverty, which may also become barriers to accessing formal or specialized supports for IPV. Moreover, cultural barriers such as the shame of being a "victim" of IPV or preferring to keep family concerns such as IPV from outsiders may discourage women from seeking assistance (Bent-Goodley, 2007). Findings from the literature also suggest that a broader definition of intimate partner violence needs to be considered for women living with HIV. This definition would consider verbal threats that threaten a women's social stability and reconceptualize IPV to include "situational abuse" or threats to one's social stability, such as threats of deportation, financial security, or the shame of being abused as being exacerbated by their HIV status (Moreno, 2007). This confirms our own findings regarding the way that IPV enters into the mothers' experiences and provides particularly strong examples of how gender inequity and HIV-related stigma oppresses HIV-positive mothers within their own homes, which subsequently impacts their overall mental health. This suggests that there is a need to further theorize risk and safety in the contexts in which HIV-positive women and mothers leave, locate, access, and reside in the various housing situations they find themselves living in.

THE WAY FORWARD

The range of housing and housing-related issues highlighted here requires that researchers, policy-makers, and practitioners work "outward from the circumstances and narrated experiences of women" (Robertson, 2007, p. 530) in order to develop housing programs and policies that are both preventative and intervention-based. This is echoed by Sikkema et al. (2000), who argue that although most conceptual models of HIV risk reduction emphasize individual interventions that focus on changing behaviour through education and support, there is also an opportunity to create change at the community level through developing neighbourhood-based programs. This has promising implications in the area of prevention because HIV prevention and care strategies will not succeed without addressing structural barriers such as homelessness and housing instability (Shubert, 2010). Within the context of HIV-positive mothers from African and Caribbean communities, this suggestion must be taken further so that the issues presented here are reflected in these programs and policies. In turn, this must include cultural, ethnic, and gendered perspectives and experiences that situate the needs of HIV-positive mothers and their children at the centre of their development. Such programs would be based on the recognition of motherhood as (1) a cultural and identity position that, like gender, race, and class, shapes women's experiences of illness in frequently contradictory ways; (2) a social and discursive practice; (3) a buffer against the sequelae of disease; and (4) a protest against stigmatization (Radtke & Van Mens-Verhulst, 2001). Such programs of care would be directed toward acknowledging the centrality of motherhood—whether conceived empirically or discursively—to the very physical and social survival of HIV-positive mothers and toward maximizing the benefits and minimizing the burdens of motherhood both for HIV-positive women and for their children.

One practical way that prevention strategies can start to tackle these issues is to develop coordinated program planning and increased communication within and between service sectors in order to influence system change. This could be achieved by developing avenues for increased cross-sectoral work with housing, immigration, mental health, child and family services, and education that would include mobilizing multiple sectors and organizations to work together to address family need at both the societal and structural level (Stewart et al., 2006). On a micro level of practice, family support interventions would also have a key role to play in supporting families who are at risk of homelessness and housing instability (Tischler, Karim, Rustall, Gregory, & Vostanis, 2004). Finally, there is also a call for cross-sectoral education and training on the multiple layers of oppression that are experienced by HIV-positive parents and their children, including the impact that HIV-related stigma and discrimination, racism, sexism, violence, and poverty have on the mental health of parents and their children. Hence, what is needed are housing strategies at both the practice and policy level that will lead to more appropriate and effective family-based practices on the ground, in addition to the creation of health, housing, social service, and immigration policies that reflect the multiple needs of HIV-positive parents who are living with and caring for their children.

Finally, an important learning from this research has taught us that effectively examining the unique housing needs and experiences of HIV-positive mothers requires a theoretical lens that incorporates gender consciousness and social justice approaches to the social determinants of health. In turn, there is a need to reframe community-based research processes to reflect a commitment to gender consciousness, intersectionality, addressing power imbalances, and reciprocity. This has and will continue to enable us to examine gender and societal inequalities in relation to women's health, as well as to capture the social world, multiple and intersecting identities of HIV-positive mothers, and the housing situations in which they live.

PROBLEM-BASED LEARNING CASE STUDY

HIV-positive mothers living in Toronto, Ontario, face a number of economic, social, and environmental challenges that can put them at risk for housing instability and homelessness. These challenges can be intensified for HIV-positive mothers from African and Caribbean communities due to the multiple and unique housing needs and experiences that this population continues to face. Moreover, these issues are often exacerbated for African and Caribbean newcomer HIV-positive mothers due to the ethnocentric shelter and housing practices that they experience as they attempt to navigate a new system of housing, health, and social care systems and their concerns about the impact of HIV-related stigma on their children. In the face of the intersecting issues of motherhood, poverty, sexism, immigration status, and HIV-related stigma and discrimination, a number of research, policy, and programming questions emerge as to how to develop a housing prevention strategy that will most effectively meet the needs of HIV-positive mothers and their children. Given the unique and complex issues facing African and Caribbean mothers living with HIV in Toronto, how would you approach or address the following questions?

CRITICAL THINKING QUESTIONS

1. What methodological and theoretical considerations would you attend to in developing research questions and processes that would result in suggestions for prevention-based strategies that will address the unique and multiple psychosocial, health, and housing needs of HIV-positive mothers and their children?

2. Research has shown that housing needs and experiences are differentiated by HIV status, race, gender, language, class, and so forth. At the same time, there are some overarching issues that require immediate attention in the area of housing prevention, such as HIV-related stigma, ethnocentrism, and sexism. Given the range of housing issues affecting HIV-positive mothers and their children, how would you go about using your research findings to start the process of developing housing prevention policies that attend to both the commonalities and differences in experience and need?

3. The most up-to-date research in the area of families, HIV, and housing suggests that an important piece of the puzzle in preventing homelessness and housing instability among HIV-positive mothers and their children is to promote and support an increase in cross-sectoral work. What practice sectors do you think are most relevant to HIV-positive mothers in their attempts to navigate and access appropriate housing for themselves and their children? How would you go about increasing communication and programming across these sectors, and why?

REFERENCES

Aidala, A., Cross, J. E., Stall, R., Harre, D., & Sumartojo, E. (2005). Housing status and HIV risk behaviors: Implications for prevention and policy. *AIDS and Behavior, 9*(3), 251–265.

Antle, B., Wells, L., Salter Goldie, R., Matteo, D., & King, S. (2001). Challenges of parenting for families living with HIV/AIDS. *Social Work, 46*(2), 159–169.

Benoit. C., & Shumka, L. (2007). *Gendering the Population Health Perspective: Fundamental determinants of women's health.* Final report. Vancouver, BC: Women's Health Research Network.

Bent-Goodley, T. B. (2007). Health disparities and violence against women: Why and how cultural and societal influences matter. *Trauma, Violence, & Abuse, 8*(2), 90.

Cheung, A. M., & Hwang, S. W. (2004). Risk of death among homeless women: A cohort study and review of the literature. *Canadian Medical Association Journal, 170*(8), 1243–1247.

Collins, P. H. (1998). It's all in the family: Intersections of gender, race and nation. *Hypatia, 13*(3), 62–82.

Crenshaw, K. (2001, August–September). *Mapping the margins: Intersectionality, identity politics and violence against women of color*. Paper presented at the World Conference against Racism, Durban, South Africa.

Culhane, D. P., Gollub, E., Kuhn, R., & Shpaner, M. (2001). The co-occurrence of AIDS and homelessness: Results from the integration of administrative databases for AIDS surveillance and public shelter utilization in Philadelphia. *Journal of Epidemiology and Community Health, 55*(7), 515–520.

DeMatteo, D., Wells, L. M., Salter Goldie, R., & King, S. M. (2002). The "family" context of HIV: A need for comprehensive health and social policies. *AIDS Care, 14*(2), 261–278.

Fisher, B., Hovell, M., Hofstetter, C. R., & Hough, R. (1995). Risks associated with long-term homelessness among women: Battery, rape and HIV infection. *International Journal of Health Services, 25*(2), 351–369.

Geduld, J., Gatali, M., Remis, R., & Archibald, C. P. (2003). *Estimates of HIV prevalence and incidence in Canada*. Ottawa, ON: Public Health Agency of Canada.

Greene, S., Tucker, R., Rourke, S. B., Monette, L., Koornstra, J., Sobota, M., ... & Guenter, D. (2010). "Under My Umbrella": The housing experiences of HIV-positive parents who live with and care for their children in Ontario. *Archives of Women and Mental Health, 13*(3), 223.

Hamers, F. F., & Downs, A. M. (2004). The changing face of the HIV epidemic in western Europe: What are the implications for public health policies? *The Lancet, 364*(9428), 83–94.

Hankivsky, O., & Christoffersen, A. (2008). Intersectionality and the determinants of health: A Canadian perspective. *Critical Public Health, 18*(33), 271–283.

Kappel Ramji Consulting Group. (2002). *Common occurrence: The impact of homelessness on women's health. Phase II: Community-based action research. Final report*. Toronto, ON: Sistering.

Kilbourne, A., Herndon, B., Andersen, R. M., Wenzel, S. L., & Gelberg, L. (2002). Psychiatric symptoms, health services, and HIV risk factors among homeless women. *Journal of Health Care for the Poor and Underserved, 13*(1), 49–65.

Li, P. S. (2003a). *Destination Canada: Immigration debates and issues*. Toronto, ON: Oxford University Press.

Li, P. S. (2003b). Deconstructing Canada's discourse of immigrant integration. *Journal of International Migration and Integration, 4*(3), 315–333.

Moreno, C. L. (2007). The relationship between culture, gender, structural factors, abuse, trauma, and HIV/AIDS for Latinas. *Qualitative Health Research, 17*(3), 340–352.

Ontario Advisory Committee on HIV/AIDS. (2002, June). *A Proposed HIV/AIDS strategy for Ontario to 2008*. Ottawa, ON: Ontario Ministry of Health and Long-Term Care.

Paradis, E., Novac, S., Sarty, M., & Hulchanski, J. D. (2009). Better off in a shelter? A year of homelessness & housing among status immigrant, non-status migrant, & Canadian-born families. In J. D. Hulchanski, P. Campsie, S. Chau, S. Hwang, & E. Paradis (Eds.), *Finding home: Policy options for addressing homelessness in Canada* (e-book) (Ch. 4.2). Toronto, ON: Centre for Urban and Community Studies Cities Centre, University of Toronto.

Parish, M., Burry, C., & Pabst, M. S. (2003). Providing comprehensive case management to urban women with HIV/AIDS and their families. *AFFILIA: Journal of Women and Social Work, 18*(3), 302–315.

Pequegnat, W., & Bray, J. H. (1997). Families and HIV/AIDS: Introduction to the special section, *Journal of Family Psychology, 11*(1), 3–10.

Phoenix, A., & Pattynama, P. (Eds.). (2006). Intersectionality [Special issue]. *European Journal of Women's Studies, 13*(3).

Radtke, L. H., & Van Mens-Verhulst, J. (2001). Being a mother and living with asthma: An exploratory analysis of discourse. *Journal of Health Psychology, 6*(4), 379–391.

Raphael, D. (2006). Social determinants of health: Present status, unresolved questions, and future directions. *International Journal of Health Services, 36*, 651–677.

Remis, R. S., Swantee, C., Schiedel, L., & Liu, J. (2008). *Report on HIV/AIDS in Ontario, 2006.* Toronto, ON: Ontario HIV Epidemiologic Monitoring Unit, University of Toronto.

Robertson, L. (2007). Taming space: Drug use, HIV, and homemaking in Downtown Eastside Vancouver. *Gender, Place and Culture, 14*(5), 527–549.

Rotheram-Borus, M. J. , Weiss, R., Alber, S., & Lester, P. (2005). Adolescent adjustment before and after HIV-related parental death. *Journal of Consulting and Clinical Psychology, 73*(2), 221–228.

Sandelowski, M., & Barroso, J. (2003). Motherhood in the context of maternal HIV infection. *Research in Nursing & Health, 26*(6), 470–482.

Shelton, D. (1993). Issues related to health care utilization and medical adherence among prenatal HIV seropositive African-American women in Miami: The role of the family and the extended kinship network. *Family Systems Medicine, 11*, 1–14.

Shubert, G. (2010, February). *Mobilizing knowledge: Housing is prevention and care.* Summary of research presented at the HIV and Housing Research Summit Series, Champ Strategy Lab.

Sikkema, K. J., Kelly, J. A., Winett, R. A., Solomon, L. J., Cargill, V. A., Roffman, R. A., ... & Mercer, M. B. (2000). Outcomes of a randomized community-level HIV prevention intervention for women living in 18 low-income housing developments. *American Journal of Public Health, 90*(1), 57–63.

Song, J. (2003). AIDS Housing of Washington. *AIDS Housing Survey,* 1.

Stewart, M. J., Neufeld, A., Harrison, M. J., Spitzer, D., Hughes, K., & Makwarimba, E. (2006). Immigrant woman family caregivers in Canada: Implications for policies and programmes in health and social sectors. *Health and Social Care in the Community, 14*(4), 329–340.

Suarez-Orozco, C., Todorova, I. L. G., & Louie, J. (2002). Making up for lost time: The experience of separation and reunification among immigrant families. *Family Process, 41*(4), 625–643.

Tangenberg, K. (2000). Marginalized epistemologies: A feminist approach to understanding the experiences of mothers with HIV. *AFFILIA: Journal of Women and Social Work, 15*(1), 31–48.

Tischler, V., Karim, K., Rustall, S., Gregory, P., & Vostanis, P. (2004). A family support service for homeless children and parents: Users perspectives and characteristics. *Health and Social Care in the Community, 12*(4), 327–335.

Tudiver, S., Kantiebo, M., Kammermayer, J., & Mayrak, M. (2004). Women's Health Surveillance: Implications for policy. *BMC Women's Health, 4*(Suppl. 1), S31.

Waegemakers Schiff, J. (2007). Homeless families in Canada: Discovering total families. *Families in Society, 88*(1), 131–140.

Weinreb, L., Goldberg, R., Lessard, D., Perloff, J., & Bassuk, E. (1999). HIV-risk practices among homeless and low-income housed mothers. *Journal of Family Practice, 48*(11), 859–867.

Wenzel, S. L., Tucker, J., Elliot, M., & Hambarsoomian, K. (2007). Sexual risk among impoverished women: Understanding the role of housing status. *AIDS and Behavior, 11*(2), 9–20.

Wuest, J., Merritt-Gray, M., Berman, H., & Ford-Gilboe, M. (2002). Illuminating social determinants of women's health using grounded theory. *Health Care for Women International, 23*(8), 794–808.

Yuval-Davis, N. (2006). Intersectionality and feminist politics. *European Journal of Women's Studies, 13*(3), 193–209.

Zierler, S., & Krieger, N. (2000). Social inequality and HIV infection in women. In K. Mayer & H. F. Pizer (Eds.), *The emergence of AIDS: The impact on immunology, microbiology and public health*. Washington, DC: American Public Health Association.

Chapter 7
IT'S ALL IN THE CONTEXT: STRUCTURAL AND PSYCHOSOCIAL CHALLENGES TO HIV PREVENTION WITH TRANSGENDER WOMEN

Greta Bauer

WHO ARE TRANS WOMEN IN CANADA?

Trans women come from every cultural and religious background, and traverse the full range of education and employment experience. They are doctors and lawyers, construction workers and students. They are youth and seniors; married, partnered, and single; parents and non-parents. Some live in Canada's largest cities and others outside of our tiniest towns. *Trans* is an umbrella term that unites those that may have much or almost nothing in common other than the shared experience of incongruence between the gender they know themselves to be and the biological sex they were assigned at birth.

In this chapter, the term *trans women* is used as shorthand for all those on the male-to-female or transfeminine spectrum. This includes those labelled male at birth who identify as girls or women, some of whom have socially transitioned to live in their core gender, and some who have medically transitioned through the use of hormonal and/or surgical therapies. It also includes those who may identify as two-spirit, bigender, genderqueer, or a range of other identities, who consider themselves to be gendered in a way that is both male and female, neither male nor female, or a third or alternate gender. Some of these individuals may have also transitioned socially or medically. Traditional categorical breakdowns of transsexual, transgender, and cross-dresser do not capture the full diversity of trans identities, bodies, and lived experience. In contrast to trans or transgender, the corresponding term *cisgender*, or simply *cis*, is increasingly being used to denote those whose core gender is concordant with the sex they were assigned at birth (Serano, 2007).

While trans people are often included in references to the "lesbian, gay, bisexual, and transgender community," it is important to note that gender identity is distinct from sexual orientation. Every trans person also has a sexual orientation. Trans women may identify as lesbian, bisexual, two-spirit, queer, straight, asexual, or may adopt a more personally unique identity. Some on the transfeminine spectrum who do not identify as "women" per se may express a range of sexual orientations that can include gay, bisexual, or straight male. Moreover, sexual orientation identities can be fluid, and for some, the process of socially transitioning the gender in which they live their day-to-day lives or medically transitioning through changes to their hormonal or anatomical sex can open up a period of re-exploration regarding sexual orientation. No matter how trans women may identify, assumptions cannot be made regarding who, if anyone, an individual trans woman may be sexually involved with.

PREVALENCE OF HIV IN TRANS WOMEN

While trans women can contract HIV through the same immediate routes as cisgender women—sexual contact or shared needle use—these health-related behaviours are impacted by social determinants of health. For trans women, these may include trans-specific discrimination or social exclusion, creating unique vulnerabilities. In most jurisdictions in Canada, trans women (and men) are not identified as part of routine epidemiologic tracking of the HIV epidemic, and statistics for trans women are not included in epidemiological surveillance reports, though researchers have argued that trans people warrant a separate demographic category (Nemoto, Operario, Keatley, Han, & Soma, 2004). It is therefore difficult to know to what extent trans women are impacted by HIV.

Methodological challenges exist to collecting valid data on HIV among trans women. Trans women constitute a "hidden population," one that cannot be randomly sampled. There is no sampling frame, or master list, of trans women from which to draw a probability-based sample that would produce results that are generalizable to all trans women. In addition, trans women are often not visibly identifiable, may not choose to disclose their trans status to researchers, and may in fact have a distrust of researchers based on the history of pathologizing research conducted on trans people. For these reasons, most existing studies rely on local convenience samples, though recent studies have attempted to overcome some earlier limitations by gathering larger samples over a broader geographic area, or by using probability-based non-random sampling methods such as respondent-driven sampling.

Despite these challenges, individual studies within trans communities have collected information on HIV status, and two meta-analyses, studies that quantitatively combine data from multiple previous studies, have been conducted. Herbst et al. (2008) estimated the prevalence of HIV by two assessment methods: self-reported HIV positivity and HIV positivity from serologic testing (seropositivity). They estimated self-reported HIV prevalence at 11.8% among trans women in the United States, based on combined data from 18 studies, and HIV seroprevalence at 27.7%, based on data from 4 studies. Operario, Soma, and Underhill (2008) estimated HIV seroprevalence at 27.3% among trans women sex workers internationally, and at

14.7% among trans women not engaged in sex work. They contrasted this with estimates of HIV seroprevalence of 15.1% among cisgender male sex workers, and 4.5% among cisgender female sex workers.

Higher prevalence of HIV has been identified for African-American trans women, with self-reported HIV positivity estimated at 30.8%, versus 16.1% for Hispanic trans women and 16.7% for white trans women (Herbst et al., 2008). Seroprevalence rates as high as 63% have been observed among African-American trans women (Clements-Nolle, Marx, Guzman, & Katz, 2001). Given U.S.–Canadian differences in the history of colonialism and slavery, as well as current differences in human rights policy and immigration policies and patterns, it is unclear to what extent ethnoracial inequities observed for African-Americans may apply to African, Caribbean, and other Black women in Canada. Nevertheless, given the impact of experiences of racism and their potential interaction with experiences of transphobia, HIV vulnerability among Black and other racialized groups of trans women in Canada should be a major concern. Given the established knowledge of HIV vulnerabilities among Aboriginal Canadians, the concerns of Aboriginal trans women have barely begun to be addressed. It has been estimated that in Ontario, 6% of trans women are Aboriginal (Bauer et al., 2010). Significant ethnoracial differences in HIV testing make it difficult to interpret Ontario data on self-reported prevalence, with Aboriginal trans people being the most likely to have been tested, and non-Aboriginal, racialized trans people being the least likely (Bauer, Travers, Scanlon, & Coleman, 2012). While the two meta-analyses conducted to date provide new information, they share a major weakness. The studies on which they were based were conducted using convenience samples, primarily in urban areas with high concentrations of homeless, street-involved, and sex worker participants. This limits the generalizability of these results to communities similar to those from which they were obtained. This is important for two reasons. First, it provides strong evidence that particular communities of trans women are strongly affected by HIV, with high proportions currently living with HIV and more at moderate to high risk of infection. Therefore, it is imperative that HIV prevention, testing, and treatment programs be designed (or redesigned) to remove barriers to access for these women, and to address the erasure of trans women that results in policies, protocols, and practices that do not accommodate their identities, experiences, or needs (Bauer et al., 2009).

Second, it is important to note that these studies do not provide estimates that can be generalized to trans communities broadly, particularly to trans women who live in small cities and towns, to those who are not publicly "out" in their lives, and to those who are not street active or currently engaged in sex work. While there is a common perception that trans women live primarily in urban environments, using respondent-driven sampling, Bauer et al. (2010) estimated that in Ontario, 77% of trans women lived outside of Metropolitan Toronto, a proportion similar to the population overall. In a U.S. Internet-based sample that included trans men as well as trans women, 60%

lived outside of major metropolitan areas (Rosser, Oakes, Bockting, & Miner, 2007). The health of trans women who have not been part of urban trans communities is only beginning to be examined through research.

The first broad trans population studies have recently been conducted, but research on HIV prevalence in Canadian trans women remains scarce. Self-reported prevalence of HIV was estimated at 2.9% for trans women in Ontario (Bauer et al., 2012), while a small study of 73 trans or two-spirit men and women in Manitoba and Northwestern Ontario reported 8% of participants indicating they were HIV positive (Taylor, 2006). Whether from a large population sample or a small needs assessment, self-reported estimates invariably underestimate actual HIV prevalence, in that some people who are HIV positive are not yet aware of their status. An estimated 42% of trans women in Ontario had never been tested for HIV, a proportion that is higher than in most international studies (Bauer et al., 2012). Moreover, some who are living with HIV may not wish to disclose this on a survey. These prevalences, even the lower estimates, remain substantially higher than expected for the Canadian population and likely mask an uneven distribution, with some communities having much higher prevalences.

Within Grant et al.'s large U.S. Internet study (2010), HIV prevalence was elevated among those who were non-citizens, had engaged in sex work, had annual incomes under $10,000, or had lost a job due to discrimination or were unemployed. It was also substantially higher among those who were members of racialized groups, and highest among African-Americans. Combined evidence from these studies suggests that trans women are highly heterogeneous in their individual HIV risk, and that being a member of another marginalized group (or other marginalized groups) compounds the level of vulnerability. In fact, the impact of transphobia may differ along ethnoracial lines. Levels of transphobic experience, stigma, and discrimination based on gender nonconformity have been found to vary by racial group, class, age, age of transition, outness, and HIV status (Lombardi, 2009; Sugano, Nemoto, & Operario, 2006). Nine factors contributing to HIV vulnerability among trans women are outlined below, grouped into three categories: lack of trans-appropriate and trans-accessible prevention programs, structural factors contributing to HIV vulnerability, and psychosocial factors contributing to HIV vulnerability. In considering these, the reader should keep in mind that the way these impact an individual trans woman will be affected by her socio-demographic location and the ways in which this shapes opportunities and challenges in her life.

LACK OF TRANS-APPROPRIATE PREVENTION PROGRAMS

HIV-related behavioural risks for trans women are not easily captured in cisgender concepts of HIV prevention. Existing programs most often assume that needles are used for injecting street drugs and not hormones or silicone, and that anatomy lines up neatly with one's gender. Prevention messages geared to women almost never consider that a woman could be the insertive partner in genital or anal sex, or that risks related to vaginal exposures may or may not be different for those with a natal versus a surgically constructed vagina. Social context issues for trans women, such as employment discrimination, gender-related body image issues, or the use of sex for gender validation are not typically considered. One participant in Trans PULSE, an Ontario-wide study of trans health, noted difficulties in trying to access available services in a large Ontario city:

> I know people who have gone to [an AIDS Service Organization] looking for services, and of course there are no trans programs [there] and because they felt that there was no way for them to have access to the services, either as men or women, they just quit and washed their hands. (Bauer, 2009)

Programs offered through AIDS Service Organizations (ASOs) and other community and health care organizations may exclude trans people directly, through sex-segregated programs and services that provide no clear point of entry for trans patients or clients, or through service implementation that is voyeuristically focused on gender rather than on the needs of trans clients or patients (Namaste, 2000). Thus, there is a need to revise most HIV prevention programming to make it trans-appropriate and respectful. This includes programs designed to meet the specific needs of First Nations, Métis, and Inuit communities; newcomers to Canada; youth; older adults; sex workers; and those living with HIV. Moreover, there is a need to work within local trans communities to build and implement programs appropriate to their trans-specific needs. Such HIV prevention programs have been developed in multiple U.S. cities (Bockting, Rosser, & Coleman, 2001; De Santis, Martin, & Lester, 2010; Hein & Kirk, 2001; Warren, 2001), and could be expanded or redeveloped in localized Canadian contexts.

STRUCTURAL FACTORS CONTRIBUTING TO HIV VULNERABILITY

Given the widespread lack of understanding of trans lives, and the high levels of discrimination that remain despite human rights protections, structural or social factors serve to create unique vulnerabilities. Structural factors are conceptualized as "prerequisites for health," and include income, shelter, social justice, and equity (World Health Organization, 1986). Structural factors include social determinants of health that relate to the formal and informal social systems impacting the distribution of social and economic resources (Raphael, 2004). Structural factors that have an impact on HIV vulnerability in trans women include: barriers to employment and economic stability, coupled with the high costs of transition-related care; ready markets for, and criminalization of, sex work; inaccessible health care systems; and other structural conditions such as sex-segregated prison systems that place trans women prisoners at high risk of physical and sexual assault.

Barriers to Maintaining or Finding Employment

While trans people are protected against employment discrimination on the grounds of sex under the Canadian Charter of Rights and Freedoms, the Canadian Human Rights Act, and provincial human rights codes, discrimination remains common (Bauer et al., 2011). The lack of more explicit inclusion has been critiqued since, to the extent that both employers and trans employees are not aware of legal protections, the laws fail to fully serve their role in preventing discrimination from occurring (Nussbaum, 2010).

In employment settings, discrimination can take many forms, including denial of a job or promotion; firing or constructive dismissal; on-the-job harassment, including deliberate misuse of names or pronouns; denial of appropriate bathroom use; physical or sexual assault; breach of confidentiality; and being moved away from client-contact positions (Nussbaum, 2010). While employers are required to accommodate the disability needs of employees (which may include trans employees during a period of transition), some employers further discriminate by instituting "accommodations" that are designed to preserve the comfort of clients or other employees, rather than to meet the needs of the trans employee (Nussbaum, 2010). In the U.S. National Transgender Discrimination Survey, 47% of participants reported at least one adverse job outcome, and 97% reported at least one form of on-the-job harassment (National Center for Transgender Equality & National Gay and Lesbian Task Force, 2009). While specific rates of discrimination in Canada are not yet known, the effects can be seen in the economic marginalization of trans people. In Ontario, it has been estimated that, despite high levels of education, 47% of trans women have personal incomes of less than $15,000 per year and only 23% have incomes over $50,000 (Bauer et al., 2010).

Persistent underemployment or unemployment can affect trans women not only through reduced financial resources and resulting economic instability, but also through the negative effects of exclusion from social participation through meaningful employment. Thus, employment discrimination generates financial, social, and emotional effects that may interact to create psychosocial challenges for coping, mental health, self-esteem, and daily living. For trans women who experience multiple forms of marginalization through experiences of historical or contemporary racism, or for those living with physical or mental health challenges, these conditions may interact in ways that are not yet fully understood. Nevertheless, a full understanding is not required to recognize that employment discrimination plays a major role in creating vulnerabilities not only to HIV, but also to maintaining physical and mental wellness more broadly.

High Financial and Social Cost of Transition

Both social and medical transition bring related financial costs. For trans women, social transitioning involves beginning to live as a woman or in a more feminine or less masculine gender, and often includes an investment of time and finances to change one's legal name and subsequently the name listed on such documents as school transcripts, driver's license, provincial health card, Indian Status card, and permanent resident card or passport. Moreover, reconstituting a wardrobe is expensive. For trans women who medically transition, expenses often include out-of-pocket payment for estrogen and testosterone-blocker treatment—where not covered through school, employer, or government programs—as well as for hair removal through electrolysis or laser treatment. Some trans women undergo sex reassignment surgeries. Orchiectomy (removal of testes) and vaginoplasty (creation of a vagina) are covered under some provincial plans but not others, and these plans do not cover some surgeries that may be needed, such as a tracheal shave to reduce an Adam's apple. Hormone treatment, hair removal, and surgeries can all be expensive, and this places additional demands on trans women at what is often an already stressful time. One Trans PULSE Project participant in Ontario described their response to this:

> There is a strain [on my] finances that is related to surgery which I am about to have, and it is causing huge stress in my life. And it is very important for me to function ... I am numbing out a lot. I am drinking more than usual as a way to cope because of the stress. (Bauer, 2009)

Transitioning often involves social costs as well, which create stress and require additional coping responses. Transitioning can bring new connections and friendships with other trans people or allies, allow for more honest or authentic interactions with family and friends, and reduce pre-transition relationship strain associated with hiding one's identity. However, few trans women transition without some major loss. Family and friends may have little information on what it means to be trans and may respond with stereotypes, anger, or a sense of betrayal (Lev, 2004). Some trans women who transition within marriages keep their marriages and families intact, but others have spouses who choose to end the relationship. It has been estimated that 40% of trans women in Ontario are also parents (Bauer et al., 2010). While case law has established that being trans, per se, is not grounds to terminate a parent's custody of or access to a child, conflicts around custody and access remain common. Disruptions to family and social networks are the norm, and few supportive resources exist for family members of those who transition (Lev, 2004).

Established Demand for Sex Work without Protections for Sex Workers

Commercial sex work provides a ready market with income potential for trans women. An estimated 16% of Ontario trans women have engaged in sex work or exchange sex, and 2% currently work as sex workers or escorts (Bauer et al., 2012). Engaging in sex with commercial partners may provide personal rewards, such as validation of gender and positive attention and affection, but it also presents personal risks to health, safety, and emotional well-being (Bockting, Robinson, & Rosser, 1998). While some may choose to engage in sex work for reasons of personal preference, for many it is a decision made within the context of the financial pressures they face, including those generated by the combination of employment discrimination and high transition-related costs. One Trans PULSE Project participant summarizes the situation as follows:

> I know a lot of people in the transsexual community from not being hired by anybody ... they've had to resort to prostitution in order to get the money to pay the rent, and it can be a very empowering sort of experience. I mean you're self-employed, tax free income... (Bauer, 2009)

However, engaging in sex work may put trans women at higher risk of HIV, particularly if they are unable to use condoms consistently with commercial partners. In a San Francisco study of racialized trans women, Nemoto, Operario, Keatley, and Villegas (2004) found that while most commercial sex workers did use condoms consistently, trans-specific economic and emotional needs put some at higher risk. In particular, transition-related financial needs and the emotional need for validation as women were identified as contributing to unprotected anal sex with commercial partners. A meta-analysis combining data across 25 studies internationally demonstrated higher prevalence of HIV among trans women sex workers than among either cisgender male or female sex workers, with trans sex workers having four times the risk as their cisgender female counterparts (Operario et al., 2008). It was not clear if this excess risk was directly related to sex work or to other factors that may make trans women vulnerable to HIV. Evidence has shown that similar to cisgender female sex workers, trans women who engage in commercial sex work may be at highest risk of HIV from men with whom they share an intimate relationship (Bockting et al., 1998; Nemoto, Operario, Keatley, & Villegas, 2004).

Sex work experience can traverse the range of positive to negative experiences. Trans sex workers in Canada have argued that, while they make a political contribution to improving social attitudes toward trans women through the work they do with their clients, this work is not only uncredited but vilified (Namaste, Forrester, Hamilton, & Ross, 2005). While selling sex in Canada is technically legal, the actions surrounding it, including negotiating for sex and living off the proceeds of prostitution, remain illegal. These policies have produced a situation in which a commercial sex worker is legally barred from taking the types of actions that could protect herself. This has placed trans women engaged in sex work, particularly street work, at an extremely high risk of violence without options to legally work indoors, take referrals for safe clients, or report assaults to police. It is because of imminent danger to sex workers that the Superior Court of Ontario struck down these provisions in September 2010, a decision that was appealed. Changes to laws regulating sex work have the potential to reduce work-related risks to the physical and sexual safety of trans sex workers. Moreover, decriminalization may protect against additional barriers to employment created through having a criminal record.

Barriers to Accessing Health Care Services

Erasure, the process through which trans people and trans experience are systematically rendered invisible and processes to include trans people are not incorporated into institutional practices, results in health care delivery systems that are not set up to accommodate the needs of trans patients (Bauer et al., 2009; Namaste, 2000). Within these systems, trans patients often find themselves in the position of having to educate the providers from whom they seek expert advice (Grant et al., 2010). A lack of training in medical, nursing, and other health professional curricula leaves providers at a loss in terms of both medical knowledge and cultural competency. As such, trans people will often avoid seeing a doctor where possible, even in a medical emergency, a situation that is not conducive to leveraging health care resources to maintain and promote one's health. Trans women who require transition-related medical care are forced to interface with the health care system to access hormonal and surgical therapies. This can require difficult work on the part of patients in navigating systems where transition pathways vary depending on whether a psychiatric or informed consent model is used (Hammond, 2010).

Difficulties with health care access due to sex designations on provincial health plan cards have been documented in Quebec and Ontario (Bauer et al., 2009; Namaste, 2000). Having a sex designator that is inconsistent with one's gender presentation may "out" a patient as trans, or may cause problems as staff try to make arrangements to have it corrected. However, even having a sex designator consistent with one's presentation may cause problems if receiving care involving sex-associated conditions. For example, billing a hysterectomy for a male patient or prostate-related treatment for a female patient can result in rejection of the claim as potential fraud or a clerical error. Thus, even doctors who are trans-knowledgeable and trans-friendly may be forced to work around administrative provisions that assume patients are cisgender.

Outside of primary care, transition-related, and emergency care, additional HIV-related health and social services needed by trans women include access to clean needles through doctors, pharmacies, or needle exchanges (for drugs, hormones, or silicone, each requiring a different needle gauge), as well as HIV testing. Sharing needles for injecting drugs, hormones, or silicone was uncommon among Ontario trans women, but it did occur (Hammond, Redman, Bauer, Travers, & Coleman, 2010). Unfortunately, testing for HIV was also uncommon, with 42% of trans women never having been tested. Barriers indicated by participants included gender-segregated clinics and fear that providers would be transphobic.

Physical or Sexual Assault

Trans people may be the targets of assault simply for being trans. While experiencing violence certainly has psychosocial implications, structural factors such as economic marginalization and homelessness, participation in the sex trade, and incarceration in the prison system can dramatically increase the risk of physical or sexual assault. Experiences of transphobic assaults are common. It is estimated that 20% of trans people in Ontario have survived transphobic physical or sexual assaults; an additional 34% have experienced verbal harassment or threats for being trans (Scanlon, Bauer, Travers, Boyce, & Coleman, 2010). This is consistent with U.S. estimates (Lombardi, Wilchins, Priesing, & Malouf, 2001; Xavier, Honnold, & Bradford, 2007).

Trans women within Canadian federal and provincial prison systems are particularly vulnerable to sexual assault, as those who have not had genital surgeries are placed in men's prisons. In a qualitative study of trans prisoners and former prisoners, Scott and Lines (1999) reported that rape was common; prisoners were forced to find a protector, with the expectation of sexual relations in exchange for protection. While condoms were available, sex between inmates was technically not allowed, making condom use difficult even in consensual sexual encounters.

PSYCHOSOCIAL FACTORS CONTRIBUTING TO HIV VULNERABILITY

Trans women make individual decisions regarding sexual or injecting behaviours that affect their HIV risk, but these must be understood as situated within the context of structural barriers to maintaining health, including those outlined above. The effects of structural factors on individual behavioural risks may be mediated by material factors or psychosocial factors. For example, loss of employment due to discrimination can create material risks due to financial resource depletion, and psychosocial risks due to a concomitant loss of self-esteem. While some material and psychosocial impacts were addressed above, this section outlines additional psychosocial factors that may impact individual risk behaviours. From a health perspective, psychosocial factors can be seen as those that either mediate the effects of structural factors on individual health, or are moderated by structural factors (Martikainen, Bartley, & Lahelma, 2002).

Bockting et al. (1998) have identified trans-specific psychosocial factors, including sexual identity conflict; shame, isolation, and fear over being trans; secrecy with regard to trans identities or experiences; the search for gender affirmation through sex; periods of compulsive sexual behaviour; and difficulties in talking about sex. Additional factors may include substance use as a coping strategy, and difficulties in finding an accepting and caring intimate partner.

Kammerer, Mason, Connors, & Durkee (2001) argue that psychosocial risk is best understood in terms of historical and contemporary risk structures, as this separation can advance understanding and promote the development of prevention strategies. Historical risk, as they define it, is developmental and refers to a life course understanding of trans-specific experience. Contemporary risk involves current social life, and encompasses contexts in which recent behaviours occur. Each of the psychosocial factors outlined below can contribute to HIV vulnerability in a historical or developmental role, or in terms of contemporary risk structure, depending on the timing and intensity.

Periods of Low Self-Esteem, Depression, Anxiety, Poor Body Image, or Substance Use

Most trans women and girls experience periods of low self-esteem and mental distress. This may be related to experiences of transphobic discrimination, body image issues, stress within the family, isolation, or other issues. Depression in particular has been reported at very high prevalences in trans women, for example, at 62% in San Francisco (Clements-Nolle et al., 2001), and 61% in Ontario (Rotondi et al., 2011). For trans women, a strong association has been observed between having been subjected to gender-related psychological or physical abuse and major depression (Nuttbrock et al., 2010), with the effects of gender-related abuse being greatest during adolescence, and declining later in life. At an extreme, these challenges may lead to serious consideration of suicide, attempts to commit suicide, and completed suicides. In Ontario, it has been estimated that 77% of trans people have seriously considered suicide at some point in their lives, and for most of them it was related to being trans (Scanlon et al., 2010). An estimated 43% had attempted suicide, similar to U.S. estimates (Grant et al., 2010). Recent suicidality was higher among youth up to age 24, and among those who had been targeted for physical or sexual assault because they were trans (Scanlon et al., 2010).

Shame and isolation may contribute to the use of alcohol or other drugs, which then allow for engagement in sexual activities (Bockting et al., 1998). Sugano et al. (2006) found depression, low self-esteem, and substance use each to be associated with increased sexual risk for HIV. One Trans PULSE participant explained her experience as follows: "When my self-esteem was at its very lowest, I didn't give a flying fuck. I abused and was slowly trying to kill myself with substances [and] dodgy sex" (Bauer, 2009). Kammerer et al. (2001) explain that the psychological dimensions to trans risk for both substance use and HIV must be seen as created and shaped by social pressures to conform to gender norms, coupled with practical issues in making a life as a woman a reality. This, they explain, can lead to "cycles of withdrawal and 'acting out'" that are not conducive to self-preservation and care. Substance use is a common coping strategy, yet acting on a decision to address problematic substance use can be difficult for trans women. Trans people dealing with drug or alcohol problems have reported negative experiences and trans-specific barriers to accessing treatment programs, which may impede their recovery (Lombardi, 2007). Thus, trans women encounter a cycle of continuing challenges to psychosocial well-being, coupled with structural barriers to accessing the care they need to recover.

Difficulties in Realizing Healthy Sexual or Intimate Relationships

Cisgender male partners of trans women come from every background, and can identify as any sexual orientation (Coan, Schrager, & Packer, 2005). While very little is
known about male partners of trans women, almost nothing is known about cisgender
female and trans partners. Research focusing on HIV-related risk has yet to make the
conceptual jump to addressing healthy sexual relationships more broadly. Challenges
in developing and maintaining healthy sexual relationships can originate from two
sources and their interacting effects: transphobia on the part of partners or potential
partners, and lack of sexual self-esteem and agency on the part of trans women.

The first challenge has not been explored in any depth in published research, though
trans women report anecdotally that they have faced romantic or sexual rejection from
cisgender straight men and lesbians, but less often from cisgender bisexuals of either sex
or from other trans people. The second challenge, lack of sexual self-esteem and agency,
can manifest in different ways as illustrated by the following two quotes:

> I did not see myself as somebody who could be in ... what most
> people considered "normal" relationships. So I tended to jump into
> relationships with people who couldn't give anything back or who
> were abusive... (Bauer, 2009)

> I didn't have any negative sexual behaviour like that because I felt
> that as a trans person sex wasn't a realm I was allowed to exist in.
> (Bauer, 2009)

This pair of quotes illustrates two responses to internalized transphobia with regard
to sexual relationships: unhealthy sexual interactions and avoidance. While stereotypes
of trans women often imagine a hypersexuality, the latter response is not uncommon.
In fact, an estimated 51% of Ontario trans women have not had sex in the past year
and 15% have never had sex (Bauer et al., 2012), some by choice and some by default.
While this may at first appear to be "good news" in terms of HIV-related risks, lack of
sexual engagement may create its own vulnerabilities when sexual activity is begun
or resumed. In such situations, the need for emotional and physical intimacy and for
gender validation may create psychosocial vulnerabilities that lower negotiating power
or overshadow immediate safety concerns (Bockting et al., 1998).

Sexual Exploration or Validation

Delayed recognition and acceptance of one's gender identity may result in periods of
prolonged or deferred "adolescent" sexual exploration, as one figures out one's sexual
orientation in light of one's gender (Bockting et al., 1998). Moreover, sexual activity
can play an important role in validating one's gender. One Trans PULSE Project focus
group participant noted that she had engaged in "very risky sexual behaviour, very,

in an attempt to affirm myself ... as female by using sex with men to get some type of self-legitimization" (Bauer, 2009). This woman's experience is not unique. Bockting et al. (1998) identified the search for affirmation as a key factor in HIV risk, in that being considered sexually attractive and desirable in a female role can interfere with setting limits in sexual situations. Simply put, HIV and other sexually transmitted diseases may not be the most immediate concern in everyday life and intimacy. For lesbian or bisexual trans women who have cisgender female partners, it is not clear that sexual validation in sexual situations may create any increased risk for HIV, though this area has not been explored in research.

NEW DIRECTIONS IN HIV PREVENTION FOR TRANS WOMEN: PROGRAM, POLICY, AND INFORMATION NEEDS

The structural and psychosocial factors discussed above point to the need for new directions in HIV prevention. Additional information is needed in developing best practices for HIV prevention for trans women in a Canadian context. Much of the available research comes from the U.S. or other countries, and it is unclear to what extent it applies in Canada. Some helpful first steps would include: identification of trans women (and trans men) in HIV test reporting, and publication of epidemiologic results tracking infections; identification of trans participants in population health research, and conduct of trans-specific analyses; development and inclusion of HIV-related sexual risk behaviour items in surveys that do not make assumptions about concordance between gender, genitals, and sex fluids; and qualitative analysis of the experiences of Canadian trans women living with, or at risk for, HIV. Given a historic distrust of researchers rooted in years of pathologizing research, community-based research strategies can be used to increase participation and also the relevance and uptake of results. Analyses that allow for the intersectional nature of marginalization can be used to explore the ways that trans experiences may shape HIV risk differently for those experiencing multiple marginalizations. In particular, while HIV has been a priority issue for research in Aboriginal communities in Canada (Canadian Aboriginal AIDS Network, 2009), two-spirit trans women's needs have only begun to be identified and addressed (Taylor, 2006; 2-Spirited People of the 1st Nations, 2008).

Development and implementation of HIV prevention programs specific to, or inclusive of, trans women is important, and is best done in collaboration with community members and organizations to ensure their needs are identified and met. However, traditional HIV prevention programming provides only one step toward addressing the prevention needs of trans women. Development of primary care models for trans health care is an important next step, given that access barriers to primary care have been documented (Bauer et al., 2009), and that such models can serve to address the HIV prevention needs of trans women (Melendez & Pinto, 2009; Williamson, 2010). Addressing institutional erasure in health care settings more broadly would require altering protocols and policies to accommodate trans patients and clients within sex-segregated services in reproductive and sexual health, sex-segregated hospital wards, and sex-based procedural billing protocols.

Implementation of policies that support hiring, promoting, and retaining trans employees at all levels of employment could serve to allow trans women to maintain or gain employment and financial stability. Additional structural interventions to reduce economic vulnerability include reducing high transition-related costs through increased public funding, and making explicit human rights protection for gender identity and expression. In addition, HIV risks could be addressed through the removal of surgical requirements for changing sex on legal identification; co-locating trans women with cisgender women rather than men in prisons, shelters, and other sex-segregated residential systems; and the decriminalization of sex work.

It is clear that while trans women may contract HIV through the same proximal behavioural risks as cisgender women, primarily through sexual contact and shared needle use, the HIV-related needs of trans women cannot be understood or addressed without consideration of the structural and psychosocial contexts in which these behaviours occur. Expecting individual trans women to make health-preserving decisions in the face of counteracting pressures would demand an unrealistic type of resiliency. Continued help-seeking may not be rational, if sources for the information one needs do not exist or access to services is problematic. The existence of urgent financial, social, or emotional needs may demand solutions that eclipse the prioritization of one's long-term health and well-being. Removing structural barriers provides an opportunity to create inclusive social structures within which healthy decision making will be both rational and possible.

PROBLEM-BASED LEARNING CASE STUDY

The community health centre at which you work has recently identified trans patients as a priority population. You have been named Program Director for Trans Programs, and charged with leading the development or revision of programs to better serve the needs of trans patients; HIV has been identified as one of the health issues to be addressed in the course of primary care. Your health centre employs doctors, nurses (including nurse practitioners), social workers, community health educators, a psychologist, and medical receptionists and takes an inter-professional collaborative approach to primary care. Your centre also serves as your community's local site for anonymous HIV testing, and the testing clinic employs additional nurses and HIV testing counsellors.

CRITICAL THINKING QUESTIONS

1. What are your first steps as the new Program Director to address the needs of trans patients?
2. What opportunities exist for HIV prevention for trans women within your community health centre?
3. How would you involve local trans community members in the development of your program?

GLOSSARY

Cisgender: One whose gender identity is consistent with the sex they were assigned at birth.

Gender expression: The way a person presents themselves as a man, a woman, or an alternate or blended gender.

Gender identity: The inherent sense each person has of being a man, a woman, neither a man nor a woman, or of being in some way both a man and a woman.

Genderqueer: An alternate gender identity that rejects the binary classifications of man and woman.

Sex: Refers to physiologic markers of biological sex, including aspects such as genitalia, chromosomes, and sex hormones.

Trans or transgender: A broad umbrella term encompassing those whose gender identity diverges from the sex they were assigned at birth. Trans people may identify as transgender, transsexual, two-spirit, bigender, genderqueer, or simply as a man or woman with a history of transitioning sex or gender.

Transsexual: One who lives, or desires to live, as the sex other than the one he or she was assigned at birth. Many transsexual people transition sex medically through the use of hormones and/or surgery.

Two-spirit: Aboriginal term that applies to those who have both a male and a female spirit, some of whom fit under the umbrella of "trans," and some of whom may be cisgender members of sexual minority groups such as gay, lesbian, or bisexual people.

REFERENCES

2-Spirited People of the 1st Nations. (2008). *Our relatives said: A wise practices guide, voices of Aboriginal trans people.* Retrieved from www.2spirits.com

Bauer, G. (2009, April). Trans women and HIV. In J. Gahagan (Chair), *Women and HIV in Canada: The past, the present and the future.* Pre-conference symposium at the 18th Annual Canadian Conference on HIV/AIDS Research, Vancouver, BC.

Bauer, G., Boyce, M., Coleman, T., Kaay, M., Scanlon, K., & Travers, R. (2010, July). Who are trans people in Ontario? *Trans PULSE E-Bulletin, 1*(1). Retrieved from http://transpulseproject.ca/documents/E1English.pdf

Bauer, G. R., Hammond, R., Travers, R., Kaay, M., Hohenadel, K. M., & Boyce, M. (2009). "I don't think this is theoretical; this is our lives." How erasure impacts health care for transgender people. *Journal of the Association of Nurses in AIDS Care, 20*(5), 348–361.

Bauer, G., Nussbaum, N., Travers, R., Munro, L., Pyne, J., & Redman, N. (2011, May). We've got work to do: Workplace discrimination and employment challenges for trans people in Ontario. *Trans PULSE E-Bulletin, 2*(1). Retrieved from http://transpulseproject.ca/documents/E3English.pdf

Bauer, G. R., Travers, R., Scanlon, K., & Coleman, T. A. (2012). High heterogeneity of HIV-related sexual risk among transgender people in Ontario, Canada: A province-wide respondent-driven sampling survey. Manuscript in preparation.

Bockting, W. O., Robinson, B. E., & Rosser, B. R. S. (1998). Transgender HIV prevention: A qualitative needs assessment. *AIDS Care, 10*(4), 505–526.

Bockting, W. O., Rosser, B. R. S., & Coleman, E. (2001). Transgender HIV prevention: Community involvement and empowerment. In W. O. Bockting & S. Kirk (Eds.), *Transgender and HIV: Risks, prevention, and care* (pp. 119–144). Binghamton, NY: Haworth Press.

Canadian Aboriginal AIDS Network. (2009, March). *Aboriginal strategy on HIV/AIDS in Canada II.* Retrieved from www.caan.ca/national-aboriginal-strategies/strategies/

Clements-Nolle, K., Marx, R., Guzman, R., & Katz, M. (2001). HIV prevalence, risk behaviors, health care use, and mental health status of transgender persons: Implications for public health intervention. *American Journal of Public Health, 91*(6), 915–921.

Coan, D. L., Schrager, W., & Packer, T. (2005). The role of male sexual partners in HIV infection among male-to-female transgendered individuals. In W. O. Bockting & E. Avery (Eds.), *Transgender health and HIV prevention: Needs assessment studies from transgender communities across the United States* (pp. 21–30). Binghamton, NY: Haworth Medical Press.

De Santis, J. P., Martin, C. W., & Lester, A. (2010). An educational program on HIV prevention for male-to-female transgender women in South Miami Beach, Florida. *Journal of the Association of Nurses in AIDS Care, 21*(3), 265–271.

Grant, J. M., Mottet, L. A., Tannis J., Herman, J. L., Harrison, J., & Keisling, M. (2010, October). *National Transgender Discrimination Survey report on health and health care.* National Center for Transgender Equality & National Gay and Lesbian Task Force. Retrieved from http://transequality.org/PDFs/NTDSReportonHealth_final.pdf

Hammond, R. (2010). *The social organization of health care for trans youth in Ontario* (Unpublished master's thesis). Dalhousie University, Halifax, NS.

Hammond, R., Redman, N., Bauer, G., Travers, R., & Coleman, T. (2010, November). HIV-related behavioural risk in Ontario's trans communities: Trans PULSE Project. Poster presented at the Ontario HIV Treatment Network Research Conference, Toronto, ON.

Hein, D., & Kirk, M. (2001). Education and soul-searching: The Enterprise HIV Prevention Group. In W. O. Bockting & S. Kirk (Eds.), *Transgender and HIV: Risks, prevention, and care* (pp. 101–118). Binghamton, NY: Haworth Press.

Herbst, J. H., Jacobs, E. D., Finlayson, T. J., McKleroy, V. S., Neumann, M. S., & Crepaz, N. (2008). Estimating HIV prevalence and risk behaviors of transgender persons in the United States: A systematic review. *AIDS and Behavior, 12*(1), 1–17.

Kammerer, N., Mason, T., Connors, M., & Durkee, R. (2001). Transgender health and social service needs in the context of HIV risk. In W. O. Bockting & S. Kirk (Eds.), *Transgender and HIV: Risks, prevention, and care* (pp. 39–58). Binghamton, NY: Haworth Press.

Lev, A. I. (2004). *Transgender emergence: Therapeutic guidelines for working with gender-variant people and their families.* Binghamton, NY: Haworth Press.

Lombardi, E. (2007). Substance use treatment experiences of transgender/transsexual men and women. *Journal of Lesbian, Gay, Bisexual and Transgender Health Research, 3*(2), 37–47.

Lombardi, E. (2009). Varieties of transgender/transsexual lives and their relationship with transphobia. *Journal of Homosexuality, 56*(8), 977–992.

Lombardi, E. L., Wilchins, R. A., Priesing, D., & Malouf, D. (2001). Gender violence: Transgender experiences with violence and discrimination. *Journal of Homosexuality, 42*(1), 89–101.

Martikainen, P., Bartley, M., & Lahelma, E. (2002). Psychosocial determinants of health in social epidemiology [Editorial]. *International Journal of Epidemiology*, 31, 1091–1093.

Melendez, R. M., & Pinto, R. M. (2009). HIV prevention and primary care for transgender women in a community-based clinic. *Journal of the Association of Nurses in AIDS Care, 20*(5), 387–397.

Namaste, V., Forrester, M., Hamilton, J. L., & Ross, M-S. (2005). In V. Namaste (Ed.), *Sex change, social change: Reflections on identity, institutions, and imperialism* (pp. 82–85). Toronto, ON: Women's Press.

Namaste, V. K. (2000). *Invisible lives.* Chicago, IL: University of Chicago Press.

National Center for Transgender Equality, & National Gay and Lesbian Task Force. (2009, November). *National Transgender Discrimination Survey: Preliminary findings.* Retrieved from http://transequality.org/Resources/NCTE_prelim_survey_econ.pdf

Nemoto, T., Operario, D., Keatley, J., Han, L., & Soma, T. (2004). HIV risk behaviors among male-to-female transgender persons of color in San Francisco. *American Journal of Public Health, 94*(4), 1193–1199.

Nemoto, T., Operario, D., Keatley, J., & Villegas, D. (2004). Social context of HIV risk behaviours among male-to-female transgenders of colour. *AIDS Care, 16*(6), 724–735.

Nussbaum, N. N. (2010). Human rights and common transgender employment law issues. In M. J. MacKillop & C. M. Thomlinson (Chairs), *The Six-Minute Employment Lawyer 2010* (pp. 8-1–8-17). Toronto, ON: Law Society of Upper Canada.

Nuttbrock, L., Hwahng, S., Bockting, W., Rosenblum, A., Mason, M., Macri, M., & Becker, J. (2010). Psychiatric impact of gender-related abuse across the life course of male-to-female transgender persons. *Journal of Sex Research, 47*(1), 12–23.

Operario, D., Soma, T., & Underhill, K. (2008). Sex work and HIV status among transgender women: Systematic review and meta-analysis. *Journal of Acquired Immune Deficiency Syndromes, 48*(1), 97–103.

Raphael, D. (2004). Introduction to the social determinants of health. In D. Raphael (Ed.), *Social determinants of health: Canadian perspectives.* Toronto, ON: Canadian Scholars' Press.

Rosser, B. R. S., Oakes, J. M., Bockting, W. O., & Miner, M. (2007). Capturing the social demographics of hidden sexual minorities: An Internet study of the transgender population in the United States. *Sexuality Research & Social Policy, 4*(2), 50–64.

Rotondi, N. K., Bauer, G. R., Travers, R., Travers, A., Scanlon, K., & Kaay, M. (2011). Depression in male-to-female transgender Ontarians: Results from the Trans PULSE Project. *Canadian Journal of Community Mental Health, 30*(2), 113–133.

Scanlon, K., Bauer, G., Travers, R., Boyce, M., & Coleman, T. (2010, November). Ontario's trans communities and suicide: Transphobia is bad for our health. *Trans PULSE E-Bulletin, 1*(2). Retrieved from http://transpulseproject.ca/documents/E2English.pdf

Scott, A. V., & Lines, R. (1999, May). *HIV/AIDS in the male-to-female transsexual and transgendered prison population: A comprehensive strategy* [Policy brief]. Toronto, ON: Prisoners' HIV/AIDS Support Action Network. Retrieved from www.heart-intl.net/HEART/030106/HIVAIDSintheMaletoFemale.pdf

Serano, J. (2007). *Whipping girl: A transsexual woman on sexism and the scapegoating of femininity.* Emeryville, CA: Seal Press.

Sugano, E., Nemoto, T., & Operario, D. (2006). The impact of exposure to transphobia on HIV risk behavior in a sample of transgendered women of color in San Francisco. *AIDS and Behavior, 10*(2), 217–224.

Taylor, C. (2006, October). *Nowhere near enough: A needs assessment of health and safety services for transgender and two spirit people in Manitoba and Northwestern Ontario.* Retrieved from www.turtleisland.org/healing/transgender.doc

Warren, B. E. (2001). Sex, truth, and videotape: HIV prevention at the Gender Identity Project in New York City. In W. O. Bockting & S. Kirk (Eds.), *Transgender and HIV: Risks, prevention, and care* (pp. 145–151). Binghamton, NY: Haworth Press.

Williamson, C. (2010). Providing care to transgender persons: A clinical approach to primary care, hormones, and HIV management. *Journal of the Association of Nurses in AIDS Care, 21*(3), 221–229.

World Health Organization. (1986, November). *Ottawa charter for health promotion: An international conference on health promotion.* Retrieved from www.phac-aspc.gc.ca/ph-sp/docs/charter-chartre/index-eng.php

Xavier, J., Honnold, J. A., & Bradford, J. (2007). *The health, health-related needs, and lifecourse experiences of transgender Virginians.* Retrieved from www.vdh.state.va.us/epidemiology/DiseasePrevention/documents/pdf/THISFINALREPORTVol1.pdf

Chapter 8
RAZORS, RIGS, AND RIGHTS: HIV PREVENTION AND THE CASE FOR HARM REDUCTION STRATEGIES IN WOMEN'S PRISONS

Rai Reece

INTRODUCTION

In Canada, the prevalence rates of HIV transmission among women prisoners are considerably higher than those of the general population at large (AIDS Calgary Awareness Association, 2007), and HIV and hepatitis C (HCV) prevalence for women prisoners exceeds that of male prisoners (Canadian HIV/AIDS Legal Network, 2008). The systemic disavowal of implementing community standards of HIV and HCV prevention measures for women prisoners has resulted in a lack of coordinated response. This has also led to the dismissal of the reality of HIV/AIDS and injection drug use within Canadian penal institutions for women. Globally, prison needle and syringe exchange programs (PNSEP) have been introduced in 11 countries. However, the Canadian government and correctional ministries have yet to respond to the call from activists, researchers, and prisoners in regard to the impact that HIV/HCV and injection drug use has on prisoners, their families, and their communities. Particularly among women prisoners, an often overlooked population, research has indicated that prevention and education programming grounded in harm reduction methodologies can reduce the transmission of HIV/HCV and foster an environment where prisoners are given the chance to become more proactive about their health. Using feminist epistemological methodologies, this chapter will examine the complexities of HIV/HCV prevention for incarcerated women and introduce readers to a multi-interdisciplinary approach to HIV prevention in the Canadian prison system for women.

EXACTING THE SOCIAL PROBLEM

A look at the treatment and punishment of women in prison in this country reflects attitudes of a paternalistic nature, never question-

> ing or challenging whether prisons are really a reasonable response
> to women's crime. It becomes obvious that the objective of women's
> prisons is to recreate and reinforce the subordination and submission
> of women according to the sexist [and racist] authority of patriarchy.
> (AIDS Calgary Awareness Association, 2007)

In Canada, there has been little feminist critical debate regarding the ongoing contestation of incarceration measures for incarcerated women. The punishment process in Canada takes its cues from the United States of America. The U.S. boasts a prison population that surpasses 2.3 million people (a rate of 730 per 100,000), while Canada's incarceration rate is 114 per 100,000 of the national population (International Centre for Prison Studies, 2009). American activists and scholars such as Angela Y. Davis (1971), Kimberlé Crenshaw (1989), Anne M. Butler (1997), and Nicole Hahn Rafter (1990) have explored the politics of incarceration in the American context. Their work has highlighted the importance of an intersectional analysis that takes into account key determinants of women's health, such as gender, "race," and class issues as they relate to female incarceration. Demographically, Canada and America differ in terms of population density; however, both countries have disproportionate numbers of Black and Indigenous women incarcerated. Although the percentage of women in prison is still very low compared to men, the rates are rapidly rising (Kurshan, 1999). In 2001, Black women in Canada made up 7.6% of the female prison population but accounted for less than 2% of the overall population. In America, during the same time period, Black women were three times as likely as Latina women and five times more likely than white women to be incarcerated. Moreover, the Canadian Association of Elizabeth Fry Societies (CAEFS) (2003) has documented the rising rates of admission of Black women to provincial custody in Ontario. Although this rate has been shown to be almost seven times that of white women (CAEFS, 2003), there still has not been substantial research or activist interest regarding the incarceration of Black women.

In a similar vein, the historical oppressive treatment of Indigenous people in general, and of Indigenous women specifically, has had serious implications for the policing and incarceration of Native communities. The legacy of colonialism and imperialism has ideologically informed the oppressive systemic and institutionalized oppression to which Indigenous people in Canada are subjected. In regard to punishment practices, this has led to a disproportionate number of Indigenous women serving time in Canadian prisons. According to the Canadian HIV/AIDS Legal Network (2008), "the overall incarceration rate for Aboriginal people in Canada is estimated to be 1,024 per 100,000 or almost 9 times higher for Aboriginal persons than for non-Aboriginal people." In the general Canadian population, women in prison, Black women, and Indigenous women are subgroups representing increasing rates of HIV infection (for further reading, see Canadian HIV/AIDS Legal Network, 2008; Public Health Agency of Canada, 2012).

Furthermore, this alarming situation of increasing rates of HIV transmission for women in prison disproportionately affects women of colour in the broader North American sense as well. Paula C. Johnson (2003) notes that, in America, "over two-thirds of women who are confined in local, state and federal institutions are women of color—mostly African American women" (p. 4). Similarly, Karlene Faith (1993) has argued that there are "increasing numbers of women of African heritage, from the United States and the Caribbean serving time [in Canadian prisons] on importing and trafficking convictions" (p. 184). In Canada, from 2004 to 2005, Aboriginal women accounted for 30% of women incarcerated in federal prisons (CAEFS, 2004), and in some provincial institutions, in regions such as Saskatchewan, Aboriginal women accounted for 87% of the entire women's provincial jail population (CAEFS, 2004). For both these groups of women, the trauma of incarceration is further exacerbated when HIV rates of transmission are on the rise. Therefore, North America represents a microcosmic glimpse of a wider global crisis. Canada and the United States are two countries, historically and contemporarily interconnected, where the number of incarcerated women of colour is directly affected by HIV transmission while incarcerated and is connected to their social and political locations in the broader societies. With this in mind, it stands to reason that if Black and Indigenous women represent increasing rates of HIV transmission in the general Canadian population, then within prison systems, they also make up a disproportionate number of HIV prevalence rates.

Rising rates of HIV transmission both within and outside of the prison system point to an increasing need for preventative measures that take into account ethnoracial understandings of health care, in particular how violence, poverty, racism, stigma, and discrimination impact HIV-positive racialized women. In regard to HIV transmission rates among Black and Indigenous women, a document produced by the Native Women's Association of Canada indicated that Indigenous women are three times more likely to be affected by HIV than non-Indigenous women (Native Women's Association of Canada, 2004). In a 2001 census, Black people accounted for 2.2% of Canada's population and 15.2% of AIDS cases (AVERT, 2012). The shared colonial histories of these two groups of women are indicative of the often forgotten realities of racism, classism, and cultural genocide perpetrated by the Canadian government. Moreover, this shared history is connected to our current social welfare policies that govern the provision of health care to ensure access to a minimum standard of health care for people living in poverty. Since there are a disproportionate number of Black and Indigenous women living in poverty and residing in lone-parent homes, it stands to reason that these two groups of women will have their health adversely affected by their social surroundings. In terms of poverty rates, according to a 2005 study, over 52.7% of unattached Black women are poor compared to 41.9% of all unattached women (Canadian Association of Social Workers, 2005); comparably, in 2005, the poverty rate for Indigenous women (including but not limited to Inuit, Métis, and First Nations women) was 36% (CAEFS, 2004).

According to the Canadian Human Rights Commission (CHRC) report, *Protecting Their Rights: A Systemic Review of Human Rights in Correctional Services for Federally Sentenced Women,* Indigenous women are disproportionately represented in federal prisons across Canada. Moreover, many women serving time in federal institutions in Canada are first-time prisoners, under the age of 35, and survivors of physical and sexual abuse (CHRC, 2003, p. 5). A majority of women in prison are mothers (or primary caregivers) and are struggling with substance use issues. The majority are economically disenfranchised, and poor, racialized women are often forced to make choices that detrimentally affect their lives. Therefore, the material conditions of women's lives, particularly for women of colour, intersect with a myriad of other social determinants of health both inside and outside the discursive politics of incarceration. For example, many women's economic realities are affected by underemployment or lack of employment. Gender and race, as key determinants of health, intersect with stigma and discrimination, making access to HIV prevention and treatment for women challenging at best.

As the Women's Prison Program Coordinator for a non-profit community-based agency, my work with incarcerated women for the past four years has brought significant insights, one of the most critical being the importance of building trust. In terms of HIV prevention program delivery, it is essential for community workers to work toward building trust with incarcerated women. Due to the nature of incarceration—the deprivation of liberty and the heightened reliance on surveillance and intrusion—many persons serving time in federal institutions may understandably be suspicious of outsiders who are intruding in their personal lives. Penal institutions do not adhere to the social rules of conduct or privacy that are associated with life on the outside. It is the business of prison officials to know what is going on at all times and with whom. The prison is designed to remind prisoners of their lack of social, psychological, and physical freedom. It is designed to survey and restrict. For those incarcerated, deprivation of liberty is psychically and physically determined by the prison system and defined as "normal." Michel Foucault (1977) referred to this disciplinary domain in which the human body is caught up in a system of deprivation: "What the apparatuses and institutions operate is, in a sense, a micro-physics of power, whose field of validity is situated in a sense between these great functionings and the bodies themselves with their materiality and their forces" (p. 26).

For persons who are incarcerated, deprivation of liberty may be understood in a number of ways. It can signal the end of one's freedom as understood in a capitalist society, where allegorical constraints of power and coercion are present in a covert sense—respective societies implement social and moral codes that are followed even though they may not be legislated as such. Deprivation of liberty can also mean the rearranging of power to suit life behind walls. This is what Foucault (1977) meant when he argued that power can manifest itself in a number of different and strategic ways. Within the prison system, power is diffuse; and power–knowledge relations are constituted within one another (Foucault, 1977, p. 27). The condemned body, then, is subject to "historical transformations" (Foucault, 1977, p. 28), and as the modern day gulag is set to reform the modern day "criminal," there is an investment in historical notions and understandings of punishment. That is to say, in an effort to rehabilitate the body, a historical reliance on rehabilitating the soul is paramount. Therefore the soul is "born rather out of methods of punishment, supervision and constraint" (Foucault, 1977, p. 29).

However, this chapter, grounded in feminist analysis, argues that prisons for women do not provide the resources for HIV/HCV prevention for women doing time. Traditional emphasis on "rehabilitating the soul" and "disease prevention" is based on Western patriarchal paradigms. Therefore, models of success for social reintegration and specifically HIV prevention are grounded in "abstinence-based" health care ideals. Where efforts have been made to address gender inequalities for the delivery of prison programming, harm reduction methodologies, including needle and syringe exchange programs, are not considered. A lack of harm reduction information and practical education strategies for reducing HIV/HCV transmission results in a disjuncture between the lived reality of those incarcerated and the ideological functioning of the prison as a "correctional" facility. In this sense, the reality of some prisoners' lives may involve having to deal with depression, drug use, mental health struggles, violence, racism, sexism, homophobia, and so forth. Being HIV positive or co-infected with HCV is compounded by these oppressions. However, since prisons prioritize security needs first and foremost, standards of health care are often compromised. Therefore, in many instances it becomes difficult for prisoners to feel empowered (by their own definitions) about their health while residing in carcerative spaces. Due to the lack of confidentiality, the subsequent fear of disclosure by prison officials or staff, or reprisal from other prisoners, incarcerated HIV-positive women often fear accessing services from health care staff units. This often makes the provision of HIV/AIDS education and prevention measures challenging for community workers and isolative for HIV-positive women.

Punishment Procedures for Women: How Prisons Exacerbate HIV Transmission

Incarceration processes for women in Canada have a long and sordid history. The first institution for "wayward" women in Canada was the Andrew Mercer Reformatory for Women, located in Toronto, Ontario. The reformatory, not officially called a prison, opened its doors in 1872. Using sex-gender stereotypes of women, the reform school for wayward young women and girls offered training in the area of obedience and servility. These Victorian ideals coupled with labour intensive jobs were designed to help rehabilitate "bad women" in need of reform. It is a misnomer to suggest that, as a reformatory, the Mercer institution relied on a steady diet of piety and kindness. Rather, the institution set the stage for the gendered division of labour seen in many women's prisons today, with the pretext still that of reforming "fallen women" via the confines of domestic duties. Based on these precepts, construction for the Prison for Women (P4W) in Kingston, Ontario, began in 1925. Over the years, allegations of sexual abuse and mistreatment would plague the prison. In 1938, the Archambault Commission recommended that the prison be closed. It was not until 66 years later that P4W would eventually close its doors. Having realized that P4W was not conducive to rehabilitation or social reintegration for women, the Task Force for Federally Sentenced Women was created. In 1990 they released the report *Creating Choices* and recommended that regional prisons be built for women. This document made recommendations for better care for incarcerated women who in some cases were working toward mental health, substance use recovery, and societal reintegration.

Clearly, punishment procedures for women were grounded in patriarchal definitions of "woman." What we see, then, is the creation of a system of punishment that does not take into account the particularities of women's lives. Carceral spaces are traditionally spaces created to warehouse men. The historical ideal of punishment as "reform" has contemporary ramifications for how women prisoners are treated. The number of women in prison in Canada is low compared to men; most women in prison are incarcerated for non-violent offences (CAEFS, 2004); and overall police-reported crime rates in Canada are declining (Wallace, 2009). Despite this, the number of women entering prisons is increasing (CAEFS, 2004). Moreover, although the turnover rate for women in provincial jails tends to be more frequent—due to the criminalization of sex work and drug use—the rate of recidivism for federally sentenced women is approximately 21% compared to 59% for men (Canadian Human Rights Commission, as cited in CAEFS, 2004), and approximately 1–2% of federally sentenced women return to prison for committing new crimes; of these, less than 0.5% are for a violent offence (CAEFS, 2004). Given these statistics, punishment procedures for women ought to take into account the realities of women's lives and not heterosexist ideals of reintegration based on cognitive male behavioural models.

Women prisoners should have access to the same resources, including HIV prevention resources, as their male counterparts. In addition, due to the fact that an overwhelming number of women prisoners have experienced some form of physical, mental, and emotional abuse, specific care- and community-based supports should be in place for women prisoners. For example, the United Nations Office on Drugs and Crime has argued that the majority of women in prison are members of marginalized groups experiencing oppression based on sexual orientation, race, class, substance use, violence, and so forth (Canadian HIV/AIDS Legal Network, 2008). As such, HIV-positive women require specialized services that are implemented and governed by best practice guidelines akin to the social determinants of health. This means working to increase HIV prevention and education, HIV testing, pre- and post-test counselling, and implementing harm reduction materials in concrete, systematic ways for incarcerated women.

Cost-Effective Care and Evidence-Based Research?

The Canadian government commissioned the Canadian Committee on Corrections (1969) to conduct a study of the criminal justice system (Johnson, 2003). The *Report of the Canadian Committee on Corrections* came to be known as the Ouimet Report, and it specifically outlined what direction penology in Canada should take. However, because the custody of prisoners is divided between federal and provincial governments, correctional institutions are governed under two different jurisdictions. Provincial jails and detention centres are managed by the Ministry of Community Safety and Correctional Services, and federal penitentiaries (prisons) are managed by the Correctional Service of Canada. The implementation and delivery of health care services follow different conditions and protocols: "a number of correctional programs in Canada are administered on the basis of federal/provincial agreements and cost-sharing schemes generated out of bilateral or multilateral discussions between the federal and provincial governments" (Ekstedt & Griffiths, 1988, p. 72). To "cost-share" effectively, the Ouimet Report designed a model of reformation based intrinsically on community corrections. The report (1969) stated that unless

> there are reasons to the contrary, the correction of an offender (*sic*) should take place in the community, where the acceptance of a treatment relationship is more natural, where family and social relationships can be maintained ... through involvement rather than confinement. (Cited in Ekstedt & Griffiths, 1988, pp. 100–101)

Many of the principles governing the Correctional Service of Canada were rooted in the philosophical idea of community involvement. However, this idea of "cost sharing" does not take into consideration the material conditions of women's lives. For example, many women in prison experience shame and stigma associated with having a criminal record, loss of their children to social services, and separation from family support networks. These matters are further complicated when women are serving time and attempting to prevent HIV infection, or are currently living with HIV within the prison system. Despite the findings of the Ouimet Report, harm reduction practices are not new to Canadian prisons. As outlined in a comprehensive report by the Canadian HIV/AIDS Legal Network (2008), condoms, bleach, and methadone maintenance treatment are available in Canadian federal prisons. However, despite their presence, many women in prison do not receive treatment for HIV transmission as early as incarcerated men (Canadian HIV/AIDS Legal Network, 2008). Women who are housed in smaller units inside men's prisons, who struggle with mental health issues, and who use injection drugs are often unaware of their HIV status until incarcerated. Furthermore, at the point of entry into a prison, many women are unaware that HIV testing is not mandatory. They submit to testing without prior knowledge that there is no pre- or post-test counselling in place to support them through their diagnosis and results—regardless of whether or not these results are negative or positive (Csete, 2005).

In terms of legislative policy, as of 1992 the primary legislation governing the Correctional Service of Canada and the National Parole Board is the *Corrections and Conditional Release Act* (CCRA). Under the Act, the purpose of the federal correctional system is to contribute to the maintenance of a just, peaceful and safe society by: *(a)* "carrying out sentences imposed by courts through the safe and humane custody and supervision of offenders; and *(b)* assisting the rehabilitation of offenders and their reintegration into the community as law-abiding citizens through the provision of programs in penitentiaries and in the community" (CCRA, 1992, sec. 3).

The Correctional Service of Canada (CSC) argues that one of its main functions is in the central role of risk assessment and rehabilitation in law. What is missing from this process is an understanding of the effectual realities of women's lives in regard to incarceration and harm reduction. In particular, women who inject drugs are often experiencing other chronic health conditions or conditions that impact their health, such as hepatitis C, poverty, and violence. This means that HIV testing may not be a priority for women who are struggling each day to survive. As such, women who are exposed to HIV are often unaware of their status and uninformed about testing, prevention, and counselling services available to them (Canadian HIV/AIDS Legal Network, 2008). The CSC, along with the Canadian judicial system, purports to work to protect the best interests of society. However, a critical analysis of rehabilitation and reintegration processes for women in prison examines why this is not an accurate statement. Understanding rehabilitation as grounded in harm reduction philosophy is imperative to integrating theory and praxis in working toward reducing the rates of HIV transmission in women's prisons.

Evidence-based research has indicated that HIV transmission rates among women in the general Canadian population is on the rise (Canadian HIV/AIDS Legal Network, 2008; Canadian Women's Health Network, 2005). In 2005, women accounted for approximately 27% of all new HIV infections, an increase from approximately 24% in 2002 (Boulos, Yan, Schanzer, Remis, & Archibald, 2006). As mentioned earlier, of these cases, a disproportionate number of new HIV infections are found in Black and Indigenous women. Moreover, the two most common risk factors for HIV transmission for women continue to be heterosexual contact and injection drug use.

In 2008, the HIV prevalence rate for incarcerated women was 4.71% compared to 1.6% for men (Correctional Service of Canada, 2012, as cited in PHAC, 2012). Although the disparity between rates of infection for men and women continues to be high, little attention is paid to HIV prevention and harm reduction strategies for women in prison. To address this glaring systemic omission, the Prisoner's HIV/AIDS Support Action Network (PASAN) published a document highlighting the explicit need for HIV prevention strategies and harm reduction practices to be made available for incarcerated women. The document, *Unlocking our Futures: A National Study on*

Women, Prisons, HIV and Hepatitis C (DiCenso, Dias, & Gahagan, 2003), was the first of its kind to specifically address the rising rates of HIV/HCV infection among women prisoners in Canada. Furthermore, by extensively interviewing women in prison, PASAN documented not only that the prevalence of HIV infection among incarcerated women was higher than among incarcerated men serving time in Canadian prisons, but also that women who engage in cutting or slashing and injection drug use, and who struggle with mental health needs, were at greater risk for HIV transmission behind bars. Women in the study cited lack of confidentiality, inadequate nutrition, lack of availability of doctors and nurses who specialize in HIV knowledge, no pre- or post-test counselling, and fear of disclosure as some of their central concerns regarding HIV information and support while in prison (Csete, 2005). The results from this study underscored what many in community-based health care settings already knew—that the evisceration of the social determinants of health affect the most marginal populations in our social environment, and that an emphasis on continuity of care for marginal populations (incarcerated women, racialized women, women sex workers, trans women) are minimal and discriminatory at best, and have long-term detrimental social effects on women's overall health.

HARM REDUCTION

In order to contextualize the significance of HIV prevention and harm reduction strategies for women in prison from a Canadian perspective, an analysis in a broader North American context is necessary to first examine how worldwide globalization processes detrimentally affect women in prison. According to the International Centre for Prison Studies, "[i]n 2005 … on any given date more than half a million women and girls were detained in prisons, either awaiting trial or serving sentences" (United Nations Office on Drugs and Crime, 2008). Furthermore, it has been noted by the Canadian Association of Elizabeth Fry Societies that "the fastest growing prison population worldwide is women, and in particular racialized, young poor women and women with mental disabilities" (CAEFS, 2004). Incarceration of women in Canada and the United States has risen to an alarming rate, with nearly the majority of those incarcerated being women of colour. Specifically, in the U.S. a report released by the Justice Department stated that "the number of women in state and federal prisons is at an all-time high and growing fast, with the rate of increase nearly twice that of men" (Greenfield & Snell, 1999). Globalization processes have affected women's economic sustainability in detrimental ways, leaving many women poverty-stricken. As such, the pervasive economic and social conditions that contribute to high incarceration rates, such as poverty, violence against women, and mental health issues, should not be ignored. Moreover, the Canadian Association of Elizabeth Fry Societies notes that an increase in the numbers of incarcerated women "is clearly linked to the evisceration of health, education, and social services" (CAEFS, 2004). Thus, in our current global environment, the marginalized position of women in regard to their lack of economic, political, and social resources can be seen as a contributing factor related to the disproportionate number of incarcerated women.

In response to these issues faced by women in prison, harm reduction approaches show great promise in mitigating HIV/HCV infection rates. Harm reduction refers to the philosophical understanding that people have the right to make choices and control their involvement in activities in regard to their health and well-being. Specifically, harm reduction practices respect the right of people to choose when and how they reduce harm while engaging in particular activities, such as drug use or sexual activity. Providing people with information about safer sex rather than abstinence-based knowledge is one example of how harm reduction can work. Another example is respecting someone's right to use drugs, and equipping them with unused syringes or needles and providing a safe way to dispose of them. Harm reduction practices and principles are enacted without judgment about the choices people make in their lives. Moreover, harm reduction philosophies recognize that the particularities of people's lives may not make room for abstinence.

Understanding the practicality of harm reduction principles and practices as particular to the realities of incarcerated women warrants further study, not only because HIV rates of transmission tend to be higher for women in prison than for men, but also because the prevalence rates of hepatitis C also tend to be higher among incarcerated women (Canadian HIV/AIDS Legal Network, 2008). As noted above, a lack of education about HIV transmission and the implementation of harm reduction strategies negatively affects two groups of women already disproportionately represented in Canadian prisons, namely Aboriginal and Black women. Since Health Canada has identified these two groups of women as particularly vulnerable to HIV transmission, and because these two groups of women are disproportionately affected by incarceration, they are in turn increasingly at risk for HCV transmission as well.

Reducing Harm: A Brief Examination of Community-Based Harm Reduction Services

Community-based AIDS Service Organizations (ASOs) began to notice the disturbing trend of HCV co-infection with HIV particularly among injection drug users (IDUs) in the general Canadian population. The Correctional Service of Canada has also noted the particularly high HCV prevalence rate among prisoners, and co-infection rates of HIV and HCV tend to be higher for people injecting drugs in prison (Canadian HIV/AIDS Legal Network, 2008). Many incarcerated women may not be familiar with safety precautions regarding safer injection use, since it is not uncommon for women who inject drugs to be sharing needles or syringes with their male partner or to have their male partner inject drugs for them. A history of assisted injection outside of prison detrimentally affects women's drug use in prison, since many women may not be aware of the associated risks for HIV/HCV transmission behind prison walls. Due to the high prevalence of HCV and HIV/HCV co-infection rates among prisoners, there is a need for the implementation of harm reduction strategies in prisons to address both HIV and HCV transmission. Access to HIV prevention and education differs for women inside and outside of prison.

Outside of prisons, harm reduction resources can be found in community health centres, ASOs, or street health services. These resources can range from distribution of safer crack kits, unused (clean) needles and syringes, condoms, and dental dams, to literature that details how and where to safely inject on one's body, and how to treat and take care of veins and/or abscesses if they occur. Although drug use is still criminalized in Canada, a move toward safer injection sites for IDUs has been called for (for further reading, see Elliot, Malkin, & Gold, 2002; Kerr & Palepu, 2001). In Vancouver, British Columbia—a city that at one time had the highest reported rate of new HIV infections for IDU (Broadhead, Kerr, Grund, & Altice, 2002), North America's first supervised injection site, InSite, opened its doors. Although InSite operates under federal rules that allow it to function as a research project (Drucker, 2006), the facility offers a health-focused space where IDUs can inject drugs safely and also connect with health care services such as addictions counselling and treatment for disease and infection (Vancouver Coastal Health, n.d.). Also referred to as safer injection facilities (SIFs), there are SIFs operating in a number of countries: "Germany with 13 SIFs operating in 4 cities; The Netherlands with 16 SIFs operating in 9 cities; Switzerland with 17 SIFs operating in 12 cities; Spain with 1 SIF operating in Madrid" (Broadhead et al., 2002, p. 331). There are 19 SIFs operating in Western Europe and, in 2001, an SIF opened in Sydney, Australia (Broadhead et al., 2002). Researchers have argued that governmentally sanctioned SIFs add an additional societal health service connected to "much larger comprehensive public health approaches to reduce drug-related harm" (Broadhead et al., 2002, p. 332). Canada has one of the highest rates of new HIV infections among IDUs. Proponents argue that SIFs can provide greater services to IDUs in areas where street outreach and needle exchange programs fall short, such as in "(1) reducing rates of drug injection and related-risks in public spaces; (2) placing injectors in more direct and timely contact with medical care, drug treatment, counseling, and other social services; (3) reducing the volume of injectors' discarded litter in, and expropriation of, public spaces" (Broadhead et al., 2002, p. 329).

While SIFs can greatly reduce the harm associated with injecting, the facilities may fall short in continuity of care for women IDUs. While some facilities may provide gynecological and prenatal health care for women injectors (Broadhead et al., 2002), Vancouver's SIF does not allow for assisted injecting (Csete, 2005). Women with a history of assisted injecting are reluctant to use a facility where this is prohibited, putting them at risk for unsafe injection use (Kerr, Wood, Small, Palepu, & Tyndall, 2003). In addition, Boyd and Faith (1999) assert that women drug users who are pregnant may be reluctant to access medical care for fear of being reported to law enforcement authorities or children's services (Csete, 2005). In light of this, SIFs should take into account gender-variant and gender-based program requirements and delivery of service. In order for harm reduction services to work, they must take into account the particularities of women's lives as connected to the social determinants of health and be ethnoracially relevant to women's lives.

Razors and Rigs: Harm Reduction Practices Inside Prisons

Inside federal prisons in Canada, harm reduction materials in the form of condoms, dental dams, and bleach have been made available. In provincial institutions, there are restrictions around access and use of these items. For example, there is no access to bleach for persons housed in provincial institutions, and access to dentals dams (in women facilities only) and condoms and lubricant (in both men's and women's facilities) is administered by the health care unit. Due to the fact that sexual activity is prohibited in provincial and federal institutions, and homophobia is rampant, prisoners are often reluctant to request these items. Furthermore, due to the fear of being labelled an IDU inside prison, many women and men do not ask for bleach. Many who do access bleach do not know that, due to the potency of HCV, bleach will not kill the virus.

Activities inside prisons that can transmit HIV and HCV include unprotected sexual intercourse, injection drug use, cutting and slashing, tattooing, and sharing razors, needles (rigs), and/or nail clippers. These activities are prohibited in prisons, and many are performed with discretion. Due to a lack of information around HIV/HCV transmission, prisoner knowledge is often not transferable in terms of practicality. For example, due to the relatively small numbers of incarcerated women, and for women housed in smaller units inside men's institutions, access to HIV/HCV prevention information is not prioritized. Therefore, the knowledge of HIV/HCV prevention for women who might engage in cutting and slashing may be inaccurate, putting them at risk for transmission. Furthermore, for HIV-positive women doing time, fear of rejection by other prisoners, and fear of disclosure by prison authorities about their HIV/HCV status, make it difficult for them to access medical care in a confidential manner.

Harm reduction practices in prison do not take into account the fact that the majority of women prisoners are doing time for drug-related charges. Addictions are a health issue, and prisoner health is a public health issue. For women in prison, the intersection of multiple oppressions, such as racism, sexism, violence, and mental health issues, makes it difficult to access harm reduction information. For women outside of prison, chronic health conditions cannot be combatted when women live in poverty and the social determinants of health cannot be met. In Canada, our current social welfare system still penalizes women who use drugs in terms of their access to shelters or treatment facilities, since harm reduction practices are often not allowed (Csete, 2005). In addition, the criminalization of sex work and drug use targets women who use drugs, and makes them more vulnerable to discriminatory treatment by the legal system. This may result in women isolating themselves from community services that can assist them in regard to HIV/HCV prevention, treatment, and self-care.

Coordinating Services for HIV/AIDS

The Public Health Agency of Canada (PHAC) is responsible for coordinating the federal initiative to address HIV/AIDS in Canada (PHAC, 2012). In terms of partnerships, the CSC receives money from the federal initiative on HIV/AIDS to address and combat the rising rates of HIV transmission in prisons. It was estimated that the CSC was to receive an annual budget of about $4.2 million for HIV/AIDS programs in federal prisons by 2009 (Csete, 2005). As part of the mandate of this initiative, PHAC will be developing a status report to guide policy, research, and programming, as well as focusing on HIV prevention services (PHAC, 2012). To address the disconnect between policy and practice in relation to HIV prevention for prisoners, PHAC has partnered with community agencies to work toward effective coordination of services for the incarcerated and formerly incarcerated. One such community-based agency working with HIV-positive and co-infected prisoners and ex-prisoners is the Prisoners HIV/AIDS Support Action Network (PASAN). PASAN is currently the only AIDS Service Organization in Canada working exclusively with HIV-positive prisoners and ex-prisoners. The agency's philosophy around working with prison populations is grounded in harm reduction practices. Of particular note is the fact that PASAN has been around for over 20 years and is not funded by the Correctional Service of Canada. Because PASAN is an HIV advocacy, prevention, and human rights organization, receiving program funding from the CSC would prove contentious and be a conflict of interest in terms of the work that the agency does. Moreover, given the connections that PASAN staff make with prisoners while working with them one-on-one or in groups, educational settings would be compromised if the agency were fiscally tied to the CSC. With funding from PHAC, the Canadian HIV/AIDS Network and PASAN published a seminal document called *Hard Time: HIV and Hepatitis C Prevention Programming for Prisoners in Canada*. Published in December 2007, the document outlines best practice prison-based programming for the prevention of HIV and HCV transmission (Canadian HIV/AIDS Network & PASAN, 2007).

As part of the federal initiative, Correctional Services Canada also has a mandate to partner with community-based agencies that address the need for HIV prevention and support services (PHAC, 2012). In this regard, PASAN has been accessing federal institutions to provide HIV/HCV prevention education and intervention to prisoners. It should be noted that PASAN also has a long-standing partnership with the Ministry of Community Safety and Correctional Services to provide HIV/HCV education and information in provincial institutions as well. In my capacity as the Women's Prison Program Coordinator at PASAN, I facilitate group and one-on-one HIV/AIDS/HCV sexual health education workshops in provincial and federal women's institutions.

I conduct these education workshops on a regular basis in an effort to address many of the salient issues that affect incarcerated women, as well as those who are ex-prisoners. The educational workshops that I facilitate provide incarcerated women with the opportunity to engage in open and frank discussions about HIV/AIDS/HCV and allow women to engage in a participatory manner regarding their health needs. Most importantly the workshops are conducted without the presence of correctional staff, as this deters women from participating fully in the workshops. The goals of the workshops are to provide women-specific/identified HIV/HCV prevention education and information in regard to harm reduction for women while incarcerated and also post-release.

My experience in working with incarcerated women has highlighted the exigent need for a more coordinated response to their needs around HIV/HCV prevention. In many cases, women are not only dealing with HIV diagnosis while incarcerated, but their fears around HIV in particular are exacerbated by other social conditions in their lives. For women who may receive an HIV-positive diagnosis while behind bars, a myriad of questions arise: Will access to my child/ren be restricted? Will my status be revealed? Will I be subject to violence inside prison or upon my release? These are just some of the salient concerns that affect women diagnosed with HIV in prison. Furthermore, with the increasing emphasis on the criminalization of HIV non-disclosure, women are either less likely to be tested for HIV, or, for those who may be HIV positive, to reveal their status to other prisoners or prison staff. This results in a lack of support and access to health care due to the possible backlash of stigma and discrimination.

Under the *Corrections and Conditional Release Act* (CCRA), the CSC is responsible for providing "every inmate (*sic*) with essential health care and reasonable access to non-essential mental health care that will contribute to the inmate's (*sic*) rehabilitation and successful reintegration in the community" (Correctional Service of Canada, 2010). However, the provision of services in regard to HIV prevention for women in prison requires specific attention. Federal initiatives that seek to address the rising rates of HIV/HCV transmission for women ought to implement more programs and education for women that specifically addresses HIV prevention (Csete, 2005) and harm reduction strategies. The reality for some women in prison does include drug use and cutting and slashing. To negate and/or ignore this is akin to violating fundamental human rights. Women prisoners who are given the opportunity to become decision makers in regard to their health in turn become more proactive and knowledgeable about their health care needs. This also means that once women return to their respective home communities, they take that knowledge with them.

A Brief Look at Prison Needle and Syringe Exchange Programs (PNSEPs)

Unfortunately, many prison administrators view harm reduction strategies such as prison needle and syringe exchange programs (PNSEPs) as drug promotion, which may lead to security risks. Globally, as of February 2009, PNSEPs have been introduced in over 60 prisons in at least 11 countries: Switzerland, Belarus, Germany, Armenia, Spain, Luxembourg, Moldova, Iran, Portugal, Romania, and Kyrgyzstan (Lines et al., 2006). To date there has not been any report of needles or syringes being used as weapons, or any other negative occurrences related to the implementation of these programs. However, Canada lags behind in terms of the implementation of PNSEPs. Unfortunately, the relationship between injection drug use and prison is a close one for people who use injection drugs, due to the criminalization of drug use; many IDUs have had some experience with the Canadian criminal justice system. For women who engage in sex work and/or who use drugs, the reality of incarceration means that they are further caught up in a system of restraints that make them vulnerable to HIV transmission. Some women who have injected drugs prior to incarceration will continue to do so, while women who may have never used drugs outside of prison may begin to inject once incarcerated (United Nations Office on Drugs and Crime, 2008).

PNSEPs in other countries have been shown to greatly reduce the incidence of HIV/HCV transmission and to be a proven prevention strategy for HIV/HCV. The document *Clean Switch: The Case for Prison Needle and Syringe Programs in Canada* offers a compelling argument for the implementation of PNSEPs in Canadian prisons (Chu & Elliot, 2009). Citing section 7 of the Canadian Charter of Rights and Freedoms, the authors demonstrate that the Canadian government has a duty and obligation under the Charter to protect everyone's right to life, liberty, and security of the person. The Charter protects everyone's right to "life, liberty and security of the person and the right not to be deprived thereof except in accordance with the principles of fundamental justice" (Chu & Elliot, 2009, p. 13) and this right extends to persons who are incarcerated. Although in prison, people still retain all Charter rights afforded to them. However, with increasing political law-and-order agendas, there has been a conservative shift toward amending the Charter to quash the rights of federally incarcerated prisoners.

Using evidence-based research, Chu and Elliot (2009) also claim that the Correctional Service of Canada spent more money from 1998–2007 than in prior years preventing drugs from entering prisons, yet drug use declined less than 1% during that period (p. 2; see also Correctional Investigator Canada, 2007). Clearly, a more coordinated response to drug use in prison is required. The call, then, is for the Canadian government to refrain from viewing prisons as spaces of rehabilitation. In the Canadian criminal justice system, particularly in the court system, the trend has been to sentence people with substance use issues to "jail time" in order for them to receive drug treatment. Many judges, lawyers, and other key stakeholders mistakenly believe that penal institutions provide effective drug rehabilitation programs for people struggling with substance use. In actuality, incarcerative spaces do not provide for short- or long-term drug treatment, because prison-based substance use programs (1) do not address HIV/HCV prevention; (2) do not always address the realities of why people use drugs; (3) are abstinence-based; (4) are cognitively gender-neutral; (5) are not ethnoracially specific; and (6) are individual-based and not family integrative (when people in general and women specifically do time, so do their families—with children bearing the greatest burden of the absence of a parent who is incarcerated). Accordingly, a more coordinated response to drug use in prison would take into account the rising rates of HIV/HCV transmission and develop long-term strategies to effectively deliver consistent programs in consultation with community-based agencies working in the area of HIV prevention, treatment, counselling, and care.

CONCLUSION

What will the next wave of HIV/HCV primary and secondary prevention look like for incarcerated women? To begin with, more attention needs to be paid to prison health as a fundamental human right. The standards of community care for HIV-positive women simply do not exist for women in prison. And even the delivery of adequate HIV prevention and care in community-based settings is compromised by discrimination and stigma. In particular, for Indigenous and Black women, the legacy of colonialism impacts women of colour who seek health care services in general and HIV prevention, treatment, and care services in particular. It should also be noted that women entering Canada from countries where HIV is endemic also face a difficult time in accessing HIV services, particularly when immigration and refugee and detention protocols that are currently in place discourage women from disclosing their status and in turn accessing health care services.

In January 2011, the federal government announced that it has committed to a five-year, $2.1-billion plan to increase capacity at federal institutions in Canada (CBC News, 2011). Coupled with this announcement is the passing of Bill S-10 (Proposed New Mandatory Sentences for Serious Drug Offences), which gives judges less discretion in sentencing dispositions for drug charges, and follows three-strike penalties for drug offences. Although crime rates are declining, more women are being warehoused in penal institutions for drug-related charges. Because capitalism is connected to social disenfranchisement, prison expansion is a profitable venture even though the fiscal costs of incarceration are extremely high. The cost of imprisoning a woman in a federal prison is estimated by CSC to average $175,000 per year (CAEFS, 2004), and in 2004/2005, CSC expenditures totalled $2.8 billion, up 2% from 2003/2004, with federal prisons accounting for the largest proportion (71%) of the expenditures (Statistics Canada, 2004/2005). The move toward prison expansion means a move toward increased police budgets, more surveillance practices, and essentially higher incarceration rates. Prisons are a business—the regulation of work at substandard pay, and the absence of sick days and union support increases precarious labour risks for women and men in prison, and provides greater profit accumulation for companies that initiate contracts with prisons for the use of deregulated prison labour.

Future imperatives for HIV prevention for incarcerated women include decriminalizing sex work, initiating and maintaining connections between community-based ASOs and women in prison for long-term care and support, the creation of substantive ethnoracial HIV prevention programs, the removal of barriers of access to health care services for immigrant and refugee HIV-positive women, access to harm reduction resources in every federal and provincial prison—without the worry of reprisal from correctional staff—and working toward prosecutorial guidelines that protect HIV-positive women from criminalization in HIV non-disclosure cases.

This chapter has sought to highlight some of the significant issues regarding HIV prevention initiatives for incarcerated women in Canada. As mentioned earlier, women in prison represent a forgotten population in the larger Canadian society. In many respects, those of us who work in the field of HIV prevention, care, treatment, and support for incarcerated women are still waiting for evidence of tangible, concrete results. As such, my work at PASAN is strengthened by the courageous HIV-positive women that I work with in federal and provincial institutions in Ontario. I am reminded on a regular basis that endurance for incarcerated women in general and for HIV-positive women specifically is often critical and enmeshed with other social determinants of life. I am reminded that the things I take for granted are essential for their survival, and somehow women in prison, who are isolated and separated from their families, manage to rise each day and breathe in the most stifling of circumstances. I am reminded of hope, alternatives to incarceration for women, and the possibility of restorative justice. This work is important because it underscores the continual need to strive toward the implementation of policy and procedures that will eradicate human rights injustices and violations for incarcerated women in Canada that contribute to HIV.

PROBLEM-BASED LEARNING CASE STUDY

As a community-based worker for the local AIDS Service Organization, you receive a call from a client incarcerated in a women's penal institution. After agreeing to an HIV test initiated through the prison health care unit, the client has just found out that she has tested positive for HIV. She does not know much about the virus and, seeking support, confided in another woman also serving time in the institution. The other woman disclosed her status to several others and now your client is being discriminated against by several women in her unit. Feeling alone and isolated, she has refused to access any future services from the medical unit.

CRITICAL THINKING QUESTIONS

1. What steps would you take in working with this woman, and how would you work to resolve the stigma and discrimination that she is experiencing in the prison?
2. What HIV prevention strategies would be useful in this situation?

REFERENCES

AIDS Calgary Awareness Association. (2007). HIV/AIDS and prison populations. Retrieved from www.aidscalgary.org/resources/publications.cfm

AVERTing HIV and AIDS. (2012). Trends in AIDS diagnoses. Retrieved from www.avert.org/canada-aids.htm

Boulos, D., Yan, P., Schanzer, D., Remis, R. S., & Archibald, C. P. (2006). Estimates of HIV prevalence and incidence in Canada–2005. *Canadian Communicable Disease Report, 32*(15), 165–174.

Boyd, S., & Faith, K. (1999). Women, illicit drugs and prison: Views from Canada. *International Journal of Drug Policy, 10*(3), 195–207.

Broadhead, R. S., Kerr, T. H., Grund, J-P. C., & Altice, F. L. (2002). Safer injection facilities in North America: Their place in public policy and health initiatives. *Journal of Drug Issues, 32*(1), 329–355.

Butler, A. M. (1997). *Gendered justice in the American West: Women prisoners in the men's penitentiaries.* Urbana and Chicago: University of Illinois Press.

Canadian Association of Elizabeth Fry Societies. (2011). *Human and fiscal costs of prison.* Retrieved from www.elizabethfry.ca/eweek2011e/factsht.htm

Canadian Association of Elizabeth Fry Societies. (2003). *Submission of the Canadian Association of Elizabeth Fry Societies (CAEFS) to the Canadian Human Rights Commission for the Special Report on the Discrimination on the Basis of Sex, Race and Disability Faced by Federally Sentenced Women.* Retrieved from www.elizabethfry.ca/submissn/specialr/specialr.pdf

Canadian Association of Elizabeth Fry Societies. (2004). *Women in prison–CAEFS fact sheets.* Retrieved from http://dawn.thot.net/election2004/issues32.htm

Canadian Association of Social Workers. (2005). *Income of Black women in Canada.*

Canadian Committee on Corrections. (1969). *Report of the Canadian Committee on Corrections—Toward unity: Criminal justice and corrections* (Ouimet Report). Ottawa, ON: Queen's Printer.

Canadian HIV/AIDS Legal Network. (2008). *HIV and hepatitis C in prisons: The facts.* Info sheet: Women in prison. Retrieved from www.aidslaw.ca/publications/publicationsdocEN.php?ref=842

Canadian HIV/AIDS Legal Network & PASAN. (2007). *Hard time: HIV and hepatitis C prevention programming for prisoners in Canada.* Retrieved from www.aidslaw.ca/publications/interfaces/downloadFile.php?ref=1217

Canadian Human Rights Commission. (2003). *Protecting their rights: A systemic review of human rights in correctional services for federally sentenced women.* Retrieved from www.chrc-ccdp.ca/legislation_policies/chapter1-en.asp

Canadian Women's Health Network. (2005). HIV/AIDS on rise for Canadian women. Retrieved from www.cwhn.ca/en/node/39481

CBC News. (2011, January 10). *More prisons to be expanded.* Retrieved from www.cbc.ca/canada/story/2011/01/10/tories-prison-infrastructure.html#ixzz1BBipLXyd

Chu, S. K. H., & Elliot, R. (2009). *Clean switch: The case for prison needle and syringe programs in Canada.* Canadian HIV/AIDS Legal Network. Retrieved from www.aidslaw.ca/publications/publicationsdocEN.php?ref=948

Constitution Act, 1982 [en. by the Canada Act 1982 (U.K.), c. 11, s. 1], pt. I (Canadian Charter of Rights and Freedoms).

Correctional Investigator Canada. (2007). *Annual Report of the Office of the Correctional Investigator 2006–2007.* Minister of Public Works and Government Services Canada. Retrieved from www.oci-bec.gc.ca/reports/AR200607_e.asp

Corrections and Conditional Release Act. (S.C. 1992, c. 20). Section 3. Retrieved from the Department of Justice Canada website: http://laws-lois.justice.gc.ca/eng/acts/C-44.6/page-2.html

Correctional Service of Canada. (2010). *CSC health services.* Retrieved from www.csc-scc.gc.ca/text/hlth/index-eng.shtml

Correctional Service of Canada. (2012). Preliminary unpublished data. CSC Infectious Disease Surveillance System (IDSS).

Crenshaw, K. (1989). Demarginalizing the intersection of race and sex: A Black feminist critique of antidiscrimination doctrine, feminist theory and anti racist politics. *The University of Chicago Legal Forum 1989,* 139–167.

Csete, J. (2005). *Vectors, vessels and victims: HIV/AIDS and women's human rights in Canada.* Toronto, ON: Canadian HIV/AIDS Legal Network. Retrieved from www.aidslaw.ca/publications/interfaces/downloadFile.php?ref=529

Davis, A. Y. (1971). *If they come in the morning: Voices of resistance.* New York: Third Press.

DiCenso, A. M., Dias, G., & Gahagan, J. (2003). *Unlocking our futures: A national study on women, prisons, HIV and hepatitis C.* Toronto, ON: Prisoners' HIV/AIDS Support Action Network.

Drucker, E. (2006). InSite: Canada's landmark safe injecting program at risk. *Harm Reduction Journal, 3,* 24. Retrieved from www.harmreductionjournal.com/content/3/1/24

Elliot, R., Malkin, I., & Gold, J. (2002). *Establishing safe injection facilities in Canada: Legal and ethical issues.* Canadian HIV/AIDS Legal Network. Retrieved from www.aidslaw.ca/publications/interfaces/downloadFile.php?ref=776

Ekstedt, J., & Griffiths, C. (1988). *Corrections in Canada: Policy and practice.* Toronto, ON: Butterworths.

Faith, K. (1993). *Unruly women: The politics of confinement and resistance.* Vancouver, BC: Press Gang Publishers.

Foucault, M. (1977). *Discipline and punish: The birth of the prison* (Trans. Alan Sheridan). New York: Vintage.

Greenfield, L. A., & Snell, T. L. (1999). *Women offenders* (p. 8, Table 20). Bureau of Justice Statistics. Washington, DC: U.S. Department of Justice. Retrieved from http://bjs.ojp.usdoj.gov/content/pub/pdf/wo.pdf

International Centre for Prison Studies. (2009). World prison brief: Canada. Retrieved from www.prisonstudies.org/info/worldbrief/wpb_country.php?country=188

Johnson, P. C. (2003). *Inner lives: Voices of African American women in prison.* New York and London: New York University Press.

Kerr, T., & Palepu, A. (2001). Safe injection facilities in Canada: Is it time? *Canadian Medical Association Journal, 165*(4), 436–437. Retrieved from www.cmaj.ca/cgi/content/165/4/436.full.pdf

Kerr, T., Wood, E., Small, D., Palepu, A., & Tyndall, M. W. (2003). Potential use of safer injecting facilities among injection drug users in Vancouver's Downtown Eastside. *Canadian Medical Association Journal, 169*(8), 759–763.

Kurshan, N. (1999). *Women and imprisonment in the U.S.: History and current reality.* Available from http://zinedistro.org/zines/18/women-and-imprisonment-in-the-us/by/nancy-kurshan

Lines, R., Jürgens, R., Betteridge, G., Stöver, H., Laticevschi, D., & Nelles, J. (2006). *Prison needle exchange: Lessons from a comprehensive review of international evidence and experience* (2nd ed.). Toronto, ON: Canadian HIV/AIDS Legal Network.

Native Women's Association of Canada. (2004, October). Background paper for Aboriginal Women's Health Canada—Aboriginal Peoples Roundtable Health Sectoral Session. Ohsweken: Native Women's Association of Canada.

Public Health Agency of Canada. (2012). Fact sheet: People in prison. Retrieved from www.phac-aspc.gc.ca/aids-sida/pr/sec4-eng.php

Rafter, N. H. (1990). *Partial justice: Women, prisons, and social control.* New Brunswick, NJ: Transaction Publishers.

Statistics Canada. (2004/2005). Adult correctional services in Canada. Retrieved from www.publications.gc.ca/Collection-R/Statcan/85-002-XIE/85-002-XIE2006005.pdf

Task Force on Federally Sentenced Women. (1990). *Creating choices: The report of the Task Force on Federally Sentenced Women.* Retrieved from www.csc-scc.gc.ca/text/prgrm/fsw/choices/toce-eng.shtml

United Nations Office on Drugs and Crime (UNODC). (2008). *UNODC/UNAIDS publication on women and HIV in prison settings.* Retrieved from www.unodc.org/unodc/en/hiv-aids/publications.html

Vancouver Coastal Health. (n.d.). *InSite—Supervised injection site.* Retrieved from http://supervisedinjection.vch.ca/

Wallace, M. (2009, July). *Police-reported statistics in Canada, 2008.* Retrieved from www.statcan.gc.ca/pub/85-002-x/2009003/article/10902-eng.htm

Chapter 9

CRIMINAL PROSECUTIONS FOR HIV NON-DISCLOSURE: PROTECTING WOMEN FROM INFECTION OR THREATENING PREVENTION EFFORTS?

Patricia Allard, Cécile Kazatchkine, and Alison Symington

> When public health endeavours fail to provide adequate protection to individuals like the complainants, the criminal law can be effective. It provides a needed measure of protection in the form of deterrence and reflects society's abhorrence of the self-centered recklessness and the callous insensitivity of the actions of the respondent and those who have acted in a similar manner ... The risks of infection are so devastating that there is a real and urgent need to provide a measure of protection for those in the position of the complainants. If ever there was a place for the deterrence provided by criminal sanctions it is present in these circumstances. It may well have the desired effect of ensuring that there is disclosure of the risk and that appropriate precautions are taken.
>
> —*R. v. Cuerrier*, 1998[1]

Since the Supreme Court of Canada's 1998 decision in the *Cuerrier* case, people living with HIV (hereinafter "PLWHIV") can be prosecuted for not disclosing their HIV-positive status to sexual partners before engaging in an activity that represents a "significant risk" of HIV transmission. To date, more than 130 people in Canada have been charged for not disclosing their status to sexual partners and the vast majority of those convicted have been sent to jail.[2]

The criminalization of HIV exposure without disclosure of HIV-positive status was put forth by the Supreme Court as a tool for prevention. Justice Cory, writing for the majority of the Court in the *Cuerrier* decision, indicated that there is a role for the criminal law to play in the response to the HIV epidemic, noting that "[t]hrough deterrence it will protect and serve to encourage honesty, frankness and safer sexual practices."[3] In theory, then, criminal prosecutions should be one tool in the cache of HIV prevention strategies that can protect women from HIV infection, particularly where other public health approaches to behaviour change are failing. In this chapter, we will interrogate these claims in relation to developments since *Cuerrier* was decided more than a decade ago, and demonstrate how Justice Cory's prediction has not come to fruition.

Indeed, there has been limited research exploring the impact of criminalization of HIV non-disclosure on prevention, especially as it relates to protecting women's health needs. The limited data that does exist, together with abundant anecdotal evidence, suggests that criminalization is not only an *ineffective* prevention tool, but that it is also *counterproductive* as it undermines prevention measures, especially those targeting women. Moreover, applying charges of aggravated assault and aggravated sexual assault to HIV non-disclosure, as is currently done in Canada, is a severe response, compounding the challenges of living with HIV, undermining positive prevention, and resulting in injustices. We would therefore suggest that criminalization of HIV non-disclosure has a detrimental impact on the lives of women (HIV negative, positive, and of unknown HIV status) by undermining prevention efforts that could reduce the risks of HIV transmission and, at times, also exacerbating vulnerabilities to socio-economic insecurity and/or violence. This chapter therefore calls for a critical analysis of the use of the criminal law in relation to HIV prevention to advance research, policy, and practice that contribute meaningfully to an effective and gender-sensitive approach to HIV prevention in the future.

This chapter begins with a brief description of the current state of the criminal law in Canada as it applies to sexual HIV exposure. It then discusses why criminalization of HIV non-disclosure is an ineffective tool for HIV prevention. Next, it presents some of the ways in which criminalization might in fact undermine HIV prevention efforts. Finally, it looks at the impact of non-disclosure on women living with HIV in Canada. Based on these different elements, we conclude that the criminalization of HIV non-disclosure is ineffective and inappropriate for HIV prevention. The use of the criminal law with respect to HIV exposure must be strictly limited in order that more responsive, supportive, and empowering HIV prevention initiatives succeed.

THE LAW

Current Canadian law with respect to HIV non-disclosure has its origins in the *Cuerrier* case, mentioned above. The case arose because two women were exposed to the risk of HIV infection through sexual relations with Mr. Cuerrier, a man who had been diagnosed as HIV positive in 1992. He had been counselled by a public health nurse to use condoms for sex and to tell his sexual partners about his HIV-positive status. However, he did not disclose or use condoms consistently.[4] In this case, a majority of the Supreme Court held that a PLWHIV may be guilty of a crime of assault for not disclosing his or her HIV-positive status before engaging in sexual activities that pose a "significant risk" of HIV transmission. In a key section of the decision, the court sets out what became the benchmark as to when HIV disclosure will be legally required in Canada.

> Yet it cannot be any trivial harm or risk of harm that will satisfy this requirement in sexual assault cases where the activity would have been consensual if the consent had not been obtained by fraud … [T]he Crown will have to establish that the dishonest act (either falsehoods or failure to disclose) had the effect of exposing the person consenting to a *significant risk of serious bodily harm.* [emphasis added][5]

The Supreme Court, however, did not define what in particular constitutes a "significant risk." The interpretation and application of the "significant risk" test was left to lower level courts. Again, to quote the Court, "[t]he phrase "significant risk of serious harm" must be applied to the facts of each case in order to determine if the consent given in the particular circumstances was vitiated."[6]

In the *Cuerrier* case, unprotected vaginal intercourse was found to constitute a "significant risk" of HIV transmission. In subsequent cases, there has been considerable inconsistency in the application of the legal test, resulting in uncertainty in the law.[7] Many questions remain without clear answers because of inconsistent rulings and the vagueness of the Supreme Court's guidance. Is there a legal duty to disclose one's HIV-positive status before engaging in protected intercourse (i.e., where condoms are used)? Is there a legal obligation to disclose one's HIV-positive status prior to lower risk sexual activities, such as oral sex? What if the risk of transmission is minimal because the PLWHIV has a low or undetectable viral load?[8] The science related to HIV transmission and HIV disease has evolved considerably since the Supreme Court decision in *Cuerrier*; some Canadian courts have taken that into account, but it has been inconsistent across the country. At the same time, some prosecutors are challenging the limitations on prosecutions established in *Cuerrier* by arguing for different legal standards. As a result, even the assumption that unprotected intercourse always requires disclosure, and negligible risk activities never require disclosure, has come into question.[9] As there has been no authoritative ruling to date updating the *Cuerrier* standard in light of scientific and legal developments, it impossible for people living with HIV to know exactly what the law requires of them today.

THE CRIMINALIZATION OF HIV NON-DISCLOSURE: AN INEFFECTIVE TOOL FOR HIV PREVENTION

According to the majority of the Supreme Court in *Cuerrier*, "[t]he criminal law has a role to play [in HIV prevention] both in deterring those infected with HIV from putting the lives of others at risk and in protecting the public from irresponsible individuals who refuse to comply with public health orders to abstain from high-risk activities."[10] Assessing the effectiveness of criminalization of HIV non-disclosure as it relates to prevention therefore invites a closer examination of whether the specific objective of deterrence is met. If criminalization of HIV non-disclosure is to meaningfully contribute to HIV prevention objectives, it must deter behaviour that risks transmitting the virus.[11]

Despite the Court's assertion that criminalization would deter PLWHIV from exposing others to HIV, there appears to be no evidence supporting this deterrent effect. The Supreme Court did not cite any specific evidence to support the deterrent function that they envisioned. The limited evidence collected since *Cuerrier* with respect to the impact of criminalization of HIV non-disclosure also offers little backing for the deterrence premise.[12]

In our analysis, the criminalization of HIV non-disclosure falls short in terms of achieving actual deterrence in at least four ways. First, for deterrence to be effective in regulating social behaviour, people need to know that their contemplated behaviour is illegal. In Canada, the law around HIV non-disclosure is so unclear that people cannot determine with certainty which activities legally require HIV disclosure. Always disclosing before activities that pose a "significant risk" is an indefinite, confusing standard for PLWHIV to follow.[13] The term *significant* invites a personal evaluation of the importance of the HIV transmission risk and does not correspond with the language and guidance with respect to risk reduction advanced by AIDS Service Organizations (ASOs), public health, and medical professionals.[14] Moreover, as discussed above, this area of law is continually evolving through judicial decisions. As the science around HIV evolves and judges are presented with new evidence and novel legal arguments, the understanding of when disclosure is legally required will likewise change.

Second, for criminalization of HIV non-disclosure to contribute to HIV prevention efforts by deterring risky behaviour, PLWHIV would need to consider the criminal law in their sexual decision making. The criminal law, however, is unlikely to be a primary source of guidance for PLWHIV with respect to sexual matters and HIV prevention. Furthermore, if reasoned judgment is outweighed by less rational considerations (such as desire, fear, or addiction), or if a moral concern for the health of others has not already prompted a change in behaviour, then it is unlikely that a legal obligation will have much additional deterrent effect.[15]

One of the only full-scale studies to attempt to determine whether criminal laws with respect to HIV exposure influence behaviour compared people at elevated risk of HIV in Chicago and New York City—that is, in one state with a law specifically regulating the sexual behaviour of PLWHIV and in one state without such a law.[16] The study found that there were very few differences in the self-reported sexual activities among participants from the two states. Moreover, people who believed the law required PLWHIV to practise safer sex or disclose their status reported engaging in similarly risky sexual behaviours without disclosing as those who did not share the same understanding of the law.[17] This study suggests, then, that the criminal law has little impact on decision making regarding disclosure and sexual activity.[18]

In fact, many PLWHIV seem to rely on their own moral or social compass, rather than what the law requires, in making decisions about disclosing their HIV status to sexual partners. According to the preliminary findings of a large study of PLWHIV in Canada (including both men and women), a significant number of participants felt unaffected by criminalization because they always disclose their HIV-positive status in sexual encounters; they openly negotiate about serostatus, often preferring sero-concordant partners; or they feel that disclosure of HIV-positive status is the morally right thing to do regardless of the law.[19] Others took a more situational or conditional approach, assessing whether to disclose in each situation depending on whether safer sex is practised, their sense of personal safety, and the type of relationship (e.g., casual versus longer term or more committed).[20] If indeed moral conviction regarding serostatus disclosure is more important than a legal requirement, criminalizing HIV non-disclosure will not add anything to extant HIV prevention initiatives.

Third, given how HIV disease progresses and the differing levels of infectiousness, the legal disclosure obligation does not have much impact at the most critical time for prevention effectiveness. To disclose, PLWHIV must know that they are HIV positive and that HIV can be transmitted sexually. However, it is estimated that approximately one-quarter of the PLWHIV in Canada have not yet been diagnosed.[21] At the same time, scientific studies (including in Canada), show that early infection accounts for approximately half (or more) of onward transmissions.[22] Criminalization of non-disclosure can have no impact on these transmissions—if a person does not know or suspect that they are HIV positive, they have nothing to disclose. By focusing legal responses to HIV exposure on the PLWHIV who are likely involved in the minority of HIV transmission in Canada, the possible population-level prevention benefit is quite limited.[23]

Finally, in order for the criminalization of HIV non-disclosure to contribute to HIV prevention efforts, disclosure must lead to safer sex, either by causing individuals to engage in less risky sexual activities (or forego sex altogether) or to use protection for sexual activities that risk transmitting HIV. However, the relationship between the legal obligation to disclose and safer sex remains uncertain. According to existing research, emphasizing disclosure is not necessarily associated with higher rates of protected sex.[24] The decision to have protected sex may depend on many factors, including an individual's ability to negotiate the terms of sex in specific circumstances. For some women, the ability to negotiate safer sex is particularly difficult, or impossible, because of their disempowered position within a relationship, cultural norms, their social location, or their individual skills and competencies (which may include factors such as a lack of personal independence, limited communication skills, personal insecurities, a history of abuse, addictions, mental illness, etc.). For all of these reasons, then, the criminalization of HIV non-disclosure is unlikely to have any significant benefit in terms of preventing new infections.

Considering the deterrence role of the criminal law with respect to HIV prevention for diverse women in Canada, it is revealing to consider that, historically, the criminal law has often been used to police deviant, socially unacceptable, or "dangerous" sexual behaviour, often under the guise of protecting women. The particular image of women deserving of and requiring state protection is one of fragile, white, middle-class women. Following this legacy, in terms of key populations at higher risk of HIV infection in Canada, there is reason to believe that criminalization may be even less effective at protecting some women of colour, of diverse sexualities, immigrant women, and women marginalized by poverty, drug use, or sex work from HIV infection.

THE CRIMINALIZATION OF NON-DISCLOSURE UNDERMINES HIV PREVENTION EFFORTS

In addition to the lack of evidence that criminalization of HIV non-disclosure contributes to HIV prevention efforts, social scientists, human rights advocates, public health researchers, and others have cautioned that criminalization may, in fact, *undermine* HIV prevention efforts, including those targeting HIV-negative women.[25] Because criminal laws seem to contradict, rather than complement, public health and human rights efforts, a tension results between the approaches. Given that voluntary engagement of at-risk groups with health information and support services and empowerment through human rights protection are generally believed to be more effective at preventing the spread of HIV than coercive measures, the potential that the criminalization of HIV non-disclosure may undermine public health prevention techniques is indeed reason for concern.

First, the criminalization of HIV non-disclosure can conflict with public health practice by threatening the therapeutic relationship between a patient and his/her physician or between a client and his/her health service providers or counsellors. PLWHIV may be inhibited from talking openly about their risk behaviours, sexually transmitted diseases, or the challenges they may be facing around disclosure if they fear that this information could later be used against them in a legal proceeding.[26] Some may not agree to partner notification procedures if they worry that a partner might in turn have them charged for non-disclosure. Some may avoid HIV testing, counselling, education, or support services for fear of the stigma and negative ramifications they may face if their HIV-positive status becomes known, including threats of criminal charges.[27] Some women already face specific challenges in accessing services, including HIV testing, treatment, care, and support, and there are concerns that specialized, responsive services that aim to address these challenges may also be undermined by the criminalization of HIV transmission and/or exposure.[28]

This discouragement of openness in HIV prevention counselling has been documented in recent research exploring the public health impact of criminalization of non-disclosure in Canada.[29] Service providers expressed numerous concerns about how criminalization hindered their efforts to work with PLWHIV in open ways with respect to their sexual activities and disclosure practices. For example, some public health nurses were concerned that the increased use of the criminal law discouraged PLWHIV from approaching or maintaining relationships with public health, in particular because sensational media coverage of criminal cases (in which police urge sexual contacts of the accused to seek HIV testing) created an impression of close ties between public health and the police.[30] Moreover, some referred to the difficulty of maintaining a health focus in counselling, given uneasiness about criminal disclosure obligations. Others expressed uneasiness about whether or how to counsel newly infected individuals about their option to pursue charges against HIV-positive partners, and some mentioned a heightened awareness to liability issues affecting their work.[31] Similarly, front-line staff from AIDS Service Organizations and family physicians indicated that the criminal law created "a chill" in their counselling relationships with HIV-positive clients and patients, particularly the disinclination on the part of PLWHIV to discuss challenges they may be facing with respect to disclosing their HIV status to sexual partners.[32]

Moreover, given the tight-knit communities in which many immigrant women live in Canada, as well as the enduring ties to their home communities overseas, many hesitate to get tested or access support services for fear that their entire network would quickly learn about their diagnosis. According to a study conducted by Women's Health in Women's Hands, "service providers were frustrated that some women would rather sacrifice their health than sacrifice their anonymity/confidentiality."[33] Criminalization may create even more anxiety and reluctance to communicate openly for women who are already highly concerned about confidentiality.

Second, criminalization of HIV non-disclosure can further conflict with public health and individualized approaches to prevention by detracting from the safer sex messaging that has traditionally been the backbone of HIV prevention, particularly the emphasis on condom use. These approaches have tended to emphasize each person's individual agency in ensuring their own health and safety, as opposed to the criminal law approach that emphasizes exclusive PLWHIV responsibility.[34] This may undermine the effectiveness of safer sex messaging, giving women a false sense of security that criminal law will protect them from HIV infection.[35] Similarly, it may advance the idea that only "criminals" fail to disclose, so for an "average person" there is minimal risk (and hence less need to use condoms to prevent disease), unless the partner indicates that he or she is infected. Notably, the criminal law approach pays little attention to safer sex, "ultimately discounting central features of the public health response to HIV," and endorses a flawed, disclosure-based norm for promoting safety in sexual interactions.[36]

Furthermore, the uncertainty in the law may also have a negative impact on well-established public health messages.[37] For instance, prosecutions in cases where people have engaged only in protected sex clearly contradict 30 years of public health messaging by punishing people who have in fact followed key advice regarding what they should do in order to prevent onward transmission of the virus. Condoms are a very effective prevention technology, and the risks of HIV transmission through sex are generally much lower than assumed by the general public.[38] Prosecutions create misconceptions about the risk of HIV transmission, implying that the virus is easily transmitted.

Third, criminalization of HIV non-disclosure is also at odds with other prevention initiatives in that it does not seek to reduce stigma and discrimination but instead may reinforce them.[39] In this way, criminalization may potentially alienate those upon whom prevention efforts depend.[40] This impact is magnified by the fact that prosecutions for non-disclosure have almost exclusively focused on HIV.[41] Concern has therefore been expressed that criminalization of HIV non-disclosure may lead to the damaging and inaccurate public sentiment that PLWHIV are uniquely sexually irresponsible and dangerous.[42] Characterizing PLWHIV in this way is contrary to prevention because it makes it even more difficult for people to speak openly about their sexual health or to see themselves as at risk.

Fourth, criminalization of HIV non-disclosure may impede another available HIV prevention intervention, that is, the use of post-exposure prophylaxis (PEP) in cases of unexpected exposure (such as when a condom breaks or excessive alcohol or drug consumption leads to unprotected sex). In order for disclosure to take place following exposure in such circumstances, there needs to be a certain degree of openness. The risk of criminal prosecution could hamper this openness and discourage a PLWHIV who had not already disclosed from doing so in order that their partner may pursue PEP treatment.[43]

Fifth, criminalization also reinforces damaging stereotypes that women are passive and weak individuals in need of protection from the criminal justice system. It thereby discounts women's agency and coping mechanisms. Rather than recognizing their diversity and creating the conditions that allow women to protect themselves and take control of their sexual lives, criminalization casts women as naive victims at the mercy of smooth-talking men.[44] HIV prevention for women requires gender-sensitive programming that recognizes and responds to the differential needs and constraints of individuals based on their gender and sexuality.[45] Criminalization of HIV non-disclosure fails miserably in this regard.

While the public health and individual prevention efforts discussed so far are mostly voluntary in nature, it is important to note that public health law also includes coercive powers. Public health approaches to preventing HIV by addressing HIV risk behaviours form a continuum from voluntary measures (e.g., voluntary testing for sexually transmitted infections; access to HIV prevention tools such as condoms and clean drug use equipment; voluntary partner notification; and counselling, support, and referrals to other services) to coercive measures that are backed up by the threat of a penalty (e.g., mandatory reporting of cases of HIV and AIDS; behaviour orders; examination, testing, and treatment orders; court enforcement of public health authorities' orders; and offences and penalties).[46] In many jurisdictions where criminal law is being used to respond to HIV exposure, however, public health law interventions are increasingly taking a back seat.

While using coercive public health laws to address HIV risk behaviours raises some of the same concerns as the criminalization of HIV non-disclosure, public health interventions have several strengths that may make them better suited to encouraging sustained changes in HIV risk behaviour, including the following: in-person, supportive contact with public health staff is more likely to result in ongoing reductions in risk behaviour than the remote threat of criminal prosecution; case management strategies can be tailored to address the specific reasons and challenges that may be leading to HIV risk behaviours; increasingly coercive interventions can be adopted if less coercive measures fail; interventions can increase access to a range of health and social services and include protections for privacy and confidentiality; and public health law interventions can focus on the protection of the public based on the actual risk posed by the behaviours of the PLWHIV, and the coercive measure can be discontinued once the risky behaviour ceases.[47]

As pointed out by the Manitoba Court of Appeal, "[c]riminal sanctions should be reserved for those deliberate, irresponsible or reckless individuals who do not respond to public health directives and who are truly blameworthy."[48] The criminal law cannot replace comprehensive HIV prevention efforts that meet the needs and address the complex circumstances of the diverse populations of women in Canada. The criminal justice system steps in after the fact. It does not provide remedy (i.e., to tackle the HIV epidemic). It only provides punishment to the accused. In contrast, prevention measures are actively engaged before and after exposure with concrete measures intended for women to take charge of their sexual health. This is not to say that there is no role for the criminal law in cases of HIV exposure or transmission. However, given its adverse impact on PLWHIV and on HIV prevention efforts, we submit that the criminal law should be used *only* in egregious cases where other less intrusive approaches have failed and the reckless or malicious behaviour of the accused warrants criminal intervention.

WOMEN LIVING WITH HIV AND THE CRIMINAL LAW

So far, this chapter has focused primarily on HIV prevention for women who are HIV negative or do not know their HIV status. However, no consideration of women and criminalization of HIV non-disclosure would be complete without considering the impact of the law on women living with HIV. Despite the increasing proportion of women living with HIV in Canada, there have been few prosecutions against women for HIV non-disclosure; only 13 to our knowledge (as compared to over 115 against men).[49] While the media has easily depicted women as "victims" of HIV exposure—deserving of protection and redress for being exposed to the risk of infection by dishonest men[50]—women living with HIV may also find themselves on the other side of the courtroom, as the accused in a non-disclosure case.

The Complexities of HIV Disclosure for Women

While disclosing one's HIV-positive status to sexual partners can play an important role in preventing onward transmission of HIV, there are some important gender considerations with respect to disclosure that are relevant to contextualizing disclosure's place in terms of HIV prevention strategies. Revealing one's HIV-positive status is generally a difficult and complicated undertaking, often involving strategic decisions about who to tell, how, when, where, and how much information to reveal. Not only is one's HIV status an intensely personal matter, but stigma and discrimination against people living with HIV continues to be plentiful in our society, with particular gendered manifestations, and therefore women living with HIV have good reason to be cautious about revealing their status.[51]

Studies have suggested that the desire to be morally responsible toward their sexual partners and to protect their partners' health often motivates HIV-positive women to disclose their status.[52] However, research on women and HIV highlights the difficulty that many women experience in disclosing to men, especially men on whom they are dependent.

On the other hand, fear that a sexual partner may share the information with others and concern about preserving confidentiality around HIV status prevents some women from disclosing to all sexual partners. Some are also worried about the reaction of their partners.[53] They may fear violence, rejection, and abandonment. These fears can lead some women to conceal their status or delay disclosure.[54]

In addition, some women who are living with HIV fear that disclosing could open them up to false accusations of non-disclosure.[55] AIDS Service Organizations have reported that some clients in serodiscordant relationships have been blackmailed by vindictive partners. Ironically, it is the act of disclosing, of complying with one's legal requirements, that in fact makes PLWHIV vulnerable to false allegations, coercion, and even violence.[56]

By its nature, criminal law is unable to accommodate a nuanced and contextualized understanding of the challenges and complexities of HIV disclosure for women. The criminal law approach is predicated on the binary of a victim and a perpetrator, and definitive determinations that disclosure took place or it did not. The legal obligation to disclose does not invite understanding that HIV disclosure is not always a simple one-step process, nor is it necessarily "all or nothing." Disclosure may take place in stages because understanding the implications of the diagnosis take time. The decision to disclose an HIV-positive status and the timing of disclosure may also differ depending on the context and the nature of the sexual relationship. For example, disclosure may be less common with casual partners or in commercial sex, especially if condoms are used.

The case of one Ontario woman charged for non-disclosure illustrates how criminal law fails to accommodate the complexities of the disclosure process and the realities of sexual relationships and HIV prevention options. In 2009, this woman pleaded guilty to aggravated sexual assault after a single sexual encounter. She had insisted upon condom use, but the condom broke. She disclosed her status immediately afterward. Despite the fact that she practised safer sex, disclosed when the condom broke, and her partner was not infected by HIV, she was sentenced to two years of house arrest, three years of probation, and was registered as a sex offender. She was described by the sentencing judge as "a lonely woman who feared rejection" because of her HIV status.[57] That may explain, at least in part, why she chose not to disclose her HIV-positive status. As a result of the prosecution, her picture and story were published in the media. In addition to demonstrating the harshness of criminalization, this case also illustrates how the criminal law can actually undermine prevention opportunities. This woman's experience may cause other PLWHIV to question whether disclosing to a sexual partner who may have been inadvertently exposed is worthwhile, given the criminal consequence that may ensue.

Criminalized Women and HIV Prevention

While the sample size is indeed small from which to extract trends, certain commonalities emerge from the basic facts of the cases of the women who have faced charges related to non-disclosure in Canada. First, we note that most of the women who have been charged occupied marginalized positions that may have made them vulnerable to HIV infection and also made disclosure of their HIV status particularly challenging. For example, some were survivors of violence, living in socio-economic insecurity, having insecure immigration status, and/or were members of racial/ethnic minority populations.

In terms of the women who have been convicted of HIV non-disclosure in Canada, we know that several have been survivors of violence. For example, a 28-year-old Aboriginal woman in Alberta pleaded guilty to a charge of nuisance in December 2002 for not disclosing her HIV-positive status to a sexual partner. According to media reports of the proceedings, she had been molested by her accuser since she was 13 years old.[58] Another example is a woman in Quebec who was convicted in 2008 for not disclosing her HIV-positive status. According to the court materials, her partner initially had sex without her having disclosed her status to him. Her testimony was that the sex was protected; he claimed that it was not. She then disclosed her status to him and they continued in a relationship for four years. He was not infected. The end of the relationship was marked by domestic violence, and she turned to the police for protection. He then complained to the police with respect to her non-disclosure prior to their first sexual encounter. At trial, she was convicted of aggravated assault and sexual assault and sentenced to 12 month's house arrest.[59] In contrast, for his assaults, he received an absolute discharge.[60] This case is particularly troubling because the trial judge recognized that the complainant was seeking revenge following her complaint about his violence.[61] Six years after she was charged, her conviction was finally reversed by the Court of Appeal of Quebec.[62] The Crown appealed to the Supreme Court of Canada.[63]

From the perspective of HIV prevention, the prevalence of violence against women associated with criminal prosecutions for HIV non-disclosure is significant. Violence against women is a severe manifestation of gender inequality, and both a cause and a consequence of HIV. If violence is a factor in women's choices regarding disclosure, and if charges are laid as another manifestation of violence against a woman, HIV prevention is impeded by both the violence and the criminal law.

Another factor is that of social and economic instability in the lives of the women charged. For example, one of the women charged was a former sex worker. This 33-year-old Ontario woman was sentenced to four years in prison after pleading guilty to charges of criminal negligence causing bodily harm and sexual assault. According to media coverage of the case, her accuser was a former client who allegedly developed a relationship with her and helped her get off the street.[64] Similarly, at least three of the women charged were single mothers, facing all of the challenges associated with raising children on their own. And at least one woman charged had mental health issues at the time of the incident. In 2009, she pleaded guilty to aggravated sexual assault in relation to two sexual encounters. She was sentenced to two years of house arrest plus three years of probation. In the sentencing decision, the judge took into account that at the time of the encounters, she was suffering from mental disorders due to brain lesions caused by her HIV infection and aggravated by alcohol abuse, which "serve[d] to explain her behaviour."[65]

Again, when considering HIV prevention and women, the fact that women living with AIDS and facing criminal charges are in these unstable situations is cause for pause. What supports do these women require in order to undertake positive prevention? How is the possibility of criminal charges for HIV non-disclosure impacting on their disclosure and safer sex practices? Are the criminal prosecutions against them fair, proportionate, and just?

Another factor to consider is immigration status and the challenges faced by newcomers to Canada. Consider the case of an immigrant from Thailand who was found guilty of criminal negligence causing bodily harm and aggravated assault in January 2007 for not disclosing her HIV-positive status to her then-husband, who was infected with HIV.[66] She admitted that she had not revealed her HIV-positive status to her husband, but explained that she did not do so because she did not believe she was HIV positive. While she had previously tested positive for HIV at a clinic in Hong Kong, she stated that she believed that she had subsequently tested HIV negative through her immigration medical exam for entry to Canada and therefore believed herself to be HIV negative. The judge found that her "simple story does not correspond with common sense."[67] He stated that he would have expected her to seek out a second test as soon as she arrived in Canada, and he also rejected her assertion that she genuinely thought the medical test required by Citizenship and Immigration Canada included an HIV test. He found that even if she thought that a second test indicated that she was HIV negative, he would have expected her to make greater efforts to clarify the conflicting result.[68] Having decided that she knew she was HIV positive, the guilty verdict easily followed because she admitted that she had not told her husband that she was HIV positive. She has since been deported.[69]

For newcomers to Canada, the criminal law around HIV disclosure can be very difficult to understand, and anxiety around how HIV-positive status may impact one's immigration status can affect a newcomer's ability to disclose his or her HIV-positive status.[70] Furthermore, HIV-related stigma among ethnic communities in Canada is pronounced. There are a range of cultural and structural issues that may increase the risk for HIV infection, create obstacles to testing and treatment, lead to isolation and stigma, and impact on newcomer PLWHIV's ability to disclose their HIV-positive status to sexual partners, negotiate safer sex, and access testing, treatment, and support services.[71] So in terms of HIV prevention and women, and how it intersects with criminalization of HIV non-disclosure, race and immigration status are important considerations that require further analysis in terms of appropriate interventions and various impacts.

These are just a few of the intersecting factors underlying the complex and emotionally charged issue of criminalizing women who have not disclosed their positive status to a sexual partner. The criminal law is ill-equipped to deal with the multiple challenges faced by women in disclosing their status and practising safer sex. Rather than empowering women living with HIV to protect themselves and others, criminalization of HIV non-disclosure creates additional challenges, fears, and, for some, harsh prison terms. As such, this issue calls for concerted research, advocacy, and policy change in the coming years in order to ensure appropriate HIV-related services are available to women, to prevent onward transmission of the virus, and to avert injustice.

CONCLUSION: THE ROLE OF THE LAW IN SUPPORTING HIV PREVENTION

As the foregoing analysis demonstrates, criminalizing HIV non-disclosure is a blunt, punitive, inflexible approach to HIV prevention that is decidedly ineffective for women. The criminalization of HIV non-disclosure cannot take into consideration the many factors that influence women's disclosure practices and sexual behaviours, and it has possibly caused some women in some circumstances to avoid HIV testing, conceal their HIV-positive status, or avoid accessing harm reduction, prevention, and support services. Rather than deterring behaviour that risks transmitting HIV, as the Supreme Court envisioned, the criminalization of HIV non-disclosure may be creating additional barriers and burdens for women living with HIV while offering little protection to women who remain HIV negative.

If we are to learn from this lesson, the next wave of HIV prevention for women will recognize that while individual behaviour change is essential, it is not sufficient to address the full range of factors that make women vulnerable to HIV and that impede women who are living with HIV from avoiding onward transmission of the virus. The role that the law can play in terms of HIV prevention is not so much as a deterrent through criminalization, but as an instrument of empowerment, protecting rights and helping to put in place the conditions that allow people to protect themselves and others. Both to protect HIV-negative women from infection and to empower HIV-positive women to protect others from infection, laws and legal institutions can protect privacy rights, promote equality, guarantee sexual and reproductive rights, and ensure access to essential services. In this way, the law can contribute to improving the social determinants of health for all women, diminishing the need for criminal law to "protect" women and ushering in a new era of HIV prevention.

Because many would "want to know" if a sexual partner had HIV (or another sexually transmitted infection), it is tempting to think that the law should always oblige disclosure, and punish non-disclosure harshly. But as the Law Reform Commission of Canada (1976) emphasized in its report on the role of the criminal law, *Our Criminal Law,*

> we have to keep our heads, not hit out blindly, and not mistake activity for action. We must avoid being misled by fears, frustrations or false expectations, however natural they may be ... The fact is, criminal law is a blunt and costly instrument ... So criminal law must be an instrument of last resort. It must be used as little as possible. The message must not be diluted by overkill ... Society's ultimate weapon must stay sheathed as long as possible. The watchword is restraint—restraint applying to the scope of the criminal law, to the meaning of criminal guilt, to the use of the criminal trial and to the criminal sentence. (pp. 27–28)

PROBLEM-BASED LEARNING CASE STUDY

HIV prevention for women requires a focus on the full range of factors that make women vulnerable to HIV and that impede the ability of women who are HIV positive to prevent transmission of the virus. The law can and should serve as an instrument of empowerment, protecting rights and helping to ensure conditions that allow people to protect themselves and others. Specifically, laws and legal institutions can protect privacy rights, promote equality, guarantee sexual and reproductive rights, and ensure access to essential services. By doing so, the law can address the social determinants of health for all women and reduce the need for criminal law to "protect" women.

CRITICAL THINKING QUESTIONS

1. A limited number of women have been charged in relation to HIV non-disclosure in Canada, yet the criminalization of HIV non-disclosure has significant impacts for many women living with HIV. How might the possibility of criminal charges for HIV non-disclosure impact on women's disclosure and safer sex practices? What other impacts does criminalization of non-disclosure have on diverse women who are living with HIV?

2. When might criminal charges in relation to HIV non-disclosure or HIV exposure be necessary or appropriate?

3. What alternative interventions are available if a PLWHIV has not disclosed to a sexual partner(s)?

4. How might the application of the criminal law with respect to HIV non-disclosure be limited in order not to undermine HIV prevention or the rights of women living with HIV?

NOTES

1 *R. v. Cuerrier*, [1998] 2 S.C.R. 371 at para. 142. [hereinafter *Cuerrier*]

2 This estimate is based on the tracking of cases conducted by the Canadian HIV/AIDS Legal Network. See also E. Mykhalovskiy, G. Betteridge, and D. McLay, "HIV Non-Disclosure and the Criminal Law: Establishing Policy Options for Ontario" (August 2010), (Toronto: A report funded by a grant from the Ontario HIV Treatment Network), and E. Mykhalovskiy and G. Betteridge, "Who? What? Where? When? And with What Consequences? An Analysis of Criminal Cases of HIV Non-disclosure in Canada" (2012), 27 *Canadian Journal of Law and Society* 31–53. Note that the analysis in this chapter focuses on criminal prosecutions for HIV transmission or exposure in the context of consensual sexual activity (that is, consensual but for the non-disclosure of HIV-positive status). Rape and other forms of sexual violence and coercion are not addressed in this paper. Criminal charges have also been brought in relation to exposing someone to a risk, real or perceived, of HIV infection in other contexts such as biting, spitting, scratching, and threatening (e.g., with a syringe). There has also been one case in which an HIV-positive woman pleaded guilty to the offence of "failing to provide the necessaries of life" in relation to transmission to her child, *R. v. J.I.*, 2006 ONCJ 356 (Ontario Court of Justice). In theory, the criminal law could also be applied to other activities representing a risk of HIV transmission, including sharing drug injection equipment. However, to date, we are not aware of any prosecution in Canada in these circumstances.

3 *Cuerrier*, para. 147.

4 *Cuerrier*, paras. 78–82.

5 *Cuerrier*, at para. 128. For more information on the criminal law and HIV non-disclosure, see Canadian HIV/AIDS Legal Network (2011), *Criminal Law and HIV* [Info sheets], at www.aidslaw.ca/publications/publicationsdocEN.php?ref=847

6 *Cuerrier*, at para. 143.

7 Mykhalovskiy, Betteridge, and McLay, "HIV Non-Disclosure" at 19–22.

8 Viral load testing measures the amount of HIV in a bodily fluid, usually blood. Viral load measurements are reported as copies of HIV per millilitre (copies/mL), and values can range from less than 50 to over a million copies/mL. Tests currently used in Canada can measure blood plasma viral loads as low as 20 to 50 copies/mL. Below this level, viral load is said to be "undetectable." This does not mean that HIV has been eliminated from the body, but rather that it is below the level of detection of the test. The goal of antiretroviral therapy is to render viral load undetectable. See CATIE, *Viral Load Testing*, produced in partnership with the Canadian Association of HIV Clinical Laboratory Specialists (CAHCLS) (2006), and NAM/aidsmap, "Viral Load" at http://aidsmap.com/page/1044622/.

9 See further Canadian HIV/AIDS Legal Network, "Criminalization of HIV exposure: Current Canadian Law—Info Sheet 1" (2011), *Criminal Law and HIV* [Info sheets] at www.aidslaw.ca/publications/publicationsdocEN.php?ref=847. Note that in 2010 the Manitoba Court of Appeal ruled that intercourse without a condom may not require disclosure if the PLWHIV's viral load is sufficiently low that there is no longer a "significant risk" of HIV transmission, or if condoms are used carefully and consistently. See *R. v. Mabior*, 2010 MBCA 93, para. 78–97, 127–37. The Quebec Court of Appeal has also acquitted a woman who had one unprotected intercourse without prior disclosing of her HIV-positive status, on the grounds that she had an undetectable viral load and thus the risk of transmission was not significant. See *R. v. D.C.*, 2010 QCCA 2289. Appeals in both of these cases were heard by the Supreme Court of Canada on February 8, 2012; no decision had yet been issued at the time of this writing. Similarly, a trial court in British Columbia acquitted a man in relation to unprotected sex, finding that the medical evidence did not establish a "significant risk" of HIV transmission for the specific sexual activities in question. See *R. v. J.A.T.*, 2010 BCSC 766. In each of these cases, the judges considered scientific evidence about the risk of HIV transmission in the specific circumstances of the case, and were careful to note that a determination regarding risk will have to be made based on the evidence presented in each case. Moreover, at the time of this writing, several cases are before trial courts where prosecutors are arguing that they do not have to prove "significant risk" to prosecute a PLWHIV for non-disclosure under criminal offences such as sexual assault simpliciter.

10 *R. v. Cuerrier*, p. 4.

11 Arguably, there could be a minimal prevention effect in terms of "incapacitation" in the sense that putting a PLWHIV in jail might stop them from having sex with other people in the community. This effect would necessarily be small, and must be considered in light of the fact that sex does occur behind bars (often without access to condoms) and those who are imprisoned usually return to the community without any relevant rehabilitation with respect to their HIV risk behaviours.

12 See for example, S. Burris et al., "Do Criminal Laws Influence HIV Risk Behaviour? An Empirical Trial" (2007), 39 *Arizona State Law Journal* 467–520; K. J. Horvath, R. Weinmeyer, and S. Rosser, "Should It Be Illegal for HIV-Positive Persons to Have Unprotected Sex without Disclosure? An Examination of Attitudes among US Men Who Have Sex with Men and the Impact of State Law" (2010), *AIDS Care* 1–8. Z. Lazzarini, S. Bray, and S. Burris, "Evaluating the Impact

of Criminal Laws on HIV Risk Behavior" (2002), 30 *Journal of Law, Medicine & Ethics* 239–253; I. Grant, "The Boundaries of the Criminal Law" (2008), 31 *Dalhousie Law Journal* 123–180.

13 E. Mykhalovskiy, "The Problem of 'Significant Risk': Exploring the Public Health Impact of Criminalizing HIV Non-Disclosure" (2011), 73 *Social Science & Medicine* 670–677, at 672.

14 For public health purposes, the degree of risk is usually described as "high," "low," or "negligible." See for instance, Canadian Aids Society, *HIV Transmission Guidelines for Assessing Risk: A Resource for Educators, Counsellors, and Health Care Providers* (5th ed., 2005).

15 R. Elliott, Canadian HIV/AIDS Legal Network, *Criminal Law, Public Health and HIV Transmission: A Policy Options Paper* (Geneva: UNAIDS, 2002).

16 S. Burris et al., 467–520. Participants in this study were people who reported behaviour associated with an elevated risk of HIV, either men reporting sex with men or people of either gender reporting injection drug use.

17 Ibid.

18 Horvath et al. validated the findings of Burris et al. in a study of 1,725 men who have sex with men in multiple states of the United States (some with and some without HIV-related criminal laws). Like Burris, Horvath et al. concluded that HIV-related laws are not a deterrent to sexual risk-taking among MSM. K. J. Horvath, R. Weinmeyer, and S. Rosser, "Should It Be Illegal for HIV-Positive Persons to Have Unprotected Sex without Disclosure? An Examination of Attitudes among US Men Who Have Sex with Men and the Impact of State Law" (2010), 22 *AIDS Care* 1221–1228.

19 B. Adam, "Drawing the Line: Views of HIV-Positive People on the Criminalization of HIV Transmission in Canada" (June 2010), presented at the 2nd Annual Symposium on HIV, Law and Human Rights: From Evidence and Principle to Policy and Practice, Toronto.

20 Ibid.

21 At the end of 2008, an estimated 26% of the 65,000 individuals living with HIV in Canada were unaware of their infection. See Public Health Agency of Canada, *Summary: Estimates of HIV Prevalence and Incidence in Canada, 2008* (2009), at www.phac-aspc.gc.ca/aids-sida/publication/survreport/estimat08-eng.php

22 B. G. Brenner et al., "High Rates of Forward Transmission Events after Acute/Early HIV-1 Infection" (2007), 195 *The Journal of Infectious Diseases* 951–959; M. Wawer et al., "Rates of HIV-1 Transmission per Coital Act, by Stage of HIV-1, Infection in Rakai, Ugunda" (2005), 191 *The Journal of Infectious Diseases* 1403–1409; H. I. Hall et al., "HIV Transmissions from Persons with HIV Who Are Aware and Unaware of Their Infection, United States" (2012), 26 *AIDS.* doi:10.1097/QAD013e328351f73f

23 P. O'Byrne, "Criminal Law and Public Health Practice: Are the Canadian HIV Disclosure Laws an Effective HIV Prevention Strategy?" (2012), 9 *Sexuality Research & Social Policy* 70–79 at 76.

24 K. Siegel, H. M. Lekas, and E. W. Schrimshaw, "Serostatus Disclosure to Sexual Partners by HIV-Infected Women before and after the Advent of HAART" (2005), 41(4) *Women and Health* 63–85, citing J. M. Simoni and D. W. Pantalone, "HIV Disclosure and Safer Sex" (2005), 65–98, in S. Kalichman (Ed.), *Positive Prevention: Reducing HIV Transmission among People with HIV/ AIDS* (New York: Kluwer Academic/Plenum, 2005). Also, one should note that the existing

evidence has largely focused on gay and bisexual men.

25 See for example, E. Cameron, *Policy Brief: Criminalization of HIV Transmission* (Geneva: UNA-IDS, 2008); UN General Assembly, *Report of the Special Rapporteur on the right of everyone to the enjoyment of the highest attainable standard of physical and mental health*, Anand Grover, Human Rights Council, Fourteenth session, Agenda item 3, A/HRC/14/20, April 27, 2010; R. Jürgens et al., "Ten Reasons to Oppose the Criminalization of HIV Exposure or Transmission" (2009), 17(34) *Reproductive Health Matters* 163–172; C. L. Galletly and S. D. Pinkerton, "Conflicting Messages: How Criminal HIV Disclosure Laws Undermine Public Health Efforts to Control the Spread of HIV" (2006), 10 *AIDS Behavior* 451–461; R. Lowbury and G. R. Kinghorn, "HIV Transmission as a Crime: Criminal Prosecutions for HIV Transmission Threaten Public Health" (2006), 14 *Student BMJ* editorial; E. Cameron, "Criminalization of HIV Transmission: Poor Public Health Policy" (2009), 14(2) *HIV/AIDS Policy and Law Review* 63–75; Athena Network, *Ten Reasons Why Criminalization of HIV Exposure of Transmission Harms Women* (2009), at www.athenanetwork.org/index.php?id=39.

26 Prosecutors can seek evidence from medical or other records in prosecuting a client accused of exposing someone to risk of HIV infection without disclosing. Canadian law does not automatically protect counselling or medical records from being seized by police or introduced as evidence in court. See also A. MacDonald and H. Worth, "The Mad and the Bad: HIV Infection, Mental Illness, Intellectual Disability and the Law," (2005), 2(2) *Sexuality Research and Social Policy: Journal of NSRC* 51–62; Mykhalovskiy, Betteridge, and McLay, "HIV Non-Disclosure," Section 4; E. Cameron, *Policy Brief: Criminalization of HIV Transmission* (Geneva: UNAIDS, 2008).

27 Cameron, *Policy Brief: Criminalization of HIV Transmission*; International Planned Parenthood Federation et al., *Verdict on a Virus: Public Health, Human Rights and Criminal Law* (2008), at www.ippf.org/resources/publications/verdict-virus.

28 Athena Network, *Ten Reasons*; International Planned Parenthood Federation et al., *Verdict on a Virus*.

29 E. Mykhalovskiy, "The Problem of 'Significant Risk.'" See also P. O'Byrne et al., "Criminal Prosecutions for HIV Status Nondisclosure and HIV Prevention: Results from an Ottawa-Based Gay Men's Sex Survey" (in press), *Journal of the Association of Nurses in AIDS Care*.

30 E. Mykhalovskiy, "The Problem of 'Significant Risk'" at 674.

31 Ibid.

32 Ibid.

33 E. Tharao, N. Massaquoi, and S. Telcom, *Silent Voices of the HIV/AIDS Epidemic: African and Caribbean Women in Toronto 2002–2004* (Toronto, ON: Women's Health in Women's Hands Community Health Centre, 2006) at 27.

34 Note that the Supreme Court dismissed this concern in the *Cuerrier* decision:
"It was also argued that criminalizing non-disclosure of HIV status will undermine the educational message that all are responsible for protecting themselves against HIV infection. Yet this argument can have little weight. Surely those who know they are HIV-positive have a fundamental responsibility to advise their partners of their condition and to ensure that their sex is as safe as possible. It is true that all members of society should be aware of the danger and take

steps to avoid risk. However, the primary responsibility for making the disclosure must rest upon those who are aware they are infected." Para. 144.

35 Cameron, *Policy Brief: Criminalization of HIV Transmission.*

36 C. L. Galletly and S. D. Pinkerton, "Conflicting Messages: How Criminal HIV Disclosure Laws Undermine Public Health Efforts to Control the Spread of HIV" (2006), 10 *AIDS Behavior* 451–461.

37 Ibid.

38 On HIV transmission risk, see D. McLay et al., "Scientific Research on the Risk of the Sexual Transmission of HIV Infection and on HIV as a Chronic Manageable Infection" (updated December 2011), at www.aidslaw.ca/lawyers-kit. Originally published in Mykhalovskiy, Betteridge, and McLay, "HIV Non-Disclosure."

39 UN General Assembly, *Report of the Special Rapporteur.*

40 Galletly and Pinkerton, "Conflicting Messages."

41 To date we are aware of three cases that are not related to HIV in Canada. Three concern herpes, another one, hepatitis B, and the last one, hepatitis C.

42 Mykhalovskiy, Betteridge, and McLay, "HIV Non-Disclosure," *Section 4.*

43 Executive Committee on AIDS Policy and Criminal Law, *"Detention or Prevention?": A Report on the Impact of the Use of Criminal Law on Public Health and the Position of People Living with HIV* (Amsterdam, Netherlands, 2004), 21.

Also see below for a discussion of a woman charged with aggravated sexual assault for telling her sexual partner of her HIV-positive status only after the condom they were using broke *(R. v. Robin Lee St. Clair,* (20 November 2009), Metro North, Ontario (OCJ). Regarding the issue of condom breakage, note that the Court of Appeal of Manitoba has adopted a more nuanced approach. According to the Court, the careful use of a condom can be sufficient to remove the duty to disclose. However, in the case of condom breakage, there would be a duty to disclose. Based on this approach, a person should not be convicted for only disclosing his/her status right after a condom breaks. *R. v. Mabior (C.L.),* 2010 MBCA 93. This decision was appealed to the Supreme Court of Canada. At the time of this writing, a decision had not yet been issued.

44 See A. Symington, "HIV Exposure as Assault: Progressive Development or Misplaced Focus?" (2012), 639–668, in E. Sheehey (Ed.), *Sexual Assault Law, Practice & Activism in a Post-Jane Doe Era* (Ottawa, ON: University of Ottawa Press, 2012).

45 G. R. Gupta, *Approaches for Empowering Women in the HIV/AIDS Pandemic: A Gender Perspective* (2000), presented at the Expert Group Meeting on "the HIV Pandemic and its Gender Implications," November 13–17, Windhoek, Namibia.

46 Canadian HIV/AIDS Legal Network and Interagency Coalition on AIDS and Development, *Addressing HIV Risk Behaviours: A Role for Public Health Legislation and Policy,* 3 (Ottawa, 2010).

47 Ibid., at 1–2.

48 *R. v. Mabior (C.L.),* 2010 MBCA 93, para. 55.

49 This estimate is based on the tracking of cases conducted by the Canadian HIV/AIDS Legal Network. See also Mykhalovskiy, Betteridge, & McLay, "HIV Non-Disclosure" and Mykhalovskiy & Betteridge, "Who? What? Where?". While 13 cases may seem like a small number in proportion to

the number of women living with HIV in Canada, we recognize that the impacts of criminalization of HIV non-disclosure go far beyond the women who have formally been charged and, moreover, that the impacts of criminalization have likely been devastating for each of these women.

50 See for example, A. Larcher and A. Symington, "Criminals and Victims? The Impact of the Criminalization of HIV Non-Disclosure on African, Caribbean and Black Communities in Ontario," 21–22 (Toronto: The African and Caribbean Council on HIV/AIDS in Ontario, 2010) at www.accho.ca/index.aspx?page=resources.

51 For an illustration of HIV stigmatization in Canada, see EKOS Research Associates Inc., *HIV/ AIDS Attitudinal Tracking Survey 2006: Final Report* (Ottawa: Public Health Agency of Canada, 2006); J. Csete, *"Vectors, Vessels and Victims": HIV/AIDS and Women's Human Rights in Canada* (Toronto, ON: Canadian HIV/AIDS Legal Network, 2006) at 20–21.

52 B. Adam, "Effects of the Criminalization of HIV Transmission in *Cuerrier* on Men Reporting Unprotected Sex with Men" (2008), 23(1–2) *Canadian Journal of Law and Society/Revue Canadienne Droit et Société* 143–159 at 149, citing O. K. Duru et al., "Correlates of Sex without Serostatus Disclosure among a National Probability Sample of HIV Patients" (2006), 10 *AIDS and Behavior* 495–507; Siegel, Lekas, and Schrimshaw, "Serostatus Disclosure."

53 Siegel, Lekas, and Schrimshaw, "Serostatus Disclosure."

54 Siegel, Lekas, and Schrimshaw, "Serostatus Disclosure" and studies cited therein. Also Tharao, Massaquoi, and Telcom, *Silent Voices of the HIV/AIDS Epidemic.*

55 C. L. Galletly and J. Dickson-Gomez, "HIV Seropositive Status Disclosure to Prospective Sex Partners and Criminal Laws That Require It: Perspectives of Persons Living with HIV" (2009), 20 *International Journal of STD & AIDS* 613–618; Mykhalovskiy, Betteridge, and McLay, "HIV Non-Disclosure" at 51–52.

56 Mykhalovskiy, Betteridge, and McLay, "HIV Non-Disclosure."

57 *R. v. Robin Lee St. Clair,* (20 November 2009), Metro North, Ontario (OCJ), p. 23. Please see note 43 for information on recent legal developments regarding condom breakage.

58 "Woman with AIDS had unprotected sex," *Calgary Herald,* December 21, 2002.

59 *R. v. D.C.,* [2008] J.Q. 994 (QL), trial decision; *R. v. D.C,* 2010 QCCA 2289, decision of the Court of Appeal.

60 B. Myles, « De bourreau à victime; de victime à criminelle », *Le Devoir,* February 15, 2008; L. Leduc, « Condamnée pour avoir cachée sa séropositivité à son partenaire », *La Presse,* February 15, 2008.

61 *R. v. D.C.,* [2008] J.Q. 994 (QL), para. 153, where the judge indicates: "Il est vrai qu[e le plaignant] attend quatre ans après le fait pour porter plainte. Il est vrai qu'il est difficile de ne pas voir dans cette démarche une certaine vengeance pour la façon dont s'est terminée leur relation. L'amertume est palpable."

62 *R. v. D.C,* 2010 QCCA 2289. The Court acquitted her on the grounds that her viral load was undetectable at the relevant time and that based on the evidence before the court there was no significant risk of transmission.

63 The Supreme Court of Canada heard the appeal on February 8, 2012. As of the time of this writing, a decision had not yet been issued.

64 "Woman gets 4 years for not telling sex partner she was HIV positive," The Canadian Press, February 27, 2009. Retrieved from www.cp24.com/woman-gets-4-years-for-not-telling-sex-partner-she-was-hiv-positive-1.374258.

65 *R. v. J.M.*, [2005] O.J. No. 5649 (QL), para. 25.

66 *R. v. Iamkhong* (16 January 2007), Toronto (Ont. Sup. Ct. J.).

67 Ibid., at p. 15.

68 Ibid., at p. 15–17.

69 T. Godfrey, "HIV Hooker deported; Woman who infected hubby sent back to Thailand," *Toronto Sun*, August 31, 2010.

70 Larcher and Symington, "Criminals and Victims?" at 14–15.

71 See E. Lawson et al., *HIV/AIDS Stigma, Denial, Fear and Discrimination: Experiences and Responses of People from African and Caribbean Communities in Toronto* (Toronto, ON: The African and Caribbean Council on HIV/AIDS in Ontario and the HIV Social, Behavioural and Epidemiological Studies Unit, University of Toronto, 2006).

REFERENCES

Adam, B. (2008). Effects of the criminalization of HIV transmission in *Cuerrier* on men reporting unprotected sex with men. *Canadian Journal of Law and Society/Revue Canadienne Droit et Société, 23*(1–2), 143–159, citing O. K. Duru, R. L. Collins, D. H. Ciccarone, S. C. Morton, R. Stall, R. Beckman, ... D. E. Kanouse. (2006). Correlates of sex without serostatus disclosure among a national probability sample of HIV patients. *AIDS and Behavior, 10*(5), 495–507.

Adam, B. (2010). Drawing the line: Views of HIV-positive people on the criminalization of HIV transmission in Canada. Paper presented at the 2nd Annual Symposium on HIV, Law and Human Rights: From Evidence and Principle to Policy and Practice, Toronto, Ontario.

Athena Network. (2009). *Ten reasons why criminalization of HIV exposure of transmission harms women*. Retrieved from www.athenanetwork.org/index.php?id=39

Brenner, B. G., Roger, M., Routy, J. P., Moisi, D., Ntemgwa, M., Matte, C., ... Tremblay, C., for the Share Quebec Primary HIV Infection Study Group. (2007). High rates of forward transmission events after acute/early HIV-1 infection. *The Journal of Infectious Diseases, 195*(7), 951–959.

Burris, S., Beletsky, L., Burleson, J. A., Case, P., & Lazzarini, Z. (2007). Do criminal laws influence HIV risk behaviour? An empirical trial. *Arizona State Law Journal, 39*, 467–520.

Cameron, E. (2008). *Policy brief: Criminalization of HIV transmission*. Geneva: UNAIDS.

Cameron, E. (2009). Criminalization of HIV transmission: Poor public health policy. *HIV/AIDS Policy and Law Review, 14*(2), 63–75.

Canadian AIDS Society. (2005). *HIV transmission guidelines for assessing risk: A resource for educators, counsellors, and health care providers—Fifth edition*. Retrieved from www.cdnaids.ca/hivtransmissionguidelinesforassessi

Canadian HIV/AIDS Legal Network. (2011). *Criminal law and HIV* [Info sheets]. Retrieved from www.aidslaw.ca/publications/publicationsdocEN.php?ref=847

Canadian HIV/AIDS Legal Network. (2011). Criminalization of HIV exposure: Current Canadian Law — Info Sheet 1, *Criminal Law and HIV* [Info sheets]. Retrieved from www.aidslaw.ca/publications/publicationsdocEN.php?ref=847

Canadian HIV/AIDS Legal Network and Interagency Coalition on AIDS and Development. (2010). *Addressing HIV risk behaviours: A role for public health legislation and policy.* Ottawa.

CATIE. (2006). *Viral load testing.* Produced in partnership with the Canadian Association of HIV Clinical Laboratory Specialists (CAHCLS), and NAM/aidsmap, *Viral load.* Retrieved from http://aidsmap.com/page/1044622/

Csete, J. (2006). *"Vectors, vessels and victims": HIV/AIDS and women's human rights in Canada.* Toronto, ON: Canadian HIV/AIDS Legal Network.

EKOS Research Associates Inc. (2006). HIV/AIDS attitudinal tracking survey 2006: Final report, Ottawa: Public Health Agency of Canada.

Elliott, R. (2002). Criminal law, public health and HIV transmission: A policy options paper. Canadian HIV/AIDS Legal Network. Geneva: UNAIDS.

Executive Committee on AIDS Policy and Criminal Law. (2004). *Detention or prevention?: A report on the impact of the use of criminal law on public health and the position of people living with HIV.* Amsterdam, Netherlands.

Galletly, C. L., & Dickson-Gomez, J. (2009). HIV seropositive status disclosure to prospective sex partners and criminal laws that require it: Perspectives of persons living with HIV. *International Journal of STD & AIDS, 20*(9), 613–618.

Galletly, C. L., & Pinkerton, S. D. (2006). Conflicting messages: How criminal HIV disclosure laws undermine public health efforts to control the spread of HIV. *AIDS Behavior, 10*(5), 451–461.

Godfrey, T. (2010, August 31). HIV hooker deported; woman who infected hubby sent back to Thailand. *Toronto Sun.*

Grant, I. (2008). The boundaries of the criminal law. *Dalhousie Law Journal, 31*(1), 123–180.

Gupta, G. R. (2000, November). *Approaches for empowering women in the HIV/AIDS pandemic: A gender perspective.* Presented at the Expert Group Meeting on "the HIV pandemic and its gender implications," Windhoek, Namibia.

Hall, H. I., Holtgrave, D. R., & Maulsby, C. (2012). HIV transmissions from persons with HIV who are aware and unaware of their infection, United States. *AIDS, 26*(7), 893–896. doi:10.1097/QAD013e328351f73f

Horvath, K. J., Weinmeyer, R., & Rosser, S. (2010). Should it be illegal for HIV-positive persons to have unprotected sex without disclosure? An examination of attitudes among US men who have sex with men and the impact of state law. *AIDS Care, 22*(10), 1221–1228.

International Planned Parenthood Federation, GNP+, & ICW. (2008). *Verdict on a virus: Public health, human rights and criminal law.* Retrieved from www.ippf.org/resources/publications/verdict-virus

Jürgens, R., Cohen, J., Cameron, E., Burris, S., Clayton, M., Elliott, R., ... & Cupido, D. (2009). Ten reasons to oppose the criminalization of HIV exposure or transmission. *Reproductive Health Matters, 17*(34), 163–172.

Larcher, A., & Symington, A. (2010). Criminals and victims? The impact of the criminalization of

HIV non-disclosure on African, Caribbean and Black communities in Ontario. Toronto, ON: The African and Caribbean Council on HIV/AIDS in Ontario. Retrieved from www.accho.ca/index.aspx?page=resources

Law Reform Commission of Canada. (1976). *Our Criminal Law: Report.* Ottawa: Information-Canada.

Lawson, E., Gardezi, F., Calzavara, L., Husbands, W., Myers, T., & Tharao, W. (2006). *HIV/AIDS stigma, denial, fear and discrimination: Experiences and responses of people from African and Caribbean communities in Toronto.* Toronto, ON: The African and Caribbean Council on HIV/AIDS in Ontario and the HIV Social, Behavioural and Epidemiological Studies Unit, University of Toronto.

Lazzarini, Z., Bray, S., & Burris, S. (2002). Evaluating the impact of criminal laws on HIV risk behavior. *Journal of Law, Medicine & Ethics,* 30: 239–253.

Leduc, L. (2008). Condamnée pour avoir cachée sa séropositivité à son partenaire. *La Presse.*

Lowbury, R., & Kinghorn, G. R. (2006). HIV transmission as a crime. Criminal prosecutions for HIV transmission threaten public health [Editorial]. *Student BMJ,* 14.

MacDonald, A., & Worth, H. (2005). The mad and the bad: HIV infection, mental illness, intellectual disability and the law. *Sexuality Research and Social Policy: Journal of NSRC,* 2(2), 51–62.

McLay, D., Mykhalovskiy, E., & Betteridge, G. (2011). Scientific research on the risk of the sexual transmission of HIV infection and on HIV as a chronic manageable infection. (updated December 2011). Originally published in Mykhalovskiy, E., Betteridge, G., and McLay, D. (2010). *HIV non-disclosure and the criminal law: Establishing policy options for Ontario.* A report funded by a grant from the Ontario HIV Treatment Network, Toronto. Retrieved from www.aidslaw.ca/lawyers-kit

Mykhalovskiy, E. (2011). The problem of "significant risk": Exploring the public health impact of criminalizing HIV non-disclosure. *Social Science & Medicine,* 73(5), 668–675.

Mykhalovskiy, E., & Betteridge, G. (2012). Who? What? Where? When? And with what consequences? An analysis of criminal cases of HIV non-disclosure in Canada. *Canadian Journal of Law and Society,* 27(1), 31–53.

Mykhalovskiy, E., Betteridge, G., & McLay, D. (2010, August). *HIV non-disclosure and the criminal law: Establishing policy options for Ontario.* A report funded by a grant from the Ontario HIV Treatment Network, Toronto.

Myles, B. (2008). De bourreau à victime; de victime à criminelle. *Le Devoir.*

O'Byrne, P. (2012). Criminal law and public health practice: Are the Canadian HIV disclosure laws an effective HIV prevention strategy? *Sexuality Research & Social Policy,* 9(1): 70–79.

Public Health Agency of Canada. (2009). *Summary: Estimates of HIV prevalence and incidence in Canada, 2008.* Retrieved from www.phac-aspc.gc.ca/aids-sida/publication/survreport/estimat08-eng.php

R. v. Cuerrier, [1998] 2 S.C.R.

R. v. D.C, 2010 QCCA 2289, decision of the Court of Appeal.

R. v. D.C., 2008 J.Q. 994 (QL), trial decision.

R. v. Iamkhong (16 January 2007), Toronto (Ont. Sup. Ct. J.).

R. v. J.A.T., 2010 BCSC 766

R. v. J.I., 2006 ONCJ 356 (Ontario Court of Justice).

R. v. J.M., 2005 O.J. No. 5649 (QL), para. 25.

R. v. Mabior, 2010 MBCA 93

R. v. Robin Lee St. Clair, (20 November 2009), Metro North, Ontario (OCJ).

Siegel, K., Lekas, H. M., & Schrimshaw, E. E. (2005). Serostatus disclosure to sexual partners by HIV-infected women before and after the advent of HAART. *Women and Health, 41*(4), 63–85.

Simoni, J. M., & Pantalone, D. W. (2005). HIV disclosure and safer sex. In S. Kalichman (Ed.), *Positive prevention: Reducing HIV transmission among people with HIV/AIDS* (pp. 65–98). New York: Kluwer Academic/Plenum.

Symington, A. (2012). HIV exposure as assault: Progressive development or misplaced focus? In E. Sheehey (Ed.), *Sexual assault law, practice & activism in a post-Jane Doe era* (pp. 639–668). Ottawa, ON: University of Ottawa Press.

Tharao, E., Massaquoi, N., & Telcom, S. (2006). *Silent voices of the HIV/AIDS epidemic: African and Caribbean Women in Toronto 2002–2004*. Toronto, ON: Women's Health in Women's Hands Community Health Centre.

UN General Assembly. (2010, April 27). *Report of the Special Rapporteur on the right of everyone to the enjoyment of the highest attainable standard of physical and mental health*. Anand Grover, Human Rights Council, Fourteenth session, Agenda item 3, A/HRC/14/20.

Wawer, M., Gray, R. H., Sewankambo, N. K., Serwadda, D., Li, X., Laey, N., ... & Quinn, T. C. (2005). Rates of HIV-1 transmission per coital act, by stage of HIV-1, Infection in Rakai, Ugunda. *The Journal of Infectious Diseases, 191*(9), 1403–1409.

Woman gets 4 years for not telling sex partner she was HIV positive. (2009, February 27). The Canadian Press. Retrieved from www.cp24.com/woman-gets-4-years-for-not-telling-sex-partner-she-was-hiv-positive-1.374258

Woman with AIDS had unprotected sex. (2002, December 21). *Calgary Herald*.

Chapter 10

PRECONCEPTION AND PREGNANCY PLANNING FOR WOMEN LIVING WITH AND AFFECTED BY HIV AS HIV PREVENTION

Mona Loutfy and Shari Margolese

INTRODUCTION

For many years, fear has thwarted the desire of people living with and affected by human immunodeficiency virus (HIV) to have children: fear of stigma and discrimination from friends, family, and health care supports; fear of infecting their partner during conception; fear of not living long enough to see their child grow up; and, of course, the fear of HIV passing to their child.

Today, with more effective treatment, HIV-positive people in Canada are living longer, healthier lives, and the risk of a child contracting HIV has been reduced to below 1%, leading many to consider starting or enlarging their families. While optimism has begun to replace fear of early death and vertical HIV transmission between mother and child, there is still much work to be done to reduce the stigma and discrimination associated with pregnancy in the context of HIV and to provide access to services and resources to reduce the risk of horizontal HIV transmission between partners during conception.

Epidemiology of HIV-Positive People Living in Canada

Globally, heterosexual contact is the most common mode of transmission of HIV, and this trend has been steadily increasing in Canada. Because of this factor, and combined with women's increased biological susceptibility to HIV infection, women comprise over half of the prevalent cases of HIV worldwide. Globally, it is estimated that 33.4 million people are living with HIV and/or have acquired immunodeficiency syndrome (AIDS). Of those, 31.3 million are adults, and 15.7 million are women (World Health Organization & UNAIDS, 2008). Most of these HIV-positive women are of reproductive age (16–44 years) and may therefore be interested in pregnancy. In Canada, by the end of 2002, there were an estimated 56,000 people with HIV/AIDS,

7,700 of whom were women (Public Health Agency of Canada [PHAC], 2007). By the end of 2007, 64,800 positive HIV tests had been reported, where 10,514 of these were women (PHAC, 2007). Among them, at least 80% were of child-bearing age (PHAC, 2007). The proportion of heterosexual men living with HIV is also rising (Baeten & Overbaugh, 2003). By December 2007, the proportion of those who tested HIV positive in Canada and who indicated that heterosexual contact was their mode of acquisition was close to 30%, while 40% reported being men who have sex with men (PHAC, 2007). This has led to an interest in having children, not only among HIV-positive women that are of child-bearing age, but also among HIV-positive men who may wish to conceive with an HIV-negative or HIV-positive female partner, indicating a need for preconception counselling for both women and men living with and affected by HIV.

Improvement of Life Expectancy with Antiretroviral Treatment

During the past 10 years, the natural history of HIV infection has significantly changed with the advent of combination antiretroviral therapy (ART). The mortality and morbidity caused by HIV have significantly decreased, resulting in a prolonged life expectancy and improved quality of life. Prior to successful treatment, which has only been widely prescribed since 1996, an HIV-positive individual could expect to live about 10 years before developing AIDS, leading to death. This uncertainty about the future discouraged many HIV-positive people from having children. Today, the life expectancy of someone living with HIV is similar to that of the general population. Present projections estimate that a person will live 30 to 40 years from the time of HIV infection (Palella et al., 1998).

Reduction in HIV Vertical Transmission

One of the most dramatic breakthroughs in HIV treatment in the past 15 years is the ability of ART to reduce the rate of vertical transmission of HIV between an HIV-positive mother and her child. Prior to the use of ART in pregnancy, the risk of vertical transmission ranged from 20% to 30% (National Institute of Allergy and Infectious Diseases, 2008). Research initiated in the early 1990s found that the use of the antiretroviral medication zidovudine (AZT) during pregnancy could reduce the rate of vertical transmission to 8% (Connor et al., 1994). As treatments have improved, the rate of vertical transmission has continued to decline. Today, the use of ART, Caesarean section if indicated, and not breastfeeding have led to the risk of vertical transmission of HIV from an HIV-positive mother to her child being less than 1% (PHAC, 2007).

The decline in vertical transmission rates combined with an increased life expectancy has created optimism about the future for people living with HIV (PLWHIV), and many HIV-positive individuals and couples are now considering starting a family. This, in turn, leads to a consideration of issues relating to fertility and pregnancy planning, including the prevention of horizontal transmission of HIV during conception.

Epidemiology of Pregnancy to HIV-Positive Women in Canada

Increased interest in pregnancy has been confirmed by the increasing numbers of pregnancies among HIV-positive women over the past decade. In Canada, all pregnancies to HIV-positive mothers are reported through a registry created by the Canadian Paediatric AIDS Research Group. The last annual reporting, in 2008, reported that 238 children were born to HIV-positive women in Canada. In the four preceding years, the annual number of children born to HIV-positive women were 208 (2007), 194 (2006), 189 (2005), and 179 (2004), confirming the increasing trend in pregnancies of HIV-positive women (Loutfy et al., 2012b).

High Rates of Unintended Pregnancies among HIV-Positive Women

As is in the general population, many pregnancies are unplanned in the context of HIV. A sub-analysis of a 2009 fertility study revealed a high prevalence of unintended pregnancies in HIV-positive women of reproductive age in Ontario, Canada (Loutfy et al., 2012b). Among 416 HIV-positive women who had been pregnant, 56% of all pregnancies were unintended (Gogna, Pecheny, Ibarlucía, Manzelli, & López, 2009). A similar study conducted in Argentina reported that 55% of HIV-positive women had at least one pregnancy after their HIV diagnosis and that more than half of those pregnancies were unintended (Loutfy et al., 2012b). One of the goals of the Canadian National HIV Pregnancy Planning Guidelines (NHPPG), which are described later in this chapter, is to encourage health care providers to discuss pregnancy planning, including contraception, with their patients as early as possible after diagnosis to reduce the incidence of unintended pregnancy and the risk of both vertical and horizontal HIV transmission (Ogilvie et al., 2007).

Intentions and Desires of HIV-Positive Women in Canada to Conceive

Two important Canadian studies have reported on the intentions and desires of HIV-positive women to conceive. In 2006, Ogilvie et al. conducted a research study to examine the fertility intentions of women living with HIV in British Columbia, Canada. Of the 182 women studied, 25.8% expressed intentions to have children regardless of their clinical HIV status, which is close to levels in the general population (Loutfy et al., 2009a). Loutfy et al. (2009a) completed a cross-sectional study designed to assess fertility desires, intentions, and actions. This study surveyed 490 HIV-positive women of reproductive age (18–52) living in Ontario. Of the 490 participating women, 61% were born outside of Canada, 52% were living in Toronto, 47% were of African ethnicity. The median age was 38 (interquartile range, 32–43), and 74% were currently on ART. Of all respondents, 69% desired to give birth and 57% intended to give birth in the future. This study found that the significant predictors of fertility intentions were younger age (less than 40), African ethnicity, residing in Toronto, and a lower number of lifetime births (p=0.02) (Williams, Watkins, & Risby, 1996).

In the aforementioned studies, it was concluded that the desires and intentions of HIV-positive women to have children were high and that clinical HIV status did not appear to be a predictor of intention to conceive. Thus, there appears to be strong desire and intent to have children among HIV-positive women in Canada, to levels approaching the general population.

A 1996 paper published by Williams et al. reviewed the modest data available on reproductive decision making in HIV-positive women and found that knowledge of HIV infection was not associated with pregnancy termination or subsequent pregnancy prevention. This alludes to the fact that HIV-positive women are having and will continue to have children, so health professionals must be prepared to guide them in this process.

Lack of Services to Support Safe Conception

Despite the fact that many HIV-positive individuals and couples wish to have children, there is a scarcity of heath care service providers in Canada offering preconception and assisted reproductive services. Such services would include advice on the management of HIV during preconception and conception, including timing of ovulation to allow fertilization, sperm washing (a procedure designed to remove the HIV viral particles from the sperm, reducing the chance of horizontal transmission), management of individuals or couples affected by infertility issues, intrauterine insemination and in vitro fertilization, as well as basic preconception advice, such as taking folic acid to reduce the risk of neural tube defects, eating a healthy diet, and stopping or reducing alcohol and recreational drug use (Bujan et al., 2007).

In Europe, HIV-positive couples have been given reproductive assistance since the 1980s, and at least five European countries have national programs to assist people living with HIV in their pregnancy planning (Apoola, tenHof, & Allan, 2001; Myer, Morroni, & El-Sadr, 2005; Pitts & Shields, 2004; Rozenberg, Gerard, Manigart, Ham, & Delvigne, 2002). As of 2003, in the U.S., less than 5% of fertility clinics offered reproductive care to HIV-positive serodiscordant couples (Klein, Peña, Thornton, & Sauer, 2003). In Canada, Southern Ontario Fertility Technologies (SOFT) in London, Ontario, was the first fertility clinic to offer services to HIV-positive individuals, such as sperm washing, which can dramatically reduce the risk of horizontal transmission when the male partner is HIV positive. A few years after SOFT had established a precedent, the ISIS Regional Fertility Centre in Mississauga and the Mount Sinai Reproductive Biology Unit began offering assisted reproduction to HIV-positive individuals and couples (Loutfy et al., 2009a). A 2010 study by Yudin, Shapiro, and Loutfy surveyed 23 fertility clinics across eight Canadian provinces. Seventy-eight percent of these clinics (18 of 23) were willing to accept HIV-positive individuals in consultation, and 52% had actually seen at least one HIV-positive man or woman in the previous year. Clinics in every province were willing to offer infertility investigations, but clinics located in only five provinces were willing to offer fertility treatments. The most commonly available treatment was intrauterine insemination for couples in which the female partner was HIV positive (52%). Other techniques, such as sperm washing or in vitro fertilization, were less commonly offered (26% and 17% respectively). A smaller number of clinics were willing to offer risk reduction techniques in achieving pregnancy. The authors concluded that access to infertility investigations and treatments in Canada is limited and regionally dependent (Yudin et al., 2010).

Different services and treatment protocols are offered depending on the individual clinic or centre and, as a result, the costs associated with each service vary depending on the type of treatment or service and the location where it is administered. There are currently only a handful of fertility clinics in all of Canada that offer full reproductive technology services to HIV-positive individuals and couples, which would include in vitro fertilization (IVF). In addition to the lack of assisted reproductive services, there remains a scarcity of pregnancy planning, and prenatal and postnatal care information resources and programs for HIV-positive individuals and couples in Canada.

REPRODUCTIVE RIGHTS, HARM REDUCTION, AND PREVENTION IN PREGNANCY PLANNING FOR HIV-POSITIVE WOMEN

Reproductive Rights

Globally, there is a long, documented history of reproductive rights violations against HIV-positive women, including coerced abortion and surgical sterilization techniques, sometimes even without consent (Engender Health and International Community of Women Living with HIV/AIDS, 2006). Women have also reported encountering negative attitudes from health care providers when they bring up the subject of pregnancy, become pregnant, or require health care services while pregnant (Bell et al., 2007). These discriminatory actions have almost certainly discouraged some HIV-positive women from discussing reproductive health with their physicians and to miss important opportunities to discuss HIV prevention in the context of pregnancy planning. According to Amnesty International USA, "all women have the right to accessible, affordable and adequate health care ... that responds to their particular needs as women. Examples include: accurate information about HIV transmission [and] the ability to choose whether and when to get pregnant" (Amnesty International USA, 2012).

Wilcher and Cates (2009) recently published a landmark piece about reproductive choices for women living with HIV. They stressed that "access to reproductive health services for HIV-positive women is critical to ensuring their reproductive needs are addressed and their rights protected" (p. 833). In addition, they stressed that preventing unintended pregnancies in women with HIV is an essential component of a comprehensive vertical transmission prevention program. They call for stronger linkages between sexual and reproductive health, and HIV policies, programs, and services. Although limited thus far, such linkages are starting to be developed in several international organizations and countries including Canada (Wilcher & Cates, 2009).

Preconception Planning for HIV-Positive Women as Harm Reduction and Prevention Issues

As stated earlier, HIV-positive women have both strong desires and intentions to become pregnant (Chen, Philips, Kanouse, Collins, & Miu, 2001). Given this, it becomes imperative to have a discussion about strategies to reduce harm during conception and pregnancy. Preconception counselling and access to assisted reproductive technologies act as both harm reduction and prevention tools. People living with HIV who do not have access to or who cannot afford assisted conception services, or who fear stigma from accessing these services, may be more likely to attempt natural conception, which carries a risk of horizontal HIV transmission. Comprehensive reproductive health and preconception counselling, and access to assisted reproductive technologies have the potential to inform couples living with and affected by HIV about practising safer conception methods and reducing the risk of horizontal HIV transmission, which in turn could reduce the risk of vertical HIV transmission. Vertical HIV transmission is highest if an HIV-negative woman seroconverts to become infected with HIV during pregnancy. This is a real possibility for couples where the man is HIV positive and the woman is HIV negative, and they are using natural conception. Furthermore, increased access to assisted reproductive technologies and reproductive health and preconception counselling also has the potential to greatly reduce the risk of unintended pregnancy. Reducing unintended pregnancies among HIV-positive women may reduce the occurrence of voluntary pregnancy termination (VPT). A recent Italian study compared 63 cases of VPT with 334 pregnancies not ending in a VPT among HIV-positive women. They found a significant correlation between unintended pregnancy and VPT, leading the authors to conclude that improved access to pregnancy planning in the context of HIV could reduce the occurrence of VPT (Floridia et al., 2010). In conclusion, providing increased reproductive and preconception counselling and services is crucial for providing opportunities for health care providers to develop individualized management strategies to reduce harm to the fetus and uninfected partners during conception, labour and delivery, and breastfeeding.

ISSUES AT HAND WHEN CONSIDERING REPRODUCTION FOR WOMEN LIVING WITH HIV

A large gap exists between the desires, intentions, and need for support of PLWHIV to have children and the availability of necessary resources, relevant research, and support networks to do so successfully and in a medically safe manner. It is important to note that the issues at hand when considering pregnancy planning in the context of HIV are not just the prevention of vertical transmission but also the prevention of horizontal transmission from one partner to the other, encouraging a healthy preconception period and the management of potential infertility issues.

Healthy Preconception

Management of HIV in pregnancy planning requires many special considerations. First and foremost, it is important for clinicians to initiate a discussion about potential pregnancy with all HIV-positive women of child-bearing age and with all HIV-positive men. A 2009 HIV pregnancy planning study found that although 95% of HIV-positive people reported that they saw a health care provider and 63% reported that they expect a future pregnancy, only 30% reported some knowledge about available pregnancy planning services and only 30% spoke to a health care provider about this issue (Loutfy et al., 2009a).

Comprehensive preconception counselling is an important opportunity for clinicians to determine pregnancy desires and intentions among individuals, to review current medications to ensure that neither prospective parent is on potentially teratogenetic treatment, to discuss safe options for conception, and to determine overall health. During preconception counselling, it is important to remember that most general recommendations for pregnancy planning also apply to HIV-positive individuals. The National HIV Pregnancy Planning Guidelines (NHPPG), currently under development, will assist clinicians in providing comprehensive evidence-based recommendations regarding pregnancy planning to their HIV-positive patients (Loutfy et al., 2012a). Several guidelines are available to assist all women in achieving optimal health prior to conception, which also apply to HIV-positive women and HIV-negative female partners in serodiscordant relationships. Clinical practice guidelines regarding pregnancy are available from the Society of Obstetricians and Gynaecologists of Canada (SOGC) (n.d.). SOGC also offers specific guidelines for management of sexually transmitted diseases such as herpes simplex virus (HSV) (SGOC, 2008), human papilloma virus (HPV) (SGOC, 2007), and hepatitis C (SGOC, 2000), all of which have important implications during delivery. This is also important when discussing HIV prevention during conception because the risk of HIV transmission increases in the presence of sexually transmitted diseases. Health Canada is another important source of information to ensure a healthy mother, child, and family. *Eating Well with Canada's Food Guide* provides women with the information they need to eat well during pregnancy and includes specific "Advice for … Women of childbearing age" (Health Canada, 2011). The Public Health Agency of Canada (PHAC) has described alcohol use in pregnancy as "an important public health and social issue for Canadians." This is due to the increasing societal awareness of the significant personal and social costs associated with fetal alcohol spectrum disorder (PHAC, 2012). PHAC has also produced *The Sensible Guide to a Healthy Pregnancy*, which includes guidance on general nutrition, folic acid, alcohol, physical activity, smoking, and oral health (PHAC, 2011).

Vertical HIV Transmission

As we have discussed in the introduction to this chapter, the rate of vertical HIV transmission to children of HIV-positive women has witnessed a dramatic decline in the past 15 years. In addition to the impressive impact of ART on the ability to reduce vertical transmission, researchers have concluded that the choice of obstetrical practices as well as choosing not to breastfeed are also important components in the prevention of vertical transmission.

Prevention of vertical HIV transmission

The importance of the prevention of vertical HIV transmission cannot be over-emphasized. Prior work in the area of HIV and fertility has focused primarily on the clinical management of pregnancy and on the health of the unborn child. A wealth of literature on this subject has been produced, as well as clinical management guidelines for HIV-positive women during pregnancy and care of the child postpartum (AIDSinfo, n.d.). Generally, these guidelines recommend initiation of a non-terato-genetic combination ART regimen after the first trimester of pregnancy for women who have stable HIV infection and do not require ART for their own HIV treatment. Women who do require ART for their own HIV treatment would be started on a non-teratogenetic combination ART regimen as soon as possible and are usually able to continue on this treatment for the duration of the pregnancy. Decisions about HIV treatment during pregnancy should be made in consultation with an HIV specialist and take into consideration both the health of the mother and the efficacy of the treatment to prevent vertical HIV transmission. In addition to treating the HIV-positive mother with ART, the infant is also given treatment for up to 6 weeks of life, which further reduces the risk of vertical HIV transmission (AIDSinfo, 2011).

Elective Caesarean section births also play a role in the reduction of vertical HIV transmission in some cases. Specifically, a Caesarean birth has been shown to reduce the risk of vertical HIV transmission if the mother has an HIV viral load greater than 1,000 just prior to the time of delivery (Shapiro et al., 2004). Caesarean section deliveries are generally available as an option for most HIV-positive women in Canada regardless of their viral load.

Breastfeeding while HIV positive increases the risk of vertical HIV transmission by an additional 16.2% (Nduati et al., 2001) and is not recommended in Canada and other resource-rich countries where feeding alternatives such as formula are available (Canadian Paediatric Society, 2004). Many Canadian provinces offer baby formula programs, which provide free formula to HIV-positive new mothers to reduce the additional cost associated with not breastfeeding. More detailed information regarding the management of HIV-positive pregnant women and their infants can be found in the *Recommendations for Use of Antiretroviral Drugs in Pregnant HIV-1 Infected Women for Maternal Health and Interventions to Reduce Perinatal HIV-1 Transmission in the United States* (Department of Health and Human Services, 2012).

Prevention of Horizontal Transmission

In the context of HIV and pregnancy planning, prevention of horizontal HIV transmission refers to the transmission of HIV from one person to another during conception. Prevention of horizontal HIV transmission is important for both serodiscordant couples, where one partner is HIV positive and the other partner is not, and seroconcordant couples, where both partners are HIV positive.

HIV transmission between HIV discordant couples

It is important to understand the risk of HIV transmission between HIV discordant couples in order for patients to make informed choices about conception and for clinicians to optimize management of conception. In the case of an HIV-positive man who is not taking ART, the risk of HIV transmission to his uninfected female partner is quoted as 0.1% to 0.3% per act of unprotected vaginal intercourse. This assumes that the couple is in a stable relationship and that they are not participating in any other form of high-risk activity (Rozenberg et al., 2002). Without the intervention of ART, the risk of transmission from an HIV-positive woman to her uninfected male partner is reported to be 0.03% to 0.09% per act of unprotected vaginal intercourse, which is lower than male-to-female transmission (Baeten & Overbaugh, 2003). Plasma viral load is also a determining factor when discussing the risk of HIV transmission. In general, plasma viral load is concordant with the viral load of genital secretions. However, HIV-positive people and their uninfected partners should be counselled that this is not always the case. Combination ART further reduces the risk when long-term viral suppression is achieved. Normally, the viral load in semen is lower than that in blood. However, this is greatly influenced by the use of ART, which is known to have optimal penetration of the genital tract, and the absence of co-existing sexually transmitted infections (STIs), as well as the absence of drug resistance. It is possible to achieve an undetectable viral load in genital secretions with the long-term use of ART. However, this can be problematic since assays to detect genital fluid viral load are not readily available. While the presence of co-existing STIs greatly increases genital viral load, it does not increase the viral load in plasma. Treatment of the STI typically reduces the genital viral load (Baeten & Overbaugh, 2003; Bagasra et al., 1994; Barreiro, Castilla, Labarga, & Soriano, 2007; Cohen et al., 1997; Maestro & de Vincenzi, 1996; Vettore, Schecter, Melo, Boechat, & Barroso, 2006).

Vernazza, Hirschel, Bernasconi, and Flepp (2008) issued a controversial statement known as the "Swiss Statement," which suggested that HIV-infected people who fulfill a series of conditions are considered non-infectious and unable to pass the virus via sexual contact. These conditions include:

- The individual living with HIV is under the care of a treating physician and is compliant with ART.
- The viral load has been undetectable for at least six months.
- The individual living with HIV is not experiencing any other STIs.

The controversial nature of the Swiss Statement has led researchers to begin to conduct further studies to verify its validity.

HIV transmission between concordant couples

The main issue of concern regarding HIV transmission between HIV concordant couples is the risk of HIV super-infection. Ramos et al. (2002) defined super-infection as "the re-infection of an individual, after a primary HIV-1 infection, with a heterologous (foreign) strain belonging to the same subtype as the primary strain or to a different one" (p. 7444). While there is no existing literature on super-infection and fertility, it is nevertheless an important topic to consider in the context of HIV and pregnancy. Specifically, studies have shown that super-infection is a necessary first step for viral recombination to occur. Recombination may produce more virulent viruses, drug-resistant viruses, or viruses with altered cell tropism. Also, recombinant viruses and super-infection can accelerate disease progression and increase the probability of sexual transmission by increasing viral load in the blood and genital tract (Blackard, Cohen, & Mayer, 2002).

Methods of Conception

Decisions regarding a method of conception for HIV-positive women and men are generally based on which partner is HIV positive and which method provides the most effective means to prevent HIV transmission. Although more research is required to determine exactly what other factors may require consideration when deciding which conception method to use, we can hypothesize that this decision may also be influenced by availability of, access to, and cost of procedures to reduce transmission, as well as knowledge about existing resources and services.

Natural conception

It was not until recently that natural conception was seen as an option for HIV-positive people. Though not for everyone, natural conception is suitable in some circumstances, and the context of each individual case must be evaluated. Prospective parents must have a frank discussion with each other and their HIV specialist on the risks of HIV transmission and super-infection during unprotected intercourse in order to make an informed decision regarding this option. As discussed above, the relative risk involved in natural conception is dependent on whether the HIV-positive partner is taking ART, the plasma viral load of the partner living with HIV, the frequency of intercourse, the presence of STIs, and which partner is positive (Barreiro et al., 2007). More research is required regarding the motivating factors surrounding the decision to conceive naturally.

Natural conception with timed ovulation

After a thorough discussion with their HIV specialist regarding the risk of transmission, some serodiscordant couples opt to proceed with what is termed *timed unprotected intercourse* in order to conceive (Barreiro et al., 2007). Limiting the number of intercourse acts to the time of ovulation may not only further reduce the risk of HIV infection merely by reducing the number of unprotected sexual exposures, but it may also increase the likelihood of becoming pregnant. Although the risk of transmission to the uninfected partner cannot be quoted as zero, mathematical models cite a risk of 1 in 100,000 per act of unprotected intercourse if the criteria of the Swiss Statement are met. Many resources are available through health care providers and on the Internet to assist women in timing their ovulation.

Home insemination

Home insemination is a particularly popular option for conception for HIV-positive women with HIV-negative partners and for same-sex female couples and single women. The procedure involves collecting sperm from a partner or donor in a sterile container or a condom. The sperm is drawn into a needle-less syringe and then inserted into the vagina as close to the cervix as possible. Optimal results are achieved when insemination is done during ovulation. This is a particularly attractive method as it is very low cost and does not require the assistance of a fertility specialist. If home insemination is unsuccessful after three to six months, HIV-positive women should seek the assistance of a fertility specialist.

Assisted reproductive technologies

Assisted reproductive technologies play an important role in preventing horizontal HIV transmission, particularly when the man is HIV positive and the woman is not. These procedures require the services of a fertility clinic. Unfortunately, many fertility clinics do not provide service to PLWHIV and those that do are limited to certain geographic areas. While a small number of reproductive services are covered by some provinces, most are not, and they range in cost from $400 to $14,000 per ovulation cycle. Added to the cost of the assisted reproductive procedures may be the cost of travel to a fertility clinic, time away from work, and child care expenses for other children.

The use of sperm washing or donor sperm with intrauterine insemination (IUI), in vitro fertilization (IVF), or intracytoplasmic sperm injection (ICSI): Sperm washing is a well established, effective, and safe risk-reduction fertility option for both discordant couples, where the man is HIV positive and the woman is HIV negative, and concordant couples, where viral resistance has been identified. Semen is centrifuged to separate live sperm (which does not carry HIV) from seminal plasma and non-germinal cells (which may carry HIV), and the sperm is then inseminated into the female partner at the time of ovulation. According to the literature published to date, which is extensive, there have been no reported cases of infection of the female partner when sperm washing is carried out following the reported published protocols in more than 3,000 cycles of sperm washing combined with IUI, IVF, or ICSI. The results of a multi-centre retrospective analysis of 1,036 serodiscordant couples from eight European centres offering sperm washing reported 2,840 IUI cycles, 107 IVF cycles, 394 ICSI cycles, and 49 frozen embryo transfers. Six months post-treatment, there was careful HIV follow-up of the negative females. All tests recorded on the females were negative (7.1% lost to follow-up), giving a calculated probability of contamination equal to zero. Clinical pregnancy rates recorded with all forms of treatment were comparable to those found in cycles carried out in HIV-negative couples (Bujan et al., 2007). In HIV-1 positive men receiving ART who have undetectable levels of viral ribonucleic acid (RNA) in the plasma, the virus may still be present in seminal cells.

IUI, IVF, and ICSI are fertility techniques that can further reduce the risk of HIV transmission to the uninfected partner, and should be considered as options whether or not the couple or individual wishing to conceive is experiencing issues with infertility. A study by Manigart et al. (2006) to assess ART outcomes in couples affected by HIV included scenarios in which the woman was HIV positive and the man was HIV negative (serodiscordant couples), the man was HIV positive and the woman was HIV negative (serodiscordant couples), and both the man and woman were HIV positive (seroconcordant couples). A total of 85 couples affected by HIV participated in the study, and procedures such as IUI, IVF, and ICSI were performed. In total, 57 cycles of ART were initiated, which included 53 IVF or ICSI cycles, 2 transfers of thawed embryos, and 2 oocyte donations. In addition, 124 IUI cycles were performed. Of the 85 couples enrolled in the study, the man was HIV positive and the woman was HIV negative in 38 (45%) of the couples. Overall, 40% of couples with HIV-positive men, and 36% treated using IUI, obtained a clinical and ongoing pregnancy. All women and newborns were found to be negative for HIV. In this series of patients, all babies born after ART were seronegative. If a couple wishes to further reduce the risk of HIV transmission or if they have additional fertility issues, sperm washing can be combined with ovulation induction, IVF, or ICSI. Theoretically, ICSI could further reduce the chance of horizontal HIV transmission.

Some studies have in fact shown that because ICSI involves fertilization with only one sperm, the risk of possible HIV transmission in HIV-serodiscordant couples should be lower than traditional ART methods. This is because in traditional IUI, women receive millions of sperm, and in classic IVF, the eggs are exposed to thousands of sperm (Loutradis et al., 2001). A 2001 report of two cases of live births after ICSI in serodiscordant couples where the male partner was HIV positive showed that following delivery, both mother and infant were HIV negative upon testing for HIV antibodies (Loutradis et al., 2001).

Fertility Issues for Women Living with HIV

As more HIV-positive women intend to become pregnant and actually do attempt to conceive, issues relating to infertility are going to arise (Yudin et al., 2010). This is partially due to the fact that many HIV-positive women were diagnosed early in the HIV epidemic, when fewer options for safe conception and pregnancy were available and prognosis with HIV was poor. These women, while still of child-bearing age, are now older and as such are experiencing difficulty conceiving due to age. Very little research has been conducted on whether or not HIV has a direct effect on fertility. However, one study showed that HIV-positive women have a much higher prevalence of tubal factor infertility than control participants (41% versus 14%) (Frodsham, Boag, Barton, & Gilling-Smith, 2006). Other studies have related an increase of infertility issues among HIV-positive women to infection with other STIs, such as chlamydia (Askew & Berer, 2003). As discussed earlier in this chapter, access and availability of assisted reproductive technologies is very limited for PL-WHIV who wish to reduce the risk of HIV during conception. HIV-positive women who must rely on the same technologies to treat infertility issues face these same access barriers.

ABOUT THE CANADIAN HIV FERTILITY PROGRAM

The Canadian HIV Pregnancy Planning Guideline Development Team at the Women and HIV Research Program of Women's College Research Institute in Toronto, Ontario, is working to reduce the stigma and discrimination associated with HIV-positive pregnancies and increase access to preconception prevention and fertility services. The team's vision is to develop both provincial and national collaborative programs to guide and assist all people living with and affected by HIV with their pregnancy planning desires in a holistic, ethical, supportive, and medically sound manner. The program includes the execution of research to assess the needs of HIV-positive families and the resources available to help people living with and affected by HIV to plan healthy families, as well as the provision of programmatic interventions such as pregnancy planning guidelines, pamphlets, and workshops, and the creation of a network of informed, supportive care providers.

National HIV Pregnancy Planning Guidelines (NHPPG)

The NHPPG (Loutfy et al., 2012a) provide information and recommendations to health care practitioners and policy-makers to (1) reduce the risk of horizontal transmission of HIV between partners, (2) increase the rate of pregnancy planning through the provision of safer options for conception, (3) reduce the stigma associated with pregnancy and HIV, and (4) increase access to pregnancy planning and fertility services. The recommendations in these guidelines were based on evidence from a comprehensive 2009 NHPPG literature review on HIV and pregnancy planning, as well as extensive consultation with experts including infectious diseases specialists, fertility specialists, obstetrician/gynecologists, family physicians, mental health professionals, policy-makers, legal experts, community service providers, and HIV-positive men and women known as the NHPPG Development Team. The

NHPPG will be submitted to the Society of Obstetricians and Gynaecologists and the Canadian Fertility and Andrology Society for endorsement.

Theoretical framework

Conceptually, guidelines have been developed regarding women's health, sexual, and reproductive rights (Amnesty International USA, 2012). By using a human rights–based approach, the Development Team recognizes that the human rights of those living with and affected by HIV are frequently violated and often affect their intentions and desires to have children. Additionally, the Development Team recognizes the need to cultivate strong leadership among all stakeholders and to integrate these mutually agreed-upon guiding principles into all aspects of HIV pregnancy planning, fertility care, treatment, and support for all PLWHIV in Canada. Recommendations and their implementation must be evidence-based, flexible, and ethnoculturally sensitive while considering the diverse and intersecting local/population needs based on the social determinants of health.

Legal and ethical issues

Legal, ethical, and policy issues surrounding pregnancy within the context of HIV remain challenging in terms of guideline development due to the limited available data and the wide range of interpretations of this data. Considering the limited data, this section of the guidelines is based on expert consensus and on the above-stated premise of human rights that PLWHIV should be privy to the fundamental right to have a healthy pregnancy free from discrimination.

Several issues emerge in the domain of ethics and law when it comes to HIV and pregnancy, all of which have serious implications for the delivery of appropriate health care services to HIV-positive men and women seeking to start a family or to HIV-positive women who are already pregnant. Good pregnancy planning for HIV-positive people requires that they access health services to assist them in dealing with the medical and psychosocial issues involved, but this, in turn, requires disclosure. A 2004 report by the World Health Organization (Maman & Medley, 2004) summarizing barriers to HIV serostatus disclosure by women in developing countries indicates that the most common reasons for failure to disclose included fear of accusations of infidelity, abandonment, discrimination, and violence (Mocroft et al., 2003). In resource-poor countries, this is a major impediment to the delivery of treatment programs that decrease vertical transmission rates of HIV.

In the West, similar issues related to HIV disclosure abound, but the legal environment in particular has become increasingly hostile toward PLWHIV. In Canada, the Supreme Court ruled in 1998 that PLWHIV could be found guilty of serious criminal charges, such as aggravated assault, if they failed to disclose their HIV status to sexual partners in situations where transmission was considered high risk. The ruling has resulted in 70 charges to date against PLWHIV who failed to disclose and the subsequent creation of a hostile legal environment for PLWHIV (Symington, 2009). In addition, these charges are becoming increasingly serious, such as aggravated sexual assault, which carries a maximum penalty of life imprisonment, setting the stage for the possibility of escalating charges, such as first- and second-degree murder (Symington, 2009).

Although the criminalization of HIV transmission was instituted to protect HIV-negative people from being infected, ironically, no evidence to date has shown that such measures decrease HIV transmission (Chu, 2009). One study by Burris and colleagues examined the sexual behaviours of people considered to be at high risk of HIV infection with regard to condom use (Burris & Edwin, 2008). They interviewed 490 people in Illinois, which has criminalized non-disclosure by HIV-positive people to their sexual partners, and in New York, where no such law exists. The authors found no significant difference in the sexual behaviours of individuals living in either of the two states.

Interestingly, the Swiss have taken a different approach to criminalization of HIV transmission. As previously mentioned, a public statement was published in the *Bulletin des Médecins Suisses*, now known as the Swiss Statement (Vernazza et al., 2008). The report concludes that unprotected sex between an HIV-positive and an HIV-negative person does not constitute criminal negligence if certain criteria (see pages 227–228) have been met. This is in keeping with a UNAIDS policy brief that states that criminal charges against HIV-positive individuals who transmit the virus through sexual contact cannot be justified if the accused individual "took reasonable measures to reduce risk of transmission" (UNAIDS, 2008). In this case, reasonable measures would include adherence to combination ART.

Furthermore, not only is criminalization ineffective when it comes to reducing HIV transmission rates, but criminalization may, in fact, undermine public health measures that are effective. In an article outlining the negative consequences of criminal HIV disclosure laws, Galletly and Pinkerton argue that criminalization conflicts with public health prevention measures by marginalizing HIV-positive people, on whom prevention measures depend, by creating an environment that encourages people to make assumptions about the HIV status of sexual partners (Galletly & Pinkerton, 2006). This idea is echoed by UNAIDS in its 2008 Policy Brief stating that criminalization could discourage HIV testing and create an atmosphere of distrust toward health care providers who can effectively treat HIV-positive patients (UNAIDS, 2008).

There is little data available on the effects of HIV criminalization laws on pregnancy planning, but legal cases do exist. In 2006, an HIV-positive woman in Hamilton, Ontario, was charged with child neglect for hiding her HIV-positive status from doctors. Furthermore, the mother failed to provide ART to the child after birth. The child tested HIV positive at two months of age, and the mother was sentenced to six months in jail for failing to provide the necessities of life (Priest, 2006).

The environment that is being created by imposing criminal penalties on HIV-positive individuals who transmit HIV will no doubt impact negatively on HIV-positive people who might be thinking about starting a family. Although the decision to have children as an HIV-positive man or woman is not illegal in Canada, criminalization laws might act as a deterrent, marginalizing these members of our society, and resulting in unplanned pregnancies in which the risk of vertical transmission is high if health care professionals are not involved. Ideally, doctors and other members of the health care community should be involved from the start, before children are born to HIV-positive mothers, so that proper planning occurs with respect to routine prevention measures, in addition to ART to decrease transmission rates.

Psychosocial issues

All individuals or couples planning pregnancy are potentially susceptible to psychosocial and mental health issues. Within the context of HIV, additional burden is placed on the HIV-positive individual or couple due to stigma surrounding the disease. HIV-positive people considering pregnancy may be concerned with discrimination, as it intersects several aspects of the parenting continuum from preconception to breastfeeding and may include self-guilt, guilt from community and family, and peer guilt. Such discrimination manifests itself in the fear of potential loss of support. As with legal and ethical issues, little data is available on this subject, and expert consensus has been relied upon to create recommendations for psychosocial counselling for PLWHIV who are planning pregnancies to start families.

The NHPPG recommends that counselling should be performed by a knowledgeable health care professional or trained peer counsellor in a supportive, non-judgmental manner that takes into account factors specific to sexual diversity and ethnocultural or religious beliefs and practices. Additionally, counselling should include a discussion of the potential risks for both horizontal and vertical transmission and how the fear of these risks might impact on the mental health of one or both parents. HIV-positive people who intend to conceive should be aware of the potential stigma they may face from others who are less informed about the risks of vertical transmission. Further, counselling may be required to help couples and individuals cope more effectively with fear, stigma, and other psychosocial issues that may arise.

Serostatus-Based Recommendations

The options recommended by the NHPPG Development Team are highlighted in this summary. However, the recommended option may not always be the most practical or preferred option for the patient based on availability of services, cost, cultural beliefs, or personal risk evaluation. In these cases, physicians and other health care providers should provide non-judgmental support of the decision of the patient(s) involved. All HIV-positive individuals and couples should be informed of the risks and benefits of all conception options.

HIV-positive woman with HIV-negative male partner
The NHPPG recommends that serodiscordant couples where the woman is HIV posi-tive be counselled to attempt home insemination during ovulation for a period of three to six months. If home insemination is unsuccessful, couples should be referred to a fertility specialist for a complete fertility workup and appropriate treatment where necessary, including counselling on all assisted reproductive technologies.

HIV-positive single woman or HIV-positive woman in a same-sex relationship
The NHPPG recommends that single HIV-positive women or HIV-positive women in a same-sex relationship be referred to a fertility specialist and consider the option of IUI with donor sperm. This option is preferred over home insemination because of the high cost of donor sperm and the increased success rate of IUI.

HIV-negative woman with HIV-positive male partner
The NHPPG recommends that serodiscordant couples where the man is HIV-positive be referred to a fertility specialist and consider the option of sperm washing with IUI. If IUI is unsuccessful, couples may consider IVF or ICSI with either sperm washing or donor sperm.

HIV-positive woman with HIV-positive male partner
The NHPPG recommends that seroconcordant couples consider natural concep-tion with timed ovulation after careful consideration of the potential risk of super-infection. Sperm washing with intrauterine insemination is also an option for these couples.

Other Programmatic Interventions
In addition to the development of guidelines, the team has developed four other im-portant knowledge translation tools that may serve to narrow the gap between the need for pregnancy planning information in the context of HIV and the availability of resources. All of the programmatic interventions below have been developed with input from various stakeholders, including clinicians, community members, and PL-WHIV.

Pamphlets
Four new pamphlets have been created for PLWHIV to address the various issues associated with HIV and pregnancy where a gap existed. These include: (1) infor-mation for women who are diagnosed with HIV during pregnancy, (2) information for HIV-positive new moms, (3) pregnancy planning information for HIV-positive women and their partners, and (4) pregnancy planning information for HIV-positive men and their partners. The pamphlets use easily accessible language to promote understanding among community members. The information within the pamphlets

is supported by the 2009 NHPPG literature review, and the guidelines. Furthermore, the pamphlet subject matter has been tested in focus groups across the province of Ontario. These pamphlets are available from the Canadian AIDS Treatment Information Exchange, in both French and English (Canadian AIDS Treatment Information Exchange, n.d.).

Workshops

Two sets of workshops have been developed to promote knowledge translation and exchange of the recommendations contained in the NHPPG; one community workshop and one clinical/academic workshop, with the academic workshop being more science intensive. Information contained within the workshops has been developed with the contributions of infectious diseases specialists, fertility specialists, community members, and PLWHIV.

Website

The team is proposing the development of a dedicated website on pregnancy planning and fertility options in the context of HIV. This comprehensive website will host all of the other knowledge translation resources: guidelines, pamphlets, and workshops, as well as the NHPPG literature review and relevant links. Our 2009 Ontario HIV Pregnancy Planning Initiative Phase research, where focus groups were carried out across the province of Ontario with PLWHIV, showed that certain populations preferred accessing information through websites rather than through one-on-one discussion (Margolese et al., 2010). Consequently, the website will serve as a medium to allow for increased knowledge dissemination, particularly among hard-to-reach populations and in rural areas of Ontario.

CONCLUSION

Breakthroughs in HIV management over the last two decades and the wider availability of assisted reproductive technology for PLWHIV who wish to conceive have contributed to an increased range of options to prevent vertical and horizontal transmission of HIV. While these options exist, many are not accessible to all PLWHIV in Canada due to continued discrimination by some health care providers, the lack of access to information and services in many areas, particularly in smaller cities and rural areas across Canada, and the prohibitive high cost of assisted reproductive technologies. Approaching such technologies as harm reduction tools in the context of HIV may be an important strategy to encourage more health care providers and fertility centres to consider providing such care to PLWHIV in Canada. Clinicians should provide comprehensive preconception counselling to all HIV-positive people to ensure that they are fully aware of all opportunities available to them to prevent vertical and horizontal HIV transmission, ensure a healthy mother and child, and address issues of infertility that may exist. The NHPPG team asserts that health care providers ought to add a discussion about pregnancy planning, healthy preconception, and contraception into routine HIV care. The team is near the completion of the national guidelines on pregnancy planning as well as the provincial and national HIV fertility programs encompassing various knowledge translation tools. It is the team's hope that ongoing projects assist HIV-positive individuals, policy-makers, and health care providers globally to develop their programs for safer reproduction for HIV-positive individuals in their communities.

PROBLEM-BASED LEARNING CASE STUDY

Sarah is a 32-year-old married woman of African descent who lives in Ontario. Sarah tested positive for HIV in 1998. In 2000, Sarah met and married her current husband who is HIV negative. In 2002, Sarah began treatment on Atripla and quickly achieved an undetectable viral load.

CRITICAL THINKING QUESTIONS

1. Sarah and her husband would like to have a child. Which specific issues should be discussed with Sarah and her husband in preconception counselling?
2. What are Sarah's first-line options for getting pregnant?
3. Sarah and her husband have been trying to get pregnant for eight months with no success. What are the next steps Sarah and her husband could consider in order to get pregnant?
4. What are some of the barriers they may face in trying to conceive?

GLOSSARY

Assisted reproductive technologies: Services provided for women and/or couples who require the assistance of a fertility specialist to conceive a child.

Combination antiretroviral therapy: Taking three or more active antiretroviral drugs at a time to treat HIV infection.

Fertility centre/clinic: Fertility clinics are staffed medical clinics that assist couples, and sometimes individuals, who want to become parents but are unable to achieve this goal via the natural course.

Fertility specialist: An obstetrician/gynecologist who specializes in the practice of fertility.

Horizontal transmission: A term used to describe the transmission of HIV from one individual to another (except from mother to child). For example, HIV is transmitted horizontally through sexual contact or exposure to infected blood.

HIV specialist: A physician who is an accredited expert in the field of HIV and who devotes his or her career to the practice of HIV patient care and research.

Infertility: The inability of an individual to achieve a pregnancy after one year of unprotected intercourse or home insemination; the inability to carry a pregnancy to term.

Intrauterine device (IUD): A form of family planning that is inserted into the uterus. IUDs provide no protection against STI/HIV transmission.

Intrauterine insemination (IUI): The process by which sperm is injected into the uterus.

In vitro fertilization (IVF): The process by which eggs are fertilized by sperm outside of the body (in vitro), and the subsequent transfer of embryos into the uterus.

Intracytoplasmic sperm injection (ICSI): The injection of a single sperm directly into an egg to facilitate fertilization.

Preconception: The period of time before pregnancy has been achieved.

Serodiscordant: A term used to describe a couple in which one partner is HIV positive while the other partner is HIV negative.

Seroconcordant: A term used to describe a couple in which both partners are HIV positive or HIV negative.

Sperm washing: A process in which seminal fluid is separated from the sperm. The technique rests on the notion that HIV material is primarily carried in the seminal fluid, rather than in the sperm itself.

Vertical transmission: A term used to describe the transmission of HIV from mother to child through pregnancy, childbirth, or breastfeeding.

REFERENCES

AIDSinfo. (n.d.). *Panel on treatment of HIV-infected pregnant women and prevention of perinatal transmission: Recommendations for use of antiretroviral drugs in pregnant HIV-1 infected women for maternal health and interventions to reduce perinatal HIV transmission in the United States.* Retrieved from http://aidsinfo.nih.gov/contentfiles/lvguidelines/perinatalGL.pdf

AIDSinfo. (2011). *Panel on antiretroviral therapy and medical management of HIV-infected children: Guidelines for the use of antiretroviral agents in pediatric HIV infection* (pp. 1–268). Retrieved from http://aidsinfo.nih.gov/contentfiles/lvguidelines/pediatricguidelines.pdf

Amnesty International USA. (2012). *Women's health, sexual and reproductive rights.* Retrieved from www.amnestyusa.org/our-work/issues/women-s-rights/women-s-health-sexual-and-reproductive-rights

Apoola, A., tenHof, J., & Allan, P. S. (2001). Access to infertility investigations and treatment in couples infected with HIV: Questionnaire survey. *BMJ, 323*(7324), 1285.

Askew, I., & Berer, M. (2003). The contribution of sexual and reproductive health services to the fight against HIV/AIDS: A review. *Reproductive Health Matters, 11*(22), 51–73.

Baeten, J. M., & Overbaugh, J. (2003). Measuring the infectiousness of persons with HIV-1: Opportunities for preventing sexual HIV-1 transmission. *Current HIV Research, 1*(1), 69–86.

Bagasra, O., Farzadegan, H., Seshamma, T., Oakes, J. W, Saah, A., & Pomerantz, R. J. (1994). Detection of HIV-1 proviral DNA sperm from HIV-1 infected men. *AIDS, 8*(12), 1669–1674.

Barreiro, P., Castilla, J. A., Labarga, P., & Soriano, V. (2007). Is natural conception a valid option for HIV-serodiscordant couples? *Human Reproduction, 22*(9), 2353–2358.

Bell, E., Mthembu, P., & O'Sullivan, S., on behalf of the International Community of Women

Living with HIV/AIDS, & Moody, K., on behalf of the Global Network of People Living with HIV/AIDS. (2007). Sexual and reproductive health services and HIV testing: Perspectives and experiences of women and men living with HIV and AIDS. *Reproductive Health Matters, 15*(29 Suppl.), 113–135.

Blackard, J. T., Cohen, D. E., & Mayer, K. H. (2002). Human immunodeficiency virus super-infection and recombination: Current state of knowledge and potential clinical consequences. *Clinical Infectious Diseases, 34*(8), 1108–1114.

Bujan, L., Hollander, L., Coudert, M., Gilling-Smith, C., Vucetich, A., Guibert, J., Vernazza, P., Ohl, J., Weigel, M., Englert, Y., & Semprini, A. E. (2007, September). CREAThE network. Safety and efficacy of sperm washing in HIV-1-serodiscordant couples where the male is infected: Results from the European CREAThE network. *AIDS, 21*(14), 1909–1914.

Burris, S., & Edwin, C. (2008). The case against criminalization. *JAMA, 300*(5), 578–581.

Canadian AIDS Treatment Information Exchange. (n.d.). *Fact sheets & guides.* Retrieved from www.catie.ca/en/treating-hiv/treating-hiv#fs-g

Canadian Paediatric Society, Infectious Diseases and Immunization Committee. (2004). In S. King (Chair), Evaluation and treatment of the human immunodeficiency virus-1-exposed infant. *Paediatric Child Health, 9*(6), 409–417.

Chen, J. L., Philips, K. A., Kanouse, D. E., Collins, R. L., & Miu, A. (2001). Fertility desires and intentions of HIV-positive men and women. *Family Planning Perspectives, 33*(4), 144–152, 165.

Chu, S. (2009). Criminal law and cases of HIV transmission or exposure. *HIV/AIDS Policy & Law Review, 14*(2), 42–47.

Cohen, M. S., Hoffman, I. F., Royce, R. A., Kazembe, P., Dyer, J. R., Daly, C. C., ... & Eron, J. J. Jr. (1997). Reduction of concentration of HIV-1 in semen after treatment of urethritis: Implications for prevention of sexual transmission of HIV-1. AIDSCAP Malawi Research Group. *The Lancet, 349*(9069), 1868–1873.

Connor, E. M., Sperling, R. S., Gelber, R., Kiselev, P., Scott, G., O'Sullivan, M. J., ... & Balsley, J. (1994). Reduction of maternal-fetal transmission of human immunodeficiency virus type 1 with zidovudine treatment. *New England Journal of Medicine, 331*(18), 1173–1180.

Department of Health and Human Services. (2012). *Recommendations for use of antiretroviral drugs in pregnant HIV-1 infected women for maternal health and interventions to reduce perinatal HIV-1 transmission in the United States.* Retrieved from http://aidsinfo.nih.gov/guidelines/ html/3/perinatal-guidelines/0/

Engender Health and International Community of Women Living with HIV/AIDS (ICW). (2006). *Sexual and reproductive health for HIV-positive women and adolescent girls: Manual for trainers and programme managers.* Retrieved from www.engenderhealth.org/files/pubs/hiv-aids-stis/ SRH_for_HIV_Positive_Women_English.pdf

Floridia, M., Tamburrini, E., Tibaldi, C., Anzidei, G., Muggiasca, M. L., Meloni, A., ... & Italian Group on Surveillance on Antiretroviral Treatment in Pregnancy. (2010). Voluntary pregnancy termination among women with HIV in the HAART era (2002–2008): A case series from a national study. *AIDS Care, 22*(1), 50–53.

Frodsham, L. C., Boag, F., Barton, S., & Gilling-Smith, C. (2006). Human immunodeficiency virus infection and fertility care in the United Kingdom: Demand and supply. *Fertility and Sterility, 85*(2), 285–289.

Galletly, C., & Pinkerton, S. (2006). Conflicting messages: How criminal HIV disclosure laws undermine public health efforts to control the spread of HIV. *AIDS Behavior, 10*(5), 451–461.

Gogna, M. L., Pecheny, M. M., Ibarlucía, I., Manzelli, H., & López, S. B. (2009). The reproductive needs and rights of people living with HIV in Argentina: Health service users' and providers' perspectives. *Social Science & Medicine, 69*(6), 813–820.

Health Canada. (2011). *Eating well with Canada's Food Guide.* Retrieved from www.hc-sc.gc.ca/fn-an/food-guide-aliment/order-commander/index-eng.php#a1

Klein, J., Peña, J. E., Thornton, M. H., & Sauer, M. V. (2003). Understanding the motivations, concerns, and desires of human immunodeficiency virus 1-serodiscordant couples wishing to have children through assisted reproduction. *Obstetrics & Gynecology, 101*(5 Pt. 1), 987–994.

Loutfy, M. R., Hart, T. A., Mohammed, S. S., Su, D., Ralph, E. D., Walmsley, S. L., ... Yudin, M. H., for the Ontario HIV Fertility Research Team. (2009a). Fertility desires and intentions of HIV-positive women of reproductive age in Ontario, Canada: A cross-sectional study. *PLoS ONE 4*(12), e7925.

Loutfy, M., Margolese, S., Yudin, M., Mohammed, S., & Wong, J., Smieja, M., & Shapiro, H. (2009b, April). *The National HIV Pregnancy Planning Guidelines Development Team: Development of Canadian evidence-based guidelines on safe pregnancy planning for HIV-positive individuals* [Abstract]. Presented at the 18th Annual Canadian Conference on HIV/AIDS Research, Vancouver, British Columbia.

Loutfy, M. R., Margolese, S., Money, D. M., Gysler, M., Hamilton, S., & Yudin, M. (2012a). Canadian HIV pregnancy planning guidelines. *Journal of Obstetrics & Gynaecology Canada, 34*(6), 575–590.

Loutfy, M. R., Raboud, J. M., Wong, J., Yudin, M. H., Diong, C., Mohammed, S. S., ... Walmsley, S. L., for the Ontario HIV Fertility Research Team. (2012b). High prevalence of unintended pregnancies in HIV-positive women of reproductive age in Ontario, Canada: A retrospective study. *HIV Medicine, 13*(2), 107–117.

Loutradis, D., Drakakis, P., Kallianidis, K., Patsoula, E., Bletsa, R., & Michalas, S. (2001). Birth of two infants who were seronegative for human immunodeficiency virus type 1 (HIV-1) after intracytoplasmic injection of sperm from HIV-1-seropositive men. *Fertility and Sterility, 75*(1), 210–212.

Maestro, T. D., & de Vincenzi, I. (1996). Probabilities of sexual HIV-1 transmission. *AIDS, 10*(Suppl. A), 75–82.

Maman, S., & Medley, A. (2004). *Gender dimensions of HIV status disclosure to sexual partners: Rates, barriers and outcomes.* A review paper. Retrieved from www.who.int/gender/documents/en/genderdimensions.pdf

Manigart, Y., Rozenberg, S., Barlow, P., Gerard, M., Bertraind, E., & Delvigne, A. (2006). ART outcome in HIV-infected patients. *Human Reproduction, 21*(11), 2935–2940.

Margolese, S., Huyhn, L., Conway, T., Maxwell, J., Munchenje, M., O'Brien-Teengs, D., ... & Loutfy, M., for the Ontario HIV Pregnancy Planning Initiative. (2010). *Improving the quality of care in prevention, treatment, care and support by improving access to safe pregnancy planning options, information and support services for people living with HIV in Ontario, Canada.* Poster session presented at the XVIII International AIDS Conference (AIDS 2010), Vienna, Austria.

Mocroft, A., Ledergerber, B., Katlama, C., Kirk, O., Reiss, P., d'Arminio Monforte, A., ... & Lundgren, J. D., for the EuroSIDA Study Group. (2003). Decline in the AIDS and death rates in the EuroSIDA study: An observational study. *The Lancet, 362*(9377), 22–29.

Myer, L., Morroni, C., & El-Sadr, W. M. (2005). Reproductive decisions in HIV-infected individuals. *The Lancet, 366*(9487), 698–700.

National Institute of Allergy and Infectious Diseases. (2008). *HIV infection in women.* Retrieved from www.niaid.nih.gov/topics/hivaids/understanding/populationspecificinformation/pages/womenhiv.aspx

Nduati, R., Richardson, B. A., John, G., Mbori-Ngacha, D., Mwatha, A., Ndinya-Achola, J., ... & Kreiss, J. (2001). Effect of breastfeeding on mortality among HIV-1 infected women: A randomised trial. *The Lancet, 357*(9269), 1651–1655.

Ogilvie, G. S., Palepu, A., Remple, V. P., Maan, E., Heath, K., MacDonald, G., ... & Burdge, D. R. (2007). Fertility intentions of women of reproductive age living with HIV in British Columbia, Canada. *AIDS, 21*(Suppl. 1), S83–S88.

Palella, F. J. Jr, Delaney, K. M., Moorman, A. C., Loveless, M. O., Fuhrer, J., Satten, G. A., ... & Holmberg, S. D. (1998). Declining morbidity and mortality among patients with advanced human immunodeficiency virus infection. HIV Outpatient Study Investigators. *New England Journal of Medicine, 338*(13), 853–860.

Pitts, M., & Shields, P. (2004). Access to infertility investigations and treatment for HIV+ people: A survey of Australian infertility clinics. *Australia and New Zealand Journal of Public Health, 28*(4), 360–362.

Public Health Agency of Canada. (2007). *HIV/AIDS Epi Updates, November 2007.* Retrieved from www.phac-aspc.gc.ca/aids-sida/publication/epi/pdf/epi2007_e.pdf

Public Health Agency of Canada. (2009). *HIV and AIDS in Canada: Surveillance Report to December 31, 2008.* Retrieved from www.phac-aspc.gc.ca/aids-sida/publication/survreport/2008/dec/pdf/survrepdec08.pdf

Public Health Agency of Canada. (2011). *The sensible guide to a healthy pregnancy.* Retrieved from www.phac-aspc.gc.ca/hp-gs/guide-eng.php

Public Health Agency of Canada. (2012). *Fetal Alcohol Spectrum Disorder.* Retrieved from www.phac-aspc.gc.ca/hp-ps/dca-dea/prog-ini/fasd-etcaf/index-eng.php

Priest, L. (2006, August 7). Mother avoiding AZT. *The Globe and Mail.* Retrieved from http://aras.ab.ca/articles/popular/200608-Crowe-AZT.html

Ramos, A., Hu, D. J., Nguyen, L., Phan, K. O., Vanichseni, S., Promadej, N., ... & Subbarao, S. (2002). Intersubtype human immunodeficiency virus type 1 superinfection following seroconversion to primary infection in two injection drug users. *Journal of Virology, 76*(15), 7444–7452.

Rozenberg, S., Gerard, M., Manigart, Y., Ham, H., & Delvigne, A. (2002). Acceptance by Belgian physicians of in-vitro fertilization treatment in women with HIV infection. *AIDS, 16*(3), 497–498.

Shapiro, D., Tuomala, R., Pollack, H., Burchett, S., Read, J., Cababasay, M., ... & Ciupak, G. (2004, February). *Mother-to-child HIV transmission risk according to antiretroviral therapy, mode of delivery, and viral load in 2,895 US women* (PACTG 367) [Abstract 99]. Oral presentation at the 11th Conference on Retroviruses and Opportunistic Infections, San Francisco, CA.

The Society of Obstetricians and Gynaecologists of Canada. (n.d.) *Clinical practice guidelines.* Retrieved from www.sogc.org/index_e.asp

The Society of Obstetricians and Gynaecologists of Canada. (2000). *The reproductive care of women living with hepatitis C infection.* Retrieved from www.sogc.org/guidelines/index_e.asp#Infectious

The Society of Obstetricians and Gynaecologists of Canada. (2007). *Canadian consensus guidelines on human papillomavirus.* Retrieved from www.sogc.org/guidelines/index_e.asp#Infectious

The Society of Obstetricians and Gynaecologists of Canada. (2008). *Genital herpes: Gynaecological aspects.* Retrieved from www.sogc.org/guidelines/index_e.asp#Infectious

Symington, A. (2009). Criminalization confusion and concerns: The decade since the *Cuerrier* decision. *HIV/AIDS Policy & Law Review, 14*(1), 5–10.

UNAIDS. (2008). *Criminalization of HIV transmission: Policy brief.* Retrieved from http://data.unaids.org/pub/basedocument/2008/20080731_jc1513_policy_criminalization_en.pdf

Vernazza, P., Hirschel, B., Bernasconi, E., & Flepp, M. (2008). Les Personnes séropositives ne souffrant d'aucune autre MST et suivant un traitement antirétroviral efficace ne transmettent pas le VIH par voie sexuelle. *Bulletin des Médecins Suisses, 89*(5), 165–169.

Vettore, M. V., Schechter, M., Melo, M. F., Boechat, L. J., & Barroso, P. F. (2006). Genital HIV-1 viral load is correlated with blood plasma HIV-1 viral load in Brazilian women and is reduced by antiretroviral therapy. *Journal of Infection, 52*(4), 290–293.

Wilcher, R., & Cates, W. (2009). Reproductive choices for women with HIV. *Bulletin of the World Health Organization, 87,* 833–839.

Williams, H., Watkins, C., & Risby, J. (1996). Reproductive decision-making and determinants of contraceptive use in HIV-infected women. *Clinical Obstetrics and Gynecology, 39*(2), 333–343.

World Health Organization and UNAIDS. (2008). *Global Summary of the HIV/AIDS epidemic, December 2008.* Last modified 2009. Retrieved from www.who.int/hiv/data/2009_global_summary.gif

Yudin, M. H., Shapiro, H. M., & Loutfy, M. R. (2010). Access to infertility services in Canada for HIV-positive individuals and couples: A cross-sectional study. *Reproductive Health, 7,* 7.

Chapter 11

NEW PREVENTION TECHNOLOGIES: PROMISES AND PITFALLS

San Patten

Demographic, technological, socio-political, and economic change will fundamentally shape the future of the HIV/AIDS epidemic in Canada and around the world. The future of Canada's HIV epidemic will largely depend on our policy choices (e.g., criminalization versus harm reduction), the strength of government and civil society leadership, and changing demographic patterns (e.g., internal migration, immigration, aging, urbanization). The HIV epidemic will also evolve along with norms within sex and drug networks, ever-widening socio-economic inequalities, and social attitudes and levels of stigma (with respect to social inclusion/exclusion and people living with HIV, and levels of sexism, homophobia, racism). Also important will be the impact of comorbidities and co-infections (particularly as the population ages), the level of investment in programming and research, and access to services (HIV counselling and testing, prevention interventions, care, treatment and support programs, rehabilitation services). Overarching drivers for Canada's HIV epidemic will be the state of our health care system, the public health response (e.g., fragmentation versus integration of jurisdictional responsibilities), community-based responses, as well as the role of stakeholders who often fall outside the formal health or HIV-specific realms, such as the education system (Public Health Agency of Canada, 2011).

Amid these various socio-political drivers of change to Canada's HIV epidemic, one of the most significant developments over the coming decade will be the introduction of new HIV prevention technologies (NPTs). Currently there are a number of global efforts underway to develop new technologies to prevent HIV, all of which are deemed to be scientifically viable products. Research is being conducted on vaginal and rectal microbicides, vaccines, pre-exposure prophylaxis (PrEP), and HIV treatment as prevention. A microbicide is any substance that can substantially reduce the risk of acquiring or transmitting sexually transmitted infections, including HIV, when it is inserted in the vagina or rectum. Microbicides may be formulated as a gel, foam, cream, or other suppository-type product. Other forms may be a vaginal ring—a device that could slowly release the protective substance over a month—or a physical barrier, such as a diaphragm or cervical cap. Almost all microbicides in the research pipeline now are based on antiretrovirals (ARVs). The CAPRISA 004 trial showed that women using a 1% tenofovir gel within 12 hours before and after sex had a 39% lower chance of becoming HIV infected and a 51% lower risk of contracting herpes simplex type 2 (HSV-2) than those using the placebo gel (Abdool et al., 2010). A vaccine is a substance that causes a response from the immune system, producing antibodies and a stronger immune response in the event of exposure to the virus. A vaccine is not a cure, but it prevents infection or slows disease progression. PrEP is an HIV prevention strategy that would use ARVs to protect HIV-negative people from HIV infection. It is currently being tested in people who are considered to be most likely to be exposed to HIV (e.g., IDUs, sex trade workers, men who have sex with men (MSM), serodiscordant couples) to assess if a daily dose of ARVs (tenofovir and Truvada) is protective against infection. The iPrEx study (released November 2010) demonstrated that MSM who took a single daily tablet containing emtricitabine and tenofovir (FTC/TDF) experienced an average of 43.8% fewer HIV infections than those who received a placebo pill (95% CI 15.4 to 62.6%; P=0.005) (Abdool et al., 2010). Finally, HIV treatment as prevention refers to the notion that treating people with HIV reduces their viral load and thus prevents transmission between serodiscordant couples. A randomized control trial (the HPTN 052 study) of serodiscordant couples demonstrated that earlier initiation of treatment by the HIV-positive partner reduced the risk of transmission to the HIV-negative partner by 96% (Cohen et al., 2011).

While NPTs have the potential to play a critical role as part of a comprehensive HIV prevention effort, in particular for those who cannot use or rely on existing prevention methods such as condoms, they would be used as part of a prevention spectrum and not as a "magic bullet." A comprehensive approach to HIV prevention balances structural changes (such as poverty reduction and gender equality), the expansion and strengthening of existing prevention strategies (such as behavioural interventions and the distribution of male and female condoms), and integration of NPTs (such as PrEP and microbicides). Clearly, biomedical tools cannot replace women's sexual and reproductive autonomy; rather, they could provide the means by which women exercise such autonomy.

The call for female-controlled HIV prevention methods emerged in the early 1990s as it became apparent that the epidemic in developing countries was primarily driven by heterosexual transmission. Pervasive and persistent power imbalances in heterosexual relationships leave women with the need to take steps to protect their own reproductive and sexual health. Although abstinence, monogamy, and condom use can be effective HIV prevention strategies, they require the co-operation of the male partner, which is problematic for many women. A woman's decision to use any prevention product is the result of a complex process requiring the balancing of perceptions of risk, an understanding of the product's characteristics and mechanisms against the anticipation of her partner's reaction, and a woman's own ability to make autonomous decisions around her sexual and reproductive health. Socio-economic status and social and cultural norms will also influence such a decision (Woodsong, 2004). Thus, use of NPTs, while technically under a woman's control, may not be possible in the face of limited decision-making power in her health care or sexual activities. This chapter offers an overview of some of the key promises and pitfalls of biomedical technologies for HIV prevention, and provides a critical analysis of their potential as tools for augmenting HIV prevention autonomy for women.

WOMEN ARE MORE VULNERABLE

The proportion of women living with HIV has grown substantially over the last two decades. From a global perspective, young women between the ages of 15 and 24 are 1.6 times more likely to be infected with HIV than their male peers (United Nations Population Fund, 2007). In Canada, women increasingly account for a significantly larger number and proportion of people living with HIV. In 1999, women comprised 11.7% of HIV-positive tests, while in 2008, women accounted for 26.2% of all HIV-positive tests (Public Health Agency of Canada [PHAC], 2010). Particularly over-represented in Canadian HIV surveillance data are young Aboriginal women and women of African or Caribbean descent.

We know that women are more vulnerable to HIV due to a myriad of biological, social, and cultural inequities. For example, women are biologically more susceptible to HIV infection through heterosexual intercourse than men (European Study Group on Heterosexual Transmission of HIV, 1992; Nicolosi et al., 1994; O'Brien et al., 1994). Semen carries higher concentrations of HIV than vaginal secretions, and a greater mucosal surface area is exposed in the female genital tract during sexual intercourse. Women are also exposed to HIV for a longer duration, as semen remains in the body for hours following unprotected vaginal or anal sexual intercourse. Young girls are especially at risk because their cervixes and vaginal linings are not fully mature and thus are more easily damaged (Moscicki, Ma, Holland, & Vermund, 2001).

From the perspective of economic inequity, women experience lower socio-economic status, lower wages, and fewer job opportunities, and thereby face greater financial dependence in relationships, poor housing, or survival sex. As discussed extensively by Greene, Chambers, Masinde, and Mukandoli (see Chapter 6 in this volume), increasing economic inequality and eroding social support networks mean that women cannot afford to leave relationships that may put them at risk. HIV risk among young women may escalate due to contexts of risk, such as physical vulnerability, and their susceptibility to sexual violence, economic dependence, and coercion.

Canada's most vulnerable women often lack the social and economic power to enforce the use of existing HIV prevention measures, such as condoms, safer injection, abstinence, or mutual monogamy. Male and female condom use requires the tacit co-operation, if not outright participation, of a woman's male partner. Within sexual relationships, women often have less power in negotiating safer sex and safer drug injection, and are more likely to experience sexual violence. As discussed by Bauer (see Chapter 7 in this volume), trans women are particularly vulnerable to unprotected anal sex due to transition-related financial needs and the emotional need for validation as women. Coercion, violence, economic dependency, and stigma render many women unable either to negotiate condom use or to leave partners who may place them at risk for HIV infection. At the same time, cultural beliefs and expectations may place an emphasis on women's fertility and reproductive capacity, making it impossible to use condoms. Since condoms are a barrier method of contraception, women now have to choose between child-bearing and HIV prevention (Global Campaign for Microbicides, 2010). Loutfy and Margolese (see Chapter 10 in this volume) discuss that optimism has begun to replace fear of early death and vertical HIV transmission between mother and child, but there is still a need for a means of preventing horizontal HIV transmission between partners during conception.

Cultural and gender-based social norms may limit women's autonomy in decision making regarding their sexuality and fertility. Among Aboriginal women, such vulnerabilities are compounded by the multi-generational legacy of residential schools, cultural disruption, and racism. Peltier et al. (see Chapter 4 in this volume) point out that however important it may be to know one's HIV status, women may encounter negative consequences as a result of that knowledge, including discrimination, fear of violence, stigmatized views of HIV/AIDS, fear of losing children, and cultural barriers around sexuality. All of these pose significant barriers to HIV testing for women. HIV testing guidelines must ensure a safe and confidential environment and adapt pre- and post-test counselling to the particular needs and cultural backgrounds of women. Counselling must also consider the implications of test results for pregnancy and prenatal care and refer women to the appropriate services, with informed consent as a central principle. Further, HIV testing must move beyond the confines of prenatal testing to actively include men in testing.

DISTRUST OF THE MEDICAL AND PHARMACEUTICAL ESTABLISHMENT

Important questions are raised about whether NPTs help to increase women's control over their own sexual and reproductive bodies, or if they play into the medical establishment's control over women's bodies. All of the viable NPTs in late-stage clinical trials are either vaccines or ARV-based methods of prevention, such as PrEP and microbicides. As with most female contraceptive methods, NPTs will likely be obtainable only from medical professionals, they will be invasive and have side effects (some serious), and require administration and monitoring by a physician. Further study is required to understand the potential for toxicity and the dangers of HIV-negative people taking ARVs, and to understand whether users would develop resistance to ARVs if they became HIV positive while using an ARV-based microbicide or taking PrEP. In a study of HIV vaccine acceptability among Black women in Canada (Williams, Newman, Sakamato, & Massaquoi, 2009), women expressed concerns about the possibility of adverse physical effects from an HIV vaccine. These apprehensions were built on knowledge of past negative events and their mistrust of institutions that they believed had colluded against their communities in the past (e.g., the Tuskegee syphilis study, and unethical clinical trials in Africa). A history of unethical treatment by governments, health systems, and researchers has left a legacy of profound mistrust of any health innovations being offered to Black communities (Williams et al., 2009).

Colonization has left the same legacy of distrust and alienation from the medical establishment, government, and research institutions among Canada's Aboriginal peoples (Fiske & Browne, 2006; Moffitt, 2004). It should also be noted that apprehensions about biomedical technologies are not completely grounded in historical experience; many attribute the slow pace of HIV vaccine research to low investment by pharmaceutical companies that have little profit incentive in developing preventive technologies that will most benefit racial minorities, women, and people living in low-income countries (Craddock, 2007). Thus, building preparedness for biomedical prevention tools will be a major hurdle for introduction of NPTs to racialized women in Canada.

Women also have reason to mistrust pharmaceutical interventions for their reproductive health. As the women's health movement has documented, the so-called side effects from birth control pills are problematic for many women. These include blood clots, depression, nausea, fatigue, migraines, and lack of sex drive. As Arditti (1977) and others in the women's health movement have noted, these side effects were seen as unacceptable for men but tolerable for women, perhaps because those associated with mood—lower sex drive, depression, fatigue—were seen as compatible with female gender roles (Arditti, 1977).

EXPANDING THE HIV PREVENTION TOOL KIT FOR WOMEN

The United Nations' Global Coalition on Women and AIDS has identified seven key areas of action needed to address the fundamental gender inequalities that fuel HIV spread among women and girls (Global Coalition on Women and AIDS, 2010). These are:

1. Reducing violence against women
2. Protecting the property and inheritance rights of women and girls
3. Ensuring equal access by women and girls to care and treatment
4. Supporting improved community-based care, with special focus on women and girls
5. Promoting access to new prevention options, including female condoms and microbicides
6. Supporting ongoing efforts toward universal education for girls
7. Preventing HIV infection among adolescents, focusing on improved reproductive health care

No one single HIV prevention intervention or technology is sufficient to address the HIV/AIDS pandemic, particularly when considering the various social, political, and economic issues fuelling the epidemic. NPTs would be only one component of what should be a full spectrum of HIV prevention interventions (including rights-focused behaviour change, voluntary counselling and testing, sexually transmitted infection screening and treatment, male and female condoms and lubricant, treatment to prevent vertical transmission, and clean injecting equipment). A greater variety of NPTs will allow individuals to find a prevention method that best meets their needs and life circumstances and economic limitations. People vulnerable to HIV need both new tools and better access to proven existing HIV prevention tools. Existing technologies, such as condoms and needle exchange, are not accessible to all who are at risk for HIV infection in Canada, and significant efforts will have to be made to ensure NPTs are accessed.

A noted limitation of the current dominant approaches to prevention (e.g., condoms, abstinence, faithfulness) is that they tend to be controlled by a male partner or are otherwise impacted by structural determinants of health, such as gender inequality (Morris & Lacey, 2010; Moscicki, 2008, Woodsong, 2004). As Dunkle and Jewkes (2007) state, such prevention approaches for women are "not only futile but morally bankrupt. Abstinence and condom use may be impossible for women to enforce. Fidelity is of no use unless it is mutual, and men's faithfulness very often lies outside of women's control" (p. 173). There is great interest, then, in biomedical technologies to prevention that may empower individuals in sexual encounters to protect themselves, regardless of the desires and wishes of their sexual partner.

Female initiated HIV prevention options, including PrEP, microbicides, and vaccines would meaningfully expand the prevention tool kit. Prevention methods such as condoms and abstinence are not always realistic options for women, especially for those who are married, who want to have children, or who are at risk of sexual violence. A safe and effective microbicide or HIV vaccine could provide women with the option of protecting themselves from HIV infection without limiting their choices to conceive. The ability to reduce the risk of horizontal HIV transmission between partners during conception (as discussed in Chapter 10 by Loutfy and Margolese) would be a key benefit of NPTs. The expansion of the tool kit, however, does not preclude the need to change the social norms that create these power imbalances between men and women.

THE STATUS OF NEW HIV PREVENTION TECHNOLOGIES

Research into new HIV prevention technologies has a long and often discouraging history (AIDS Vaccine Advocacy Coalition [AVAC], 2010). However, recent trial results have brought renewed hope to the field. In 2009, a Thai clinical trial demonstrated proof-of-concept of an HIV vaccine, and a global collaboration led to the discovery of four new broadly neutralizing antibodies that show promise for an effective HIV vaccine. In 2010, South African researchers provided proof-of-concept for an antiretroviral-based vaginal microbicide (CAPRISA 004 trial), and PrEP was also proven effective in preventing HIV transmission among men who have sex with men (iPrEx trial) (Abdool et al., 2010).

Interest in female-initiated HIV prevention methods was bolstered by the results of the CAPRISA 004 trial, which provided proof-of-concept for prevention of HIV among women using a vaginal microbicide (consisting of 1% tenofovir gel). As noted above, the microbicide was found to be 39% effective in reducing a woman's risk of becoming infected with HIV during vaginal intercourse and 51% effective in preventing genital herpes infections in the women participating in the trial. In July 2010, at the International AIDS Conference in Vienna, Austria, lead researchers presented evidence demonstrating proof-of-concept for an antiretroviral-based vaginal microbicide. Attendees gave the researchers a tearful standing ovation, an extremely rare event in science. The excitement stemmed from the unprecedented evidence that female-controlled prevention technology was possible, that a microbicide could reduce women's risk of both HIV and HSV-2 infection, and also from the strength of the data, which showed consistent evidence of protection across a variety of statistical analyses (AVAC, 2010b).

The CAPRISA 004 trial confirmed tenofovir gel as a promising microbicide candidate. However, the trial was not designed to provide sufficient evidence to license a new drug (which would generally require a definitive phase III trial). More research is needed to confirm the effectiveness demonstrated in both the iPrEx and CAPRISA 004 trials, as well as research into different dosing strategies, formulations, and products containing other antiretrovirals or compounds. Additional research is also needed to find microbicides that are not antiretroviral-based in order to benefit women who are living with HIV, and to establish the safety and efficacy of the microbicide for rectal use.

If a future trial shows that tenofovir—or another drug—does work, another two to four years are expected for Canada's regulatory processes to approve the microbicide for distribution to women considered most at risk (e.g., Black and Aboriginal women; women who inject drugs). It is also expected that a microbicide will not be available to all Canadians at the same time; rather, it will be made available to some people and not others during introduction and scale-up. For example, efficacy for women may be determined before efficacy in men, as advanced trials to date have focused on vaginal use. Canadian regulators, HIV policy-makers, service providers, and community members will all have to work through issues of prescription guidelines, education, and prioritizing specific high-risk groups.

NPTs AS TOOLS FOR "EMPOWERMENT"?

NPTs can be seen as "empowering" for a number of groups that experience problems with safer sex negotiation. Pre-exposure prophylaxis (PrEP), for instance, has a number of characteristics that set it apart from the other technologies. It can be used by men or women; covert use may be easier because the treatment is "distant" from the risk exposure; and it may provide protection for more than one type of risk exposure (e.g., drug use and sex) (International AIDS Society, 2007). NPTs could benefit populations where condom usage is rare, particularly for men and women who either choose not to use condoms or are in situations where they do not have the agency to negotiate safer sex (United Nations Population Fund, 2007).

It is important to recognize and understand how the use of NPTs, especially microbicides and vaccines, is impacted by gender relations and broader social, political, and economic inequalities. Much of the focus in this area has been on women, and microbicides as a form of female-controlled prevention. Tolley and Severy (2006), for instance, note that the literature on the structural determinants of condom use can provide insight into some of the structural barriers that may impede microbicide use, such as the power dynamics of relationships and the meanings associated with the use of prevention methods (e.g., condoms as a sign of mistrust) (Marston & King, 2006). To this end, Severy, Tolley, Woodsong, and Guest (2005), drawing on the AIDS Risk Reduction Model, posited a framework that situates microbicide acceptability within three levels: individual, couple, and socio-cultural. At the individual level, they note how perceived susceptibility to HIV and belief in the efficacy of the product can impact acceptability and use. However, they take this further to note that the dynamics of the relationship itself can impact perceptions of susceptibility to HIV (i.e., new relationships versus established ones) and how women may find it difficult or impossible to raise the topic in some situations. (The authors assume heteronormative "relationship" status for women and do not discuss considerations for women in the sex trade or women who are street-involved to any depth.) Along similar lines, they acknowledge that structural factors, such as economic and gender-based inequalities that produce women's economic dependence on men, can influence the acceptability of microbicides, reflecting broader issues of political economy. In earlier work, Woodsong (2004) likewise noted four factors related to the acceptability of microbicide use: women's perception of risk; the characteristics of the product; partner perceptions/reactions to use; and gender relations. Many of these same issues are raised in consideration of HIV vaccine acceptability (Laird, 1994; Rudy et al., 2005; Williams et al., 2009).

Indeed, more research has been called for in understanding the "trade-offs" that exist in decisions around microbicide use; the cultural norms about intravaginal practices that may ultimately impact microbicide use; who would have access to microbicides and why or why not; and the role of gender relations in eventual microbicide acceptability and use (Mantell et al., 2005; Patten, 2008). Recent research has shown how women's use of microbicides can be impacted by the dynamics of the relationship and the perceptions of the male partners. Tanner et al. (2010), for instance, found that women in more established relationships found it easier to talk about microbicidal products than those in casual relationships, who felt more need to protect themselves (Koo, Woodsong, Dalberth, Viswanathan, & Simons-Rudolph, 2005; Short, Rosenthal, Auslander, & Succop, 2009). Other recent research has shown that women might be more likely to use microbicides with casual partners, rather than with regular partners (Hoffman et al., 2010). A trial of a simulated microbicide with high-risk women in Connecticut showed that sexual assertiveness predicted use of the product (Mosack, Weeks, Sylla, & Abbott, 2006). Research on the acceptability of vaccines echoes similar issues, where women are concerned that broaching the topic of vaccines with their male partners might signify mistrust or accusation or evidence of infidelities (Newman, Duan, Kakinami, & Roberts, 2008; Newman, Duan, Rudy, & Johnston-Roberts, 2004), or violate cultural norms (Williams et al., 2009).

YET ANOTHER RESPONSIBILITY FOR WOMEN?
The nearly ubiquitous power inequities in sexual relationships means that women around the world need strategies to protect their reproductive health and to hide these strategies from their male partners. Secret use of contraceptives is perhaps the most common of these strategies, and, increasingly, women are also seeking means of preventing HIV. As with prevention of unwanted pregnancies, women may feel that they cannot trust their male partners to take the initiative, and want to take control of protecting themselves. To this end, a review of young adults and microbicides observed that "ultimately, it may be passive acquiescence on the part of the male that will be more important than clandestine use [of a microbicide] by the female," underlining the importance of considering male partners in acceptability research and the need to continue to support women in developing sexual negotiation skills (Rupp & Rosenthal, 2003).

Despite the widespread assumption of empowerment through female-controlled prevention products, there has been criticism:

> [Microbicides for HIV prevention is] an approach erring on the side of damage control: the image is of a woman down on the floor being kicked and now we have given her some armour, with a subtle acknowledgment that we are all powerless to stop the kicking. (McNally, 2010)

McNally (2010) goes on to posit that the excitement around microbicides' proof-of-concept (in reference to the CAPRISA 004 trial) is partly fuelled by a relief that we won't have to wrestle with changing men's attitudes and sexual practices. We can abandon the work on changing attitudes toward sex, tacitly endorse the belief that male enjoyment of sex is beyond reproach, and accept that men cannot be taught how to practice safer sex.

For instance, in some cases it has been noted that if women are discovered covertly using prevention products, they could face adverse consequences from their male partners as the products might be seen as an affront to men's power and the traditional gender norms (Mantell et al., 2006; Woodsong, 2004). Even among cases where women disclose to their male partners about microbicides, an outcome could be a discontinuation of the use of condoms. This could increase women's risk of HIV and STI transmission (Woodsong, 2004) since microbicides may not be as effective at preventing HIV transmission as condoms. And if women do disclose their desire to use an NPT such as a microbicide, the discussions will be no different than those around condom use in raising doubts about fidelity and trust. Thus, even with woman-controlled methods, the consequences attached to their use can still present barriers (Williams et al., 2009). Microbicides could also further entrench women's responsibility for sexual health, rather than promoting a shared responsibility. Thus, female-controlled prevention "should not obviate the need to strive for more equitable responsibility between partners for risk reduction" (Koo et al., 2005; Woodsong, 2004).

NPTs AS A CATALYST FOR BROADER STRUCTURAL CHANGE

Female-controlled HIV prevention products are not simply the panacea for women's equality and empowerment that they are sometimes purported to be, particularly by enthusiastic advocates (Mantell et al., 2006; Woodsong, 2004). They may, however, serve as a catalyst for longer term, broader structural change to the extent that female-controlled interventions stimulate further policy and programming discussions and are introduced within multi-level interventions that address women's core HIV vulnerabilities, such as gender inequality, poverty, and other forms of discrimination (Mantell et al., 2006).

> Providing women with access to their own prevention methods might not raise their wages, cultural valuations, or reduce discriminatory legal practices, but these methods can act as a catalyst to change norms of self-care, communication and decision-making about sex and fertility, and sexual pleasure. (Mantell et al., 2006, p. 2002)

There remains, however, a call for further enhancement of "gender-transformative" or social change interventions with men to alter the social constructions of masculine sexuality that perpetuate disempowering gender norms (Dunkle & Jewkes, 2007). Efforts to change power imbalances between men and women must involve challenging the position that men hold in society and in their relationships. Men's dominance in deciding how and when sex takes place, their use of violence against women, their reluctance to pay attention to their health needs, and resistance to using condoms are among the biggest challenges to reducing HIV risk worldwide. Expanding women's HIV prevention tool kit is unlikely to lead to greater equality in relationships with men unless gender norms change.

User-initiated prevention doesn't necessarily imply covert prevention. But unlike the male or female condom, PrEP or a microbicide could be used without a partner's active co-operation at each act of intercourse, providing options for user-initiated, rather than partner-controlled, tools. Social scientists have interviewed women in several countries to explore how they felt about the possibility of a user-initiated method (Woodsong, 2004). A large proportion of respondents said that if they planned to use a microbicide in the future, they would probably discuss the issue in advance with their husbands or boyfriends. But, they said, this could be a one-time conversation and would not have to be repeated each time the couple has sex.

Some women, however, may choose to use a microbicide without any partner discussion. Microbicides may initially come in gels or creams—products that will somewhat increase vaginal lubrication. This may make their secret use a bit of a problem for women in long-term partnerships. However, microbicides that come in the form of vaginal rings and films are also being formulated. A flexible, microbicide-loaded vaginal ring, for example, could provide time-released protection with minimal lubrication change, providing another option to women who can't or don't want to discuss the issue of protection with their male partners.

There is some evidence that suggests the biomedical field is acknowledging and responding to these issues. For example, in research on microbicides, there has been a change in emphasis from pursuing products that require use at the time of the sexual encounter, to products that are more distant from the actual encounter (Sawires, Birnbaum, Abu-Raddad, Szekeres, & Gayle, 2009). This shift is based on the realization that "even a biologically successful microbicide may not provide women the sought-after protection, as it can do little if anything to encourage agency over sexuality or mitigate the social terms in which sex occurs" (Sawires et al., 2009, p. S75).

COMPARING NPTs TO THE ORAL CONTRACEPTIVE ("THE PILL")

Advocates for NPTs argue that the greater the variety of prevention tools available, the greater our chances of decreasing HIV transmission rates. The advantage of variety in NPTs is analogous to the variety of contraception methods for prevention of pregnancy. While contraceptive technologies separate sex from reproduction, NPTs allow separation of sex from HIV prevention, and would perhaps allow women to separate HIV prevention from contraception. Put another way, female contraceptives and women-initiated or -controlled NPTs give women the responsibility for ensuring sex without consequences.

In many heterosexual relationships, men have the sexual decision-making power, including over decisions regarding contraception and STI or HIV prevention (Amaro, 1995; Gomez & Marin, 1996; Pulerwitz, Gortmaker, & DeJong, 2000). Although women bear the greatest burden of bearing and raising children, in many countries reproductive decision making is controlled by men and the extended family, and men may refuse to allow their partners to use contraceptives due to their associations with sexual infidelity and the erosion of male authority (Watkins, Rutenberg, & Wilkinson, 1997). Decision making around contraceptive use is analogous to use of NPTs with respect to power imbalances within heterosexual relationships, with both influenced by factors such as intimacy, sexual enjoyment, and communication (Heise, 1997). The prevention of unintended pregnancy through covert use of contraceptives leads us to anticipate women's need for NPTs that can be used covertly for the prevention of STIs and HIV, perhaps even more so, given that it is easier to discuss pregnancy with a male partner than it is to discuss STIs (Woodsong & Koo, 1999). Ideally, microbicides would include formulations that either include contraception or allow pregnancy. Contraceptive microbicides could provide both pregnancy and STI prevention to women wishing to meet both needs with one product. The candidates furthest advanced in trials at the time of writing are all non-contraceptive, but a contraceptive component could be added. A non-contraceptive microbicide would be especially valuable to women who are living with HIV but still wish to conceive with their serodiscordant partner.

One of the goals of ensuring contraceptive availability is to increase women's power in reproductive decision making and autonomy, and to generally improve women's quality of life (Beckman & Harvey, 2005). The innovations in birth control during the last four decades have had a strong impact on modern societies. The direct effect on demography, and especially on birth rates in specific social groups, has been abundantly studied (Mehra, 1997; Hotz, Klerman, & Willis, 1996; Oltmans & Hungerman, 2007). An additional, indirect effect operates through the reduction in uncertainty faced by women and their partners due to the increased ability to plan reproduction. This fact has dramatically altered the context in which decisions regarding women's education and employment are made. Indeed, the oral contraceptive pill, or "The Pill" as it is known as a cultural icon, has come to represent women's economic and social advancement. For instance, many authors have argued that the spectacular increase in women's education and participation in the labour market since the 1960s was largely due to contraceptive innovations (Goldin & Katz, 2000, 2002, 2008; Laumann, Gagnon, Michael, & Michaels, 2000). A third, and relatively less studied consequence of increased access to contraceptive choices is the impact of the changes on the "balance of power" within heterosexual couples. After all, innovations in birth control technology, including the legalization of abortion, have a potentially huge effect on men's and women's respective decision rights within the household regarding such crucial issues as the number or timing of births. A number of sociologists (Coombs & Fernandez, 1978; Michael, 2000; Williams, 1994) have argued that a shift of such magnitude has altered the balance of powers within heterosexual relationships.

Although increasing women's range of choices and autonomy in sexual and reproductive decision making is a worthy goal, these efforts reinforce the gender norm of women having to assume the sole responsibility for contraception. NPTs such as microbicides could become another example of women having to take on the burden of protection against the negative consequences of sexual practices. Far more contraceptive agents have been developed for use by females than by males. Contraceptive options for women began to dramatically increase in the 1960s, including hormone-based contraceptives, from birth control pills to implants and injections. In that same period, male contraceptive choices remained relatively constant: condoms and vasectomies. Pharmaceutical companies and the medical establishment decided that research in the area of hormonal contraception for men would not be profitable based on the beliefs that men would be less motivated than women to use such a contraceptive and would be less willing to accept the adverse effects (Oudshoorn, 2003). Arditti (1977) argued that concern over "loss of libido" was a major factor in prohibiting research in the area of male birth control pills. Yet, she notes that the same "loss of libido" was "almost never taken into consideration when dealing with female contraception, the obvious bias being that women do not have anything to lose since the 'active' force in sexual intercourse stems from the male" (p. 123).

Despite the claims that women's liberation is partially dependent on women's ability to control their fertility, the relationship between contraception and women's emancipation is not as clear as it appears. Concerns about contraceptive technologies and practices lie both with the types of methods available and their health effects, and the lack of variety for male contraceptives. Women already bear a disproportionate burden of responsibility for prevention of pregnancy, and NPTs would add the responsibility for HIV and STI prevention, with all of the health risks associated with these biomedical interventions. This additional burden of health risks is particularly salient considering that many NPTs are ARV-based and potentially toxic. It is a matter of equity that the health risks associated with adequate contraception and HIV prevention should be shared between male and female partners.

With the limited number of male birth control methods available, and due to gender norms, men tend to relinquish the responsibility, and thus the health risks, of fertility control to women (Laird, 1994). Even though weekly testosterone injections can be a highly effective form of male contraception, men taking an active role in birth control is contradictory to notions of masculinity as stemming from virility (Kinnon, 1985). In her study of men's and women's attitudes toward a hypothetical male birth control pill and toward the current female oral contraceptive, Laird (1994) found that, given the same level of health risks, men were much less likely to be willing to take an oral contraceptive. According to the men in the study, the male pill is more against nature, more of a bother, more harmful, and goes more against their beliefs, as compared to an identical female pill. The fact that only 20% of male subjects reported that they would use an oral contraceptive is disturbing when coupled with the finding that 71% of these men would not be hesitant to have their partners use a comparable female birth control pill, indicating an apparent disregard for women's health (Laird, 1994).

Heterosexual women have few options but to bear the risks and inconveniences of contraception themselves, due not only to the lack of male methods, but ultimately because men are reluctant to use them. Laird's (1994) conclusion with respect to male birth control methods is analogous to concerns about the limitations of NPTs for HIV prevention:

> [A]dvocating the immediate, unbridled development of such methods would be misguided. Technology exists within a social context and interacts with politics, economics, religion, race and gender power relationships. Simply developing more male birth control methods [or female-controlled NPTs] will not ensure gender equality. (p. 467)

In the context of the birth control pill, a "choosing woman" is not necessarily a "liberated woman"; choosing to use an oral contraceptive is not so much the enactment of a right, but more about compromising or "making due" within a range of options bound by social expectations. Women's decision making around birth control is a relational choice (in reference to relationships with their sexual partners) rather than a purely individual one (Lowe, 2005). Women's right to choose and to have access to a range of reproductive and preventive technologies is replete with complications and paradoxes in terms of autonomous decision making, sex, sexual health, and reproduction (Granzow, 2008). Access to contraception may leave patriarchal power imbalances largely intact or may even reinforce that social order. The rhetoric of women's liberation does not acknowledge that technology works in compliance with, rather than against, a dominant paradigm. There is, therefore, a large gap between the power of the birth control pill and women's liberation, for which it is so often credited.

SEXUAL PLEASURE

Microbicide studies indicate that women place higher value on the use of a vaginal gel when they perceive it to enhance their own and their partners' sexual pleasure and performance (Hoffman et al., 2010). Tanner et al. (2010) noted that microbicide use was more likely where male partners had positive evaluations of the product, and where the product would increase the man's sexual pleasure, underlining the continuing effect of gender-based sexual norms in women's relationships (Mantell et al., 2006). Male sexual pleasure is of tantamount priority, with women's pleasure and sexual and/or reproductive health as secondary concerns. Thus, it has been suggested that marketing efforts frame microbicides as products for sexual enhancement and/or vaginal hygiene, rather than for HIV prevention, to increase their uptake (Hoffman et al., 2010).

Gel formulations of microbicides have been found to increase sexual pleasure for both women and their male partners due to the extra lubrication. Since insufficient vaginal lubrication during sex is a common problem, microbicides could improve sexual intercourse for many women (Braunstein & Van De Wijgert, 2005). Women in microbicides trials have suggested that a product that improves the sexual encounter by providing a comfortable amount of lubrication, and that also has an attractive smell, taste, or tingle, might enable them to use microbicides without disclosing their true purpose, or at least to facilitate acceptance by male partners (Woodsong, 2004). However, again it must be noted that adding another chemical substance into women's bodies, even if in the form of a pleasure-enhancing lubricant, does not address heteronormative sexual relations, nor shift the structural inequalities placing women at risk of HIV.

IMPLICATIONS FOR HIV PREVENTION AMONG WOMEN IN CANADA

Gender-based analysis of NPTs is a vital area for HIV researchers, policy analysts, and programming stakeholders. Lack of social and economic autonomy, cultural prohibitions, and other factors make it impossible for many women to insist on condom use during sex. And it is unknown how the introduction of NPTs could impact the risk and autonomy of receptive sexual partners who generally have low control over condom use by their insertive partners. Social scientists, service providers, and women's advocates need to grapple with the important questions of whether NPTs serve women's strategic gender interests and whether the new prevention tools will increase women's control over their sexual and reproductive lives.

As indicated by Gahagan et al. (see Chapter 3 in this volume), there continues to be a limited focus on the diversity of women-specific HIV prevention issues outside of "normative" contexts (i.e., prenatal) or contexts of risk (i.e., injection drug use). And most studies do not address heterosexual or opposite-sex sexual partners in HIV prevention or gender dynamics as key factors in understanding HIV prevention. Gahagan also makes the point that women's sexual and reproductive autonomy and HIV prevention capacity cannot be built in isolation from political and economic structural factors.

The next wave of HIV prevention for, by, and with women in Canada must include augmenting the focus on the diversity of women's experiences with HIV; reframing prevention policies so that they are more inclusive of women's unique experiences and recognize the complexities of women's lives and identities; and within programs, placing a greater emphasis on the uniqueness of women's HIV prevention experiences and needs. These considerations are especially important when considering the introduction of NPTs to Canada's most vulnerable women, such as young Aboriginal, African, or Caribbean women, or women who inject drugs.

There is clearly a need to revitalize a national, coordinated HIV prevention research, programming, and policy agenda that takes the lived experiences of women as the jumping off point for the development of innovative approaches to addressing the epidemic in Canada. Further intervention-focused research is needed to understand how NPTs can address both the contexts and conditions of HIV risk beyond the divisiveness of personal agency approaches in sexual negotiation. It is also crucial that the next wave of HIV prevention efforts in Canada assess the gender-based implications of NPTs in terms of autonomy, covert use, partner negotiation, and risk compensation, and to explore the mechanisms by which NPTs may serve as a catalyst for broader structural changes in gender norms.

In addition to social, cultural, and economic realities, ARV-based prevention technologies require extensive consideration of the safest and most appropriate modes of administration. As with hormonal contraception as a method to prevent pregnancy, future assessments of prevention with ARV drugs will need to focus on modes of delivery (oral, topical [vaginal, rectal], injectable); dosing regimen (daily, monthly, intermittent, or exposure-related [before and after sex]); single versus combination products; and what works in specific target populations (defined by risk, behaviour, and infection status) (Padian, Buvé, Balkus, Serwadda, & Ward, 2008).

While women and girls in Canada are continuing to become HIV positive in proportionally larger numbers, women are also leading efforts to address the enormous gender-based power imbalances that fuel this trend (Gruskina, Fergusona, & O'Malley, 2007; Human Rights Watch, 2003; Shannon et al., 2008). Given this reality, women-specific HIV prevention needs must be mobilized through national, regional, and local organizations in order to develop and deliver gender-appropriate HIV prevention programs and services. In addition, women's caregiving burden and economic and social status, gender-based violence, and poverty must be attended to in the process. Furthermore, women have a crucial role to play in all phases of NPT development and introduction, including shaping the research agenda, ensuring that community views and perspectives are included in the development of prevention policies and programs, and creating political pressure for widespread and timely access to safe and effective products. Female users of NPTs must be at the centre driving scientific innovation and not simply recipients of such efforts. In Chapter 4 of this volume, Peltier and colleagues remind us that all HIV prevention policy, research, and service design and delivery must be based on respect for self-determination (e.g., by Aboriginal women for Aboriginal women).

Between 1999 and 2008, Aboriginal women represented an increasingly higher proportion of positive HIV test reports, reaching a high of 52% of all case reports among women in 2008. This trend was also seen in Black women, with an increase in proportion from 12.2% of positive HIV test reports among women in 1999 to 26.3% in 2008 (PHAC, 2010). Women in Canada of African or Caribbean descent do not perceive themselves as being at risk for HIV transmission, and characterize people affected by HIV/AIDS as "unfaithful husbands, unfaithful wives, living in Africa and the Caribbean," or people in the sex trade, drug users, or gay men (Williams et al., 2009). Williams et al. (2009) found that, although women were able to describe sexual practices within Black communities as including serial monogamy, polygamy, and infidelity, they did not discuss the possibility of changing or ways to change these sexual dynamics. This may reflect a prevailing assumption that sexual practices are fixed, or that trying to change health and sexual practices of male partners would generate negative reactions from their partners and from their broader community (Tharao & Massaquoi, 2000). Other barriers to challenging sexual practices within the Black community include: instruction by churches to women to obey their husbands, and the desire not to violate sacred/cultural norms in the community by confronting male partners about sexual behaviours; dependence on men for financial and social support, and the fear of jeopardizing these resources by refusing unprotected sex; discomfort discussing sexual practices such as infidelity; and concerns about being suspected of immoral behaviour if they sought an NPT such as an HIV vaccine (Williams et al., 2009).

Given all of these complex interplays between personal perceptions of risk and strong implications for individual self-regard, relationship stability, and status in the community, it is unlikely that an NPT will make any dent in the overarching social vulnerabilities of many women in Canada.

The introduction of NPTs, once they become available, will be a complex process with key considerations including:

- the potential impact on contexts of risk, and concerns of "behavioural disinhibition" or "risk compensation";
- the risk of poor adherence and inadequate HIV testing, potentially leading to drug resistance with ARV-based methods;
- the challenges of communicating partial efficacy and translation of clinical trial efficacy rates to individual decision making;
- the potential for medicalization of prevention to detract from needed shifts in social, behavioural, or structural interventions;
- the decision as to which populations should be prioritized and who decides on this prioritization for a partially efficacious ARV-based product;
- the challenges of controlling off-label and community use of PrEP;
- the implications for access and cost, given the complexity of combination prevention spanning both clinical and community settings;
- the implications of NPT availability/use on standards of legally defined "significant risk" of HIV transmission in the context of sexual intercourse without a condom, and the effect on criminalization of individuals who do not disclose their HIV status before unprotected sex; and
- the evidentiary standards and minimum effectiveness necessary for Canadian regulators to make NPTs available on the market.

CONCLUSION

The distinction commonly made between socio-behavioural and biomedical approaches for HIV prevention for women remains problematic. For example, behaviour change programs depend on the existence of essential technologies—such as condoms, clean injecting equipment, and HIV testing kits—but biomedical tools will have limited impact in reducing new infections without supportive preventive behaviours. The emergence of NPTs to reduce the risk of HIV transmission offers potential opportunities to improve our understanding of human behaviour with respect to health seeking and adoption of new health technologies (Global HIV Prevention Working Group, 2008).

Hope for more tools to provide biological protection of women rests, in part, on NPTs that are initiated and controlled by receptive partners. However, this biological protection is not mutually exclusive to, nor does it negate the need for, structural changes to social norms of sexual relationships and sexual practices. Assigning greater control or greater autonomy for women over their sexual and reproductive health does not necessarily change the gender status quo. NPTs fall short of challenging the social norms whereby men hold decision-making power and use this power to control the sexuality and reproduction of their partners. NPTs simply expand options for women to exercise their sexual and reproductive rights to protect themselves, and may enhance their safer-sex bargaining power within relationships. Providing women with NPTs as means of protection within their control does not obviate the need to strive for more equitable responsibility between partners for HIV risk reduction. The introduction of NPTs (such as PrEP, vaccines, and microbicides) could result in an increase in societal expectations for women to assume primary responsibility for prevention of HIV infection, which might have the effect of exacerbating gender inequities. Essentially, NPTs can be seen to go hand in hand with dominant social norms that hold women as primarily responsible for ensuring sex without consequences, such as HIV and/or unintended pregnancies.

Effective HIV prevention for women in Canada requires a combination of behavioural, biomedical, and structural intervention strategies. Any compartmentalization (either in discourse or application) of these strategies will remain superfluous and counterproductive. The next wave of HIV prevention will not be achieved at any one level nor with any one type of stand-alone intervention. Rather, promising new HIV prevention interventions for, by, and with women must be aggregated into combination prevention approaches that cut across sectors—health, legal, political, economic, social, and so forth. The overarching goal of the next wave of HIV prevention for women in Canada must centre on evidence-based, comprehensive strategies that address women's diverse needs and complex vulnerabilities.

PROBLEM-BASED LEARNING CASE STUDY

As we have seen in this chapter on new prevention technologies, issues such as who benefits from these technologies and who has access to these advances remain central to the changing landscape of HIV prevention in Canada, as well as globally. Gender and other key determinants of health need to be considered in both the development and uptake of new prevention technologies in order to help ensure success.

CRITICAL THINKING QUESTIONS

1. Based on the evidence provided in this chapter, what are some of the keys issues to be considered in the development and uptake of new HIV prevention technologies for women in Canada? For men? At the international level?
2. What are some of the issues related to community preparedness that need to be considered throughout the prevention technology development process?
3. How can the next generation of new HIV prevention technologies take into consideration the intersections of race, class, and gender to better meet the needs of diverse populations of women in Canada?

REFERENCES

Abdool K. Q., Abdool Karim, S. S., Frohlich, J. A., Grobler, A. C., Baxter, C., Mansoor, L. E., ... & Taylor, D. (2010). Effectiveness and safety of tenofovir gel, an antiretroviral microbicide, for the prevention of HIV infection in women. *Science, 329*(5996), 1168–1174.

AIDS Vaccine Advocacy Coalition. (2010). *Advocates' network update, July 29, 2010*. Retrieved from www.avac.org/ht/d/sp/i/28566/TPL/AN/pid/28566/displaytype/iframe

Amaro, J. (1995). Love, sex and power: Considering women's realities in HIV prevention. *American Psychologist, 50*(6), 437–447.

Arditti, R. (1977). Have you ever wondered about the Male Pill? In C. Dreifus (Ed.), *Seizing our bodies: The politics of women's health* (pp. 121–130). New York: Vintage Books.

Beckman, L. J., & Harvey, S. M. (2005). Current reproductive technologies: Increased access and choice? *Journal of Social Issues, 61*(1), 1–20.

Braunstein, S., & Van De Wijgert, J. (2005). Preferences and practices related to vaginal lubrication: Implications for microbicide acceptability and clinical testing. *Journal of Women's Health, 14*(5), 424–433. doi:10.1089/jwh.2005.14.424.

Cohen, M. S., Chen, Y. Q., McCauley, M., Gamble, T. Hosseininpour, M., Kumarasamy, N., ... Fleming, T. R., for the HPTN 052 Study Team. (2011). Prevention of HIV-1 infection with early antiretroviral therapy. *The New England Journal of Medicine, 365*(6), 493–505.

Coombs, L., & Fernandez, D. (1978). Husband-wife agreement about reproductive goals. *Demography, 15*(1), 57–73.

Craddock, S. (2007). Market incentives, human lives and AIDS vaccines. *Social Science & Medicine, 64*(5), 1042–1056.

Dunkle, K. L., & Jewkes, R. (2007). Effective HIV prevention requires gender-transformative work with men. *Sexually Transmitted Infections, 83*(3), 173–174.

European Study Group on Heterosexual Transmission of HIV. (1992). Comparison of female to male and male to female transmission of HIV in 563 stable couples. BMJ, *304*, 809–813.

Fiske, J., & Browne, A. (2006). Aboriginal citizen, discredited medical subject: Paradoxical constructions of Aboriginal women's subjectivity in Canadian health care policies. *Policy Sciences, 39*(1), 91–111.

Global Campaign for Microbicides. (2010). *Microbicides: What do they mean for women?* [Fact sheet]. Retrieved from www.global-campaign.org/EngDownload.htm

Global Coalition on Women and AIDS. (2010). *Action areas.* Retrieved from http://data.unaids.org/GCWA/gcwa_backgrounder_en.pdf

Global HIV Prevention Working Group. (2008). *Behavior change and HIV prevention: (Re)Considerations for the 21st century.* Retrieved from www.globalhivprevention.org/reports.html

Goldin, C., & Katz, L. (2000). Career and marriage in the age of the pill. *American Economic Review, 90*(2), 461–465.

Goldin, C., & Katz, L. (2002). The power of the pill: Oral contraceptives and women's career and marriage decisions. *Journal of Political Economy, 110*(4), 730–770.

Goldin, C., & Katz, L. F. (2008). Transitions: Career and family life cycles of the educational elite. *American Economic Review, 98*(2), 363–369.

Gomez, C., & Marin, B. (1996). Gender, culture and power: Barriers to HIV prevention strategies. *Journal of Sex Research, 33*(4), 355–362.

Granzow, K. (2008). The imperative to choose: A qualitative study of women's decision-making and use of the birth control pill. *Social Theory & Health, 6,* 1–17.

Gruskina, S., Fergusona, L., & O'Malley, J. (2007). Ensuring sexual and reproductive health for people living with HIV: An overview of key human rights, policy and health systems issues. *Reproductive Health Matters, 15*(29 Suppl.), 4–26.

Heise, L. (1997). Beyond acceptability: Reorienting research on contraceptive choice. In T. Ravindran, M. Berer, & J. Cottingham (Eds.), *Beyond acceptability: Users' perspectives on contraception* (pp. 6–14). London, UK: Reproductive Health Matters.

Hoffman, S., Morrow, K. M., Mantell, J. E., Rosen, R. K., Carballo-Dieguez, A., & Gai, F. (2010). Covert use, vaginal lubrication, and sexual pleasure: A qualitative study of urban U.S. women in a vaginal microbicide clinical trial. *Archives of Sexual Behavior, 39*(3), 748–760.

Hotz, V. J., Klerman, J. A., & Willis, R. J. (1996). The economics of fertility in developed countries: A survey. Labor and Population Program Working Paper Series 96–09. *RAND.* Retrieved from www.rand.org/pubs/drafts/2007/DRU1422.pdf

Human Rights Watch. (2003). *Policy paralysis: A call for action on HIV/AIDS-related human rights abuses against women and girls in Africa.* Retrieved from www.hrw.org/en/node/80717/section/1

International AIDS Society. (2007, July). *Developing country-level participation and capacity for PrEP implementation.* Report on the PrEP Implementation Policy Forum, Sydney, Australia.

Kinnon, D. (1985). The birth control gap. *Healthsharing,* 15–17.

Koo, H. P., Woodsong, C., Dalberth, B. T., Viswanathan, M., & Simons-Rudolph, A. (2005). Context of acceptability of topical microbicides: Sexual relationships. *Journal of Social Issues, 61*(1), 67–93.

Laird, J. (1994). A male pill? Gender discrepancies in contraceptive commitment. *Feminism and Psychology, 4*(3), 458–468.

Laumann, E. O., Gagnon, J. H., Michael, R. T., & Michaels, S. (2000). Sex and fertility. In *The social organization of sexuality: Sexual practices in the United States* (pp. 442–473). Chicago, IL: University of Chicago Press.

Lowe, P. (2005). Contraception and heterosex: An intimate relationship. *Sexualities, 8*(1), 75–92.

Mantell, J. E., Dworkin, S. L., Exner, T. M., Hoffman, S., Smit, J. A., & Susser, I. (2006). The promises and limitations of female-initiated methods of HIV/STI protection. *Social Science & Medicine, 63*(8), 1998–2009.

Mantell, J. E., Myer, L., Carballo-Dieguez, A., Stein, Z., Ramjee, G., Morar, N. S., & Harrison, P. F. (2005). Microbicide acceptability research: Current approaches and future directions. *Social Science & Medicine, 60*(2), 319–330.

Marston, C., & King, E. (2006). Factors that shape young people's sexual behaviour: A systematic review. *The Lancet, 368*(9547), 1581–1586.

McNally, P. (2010, August 2). Men off the hook with HIV gel: A new gel designed to help prevent the spread of HIV may be used to pander to male irresponsibility over safe sex. *The Guardian.* Retrieved from www.guardian.co.uk/commentisfree/2010/aug/02/hiv-gel-men-abandon-safe-sex

Mehra, R. (1997). Women, empowerment and economic development. *The ANNALS of the American Academy of Political and Social Science, 554*(1), 136–149.

Michael, R. (2000). Abortion decisions in the U.S. In E. Laumann & R. Michael (Eds.), *Sex, love and health in America: Private choices and public policy* (pp. 377–438). Chicago, IL: University of Chicago Press.

Moffitt, P. M. (2004). Colonialization: A health determinant for pregnant Dogrib women. *Journal of Transcultural Nursing, 15*(4), 323–330.

Morris, G. C., & Lacey, C. J. N. (2010). Microbicides and HIV prevention: Lessons from the past, looking to the future. *Current Opinion in Infectious Diseases, 23*(1), 57–63.

Mosack, K. E, Weeks, M. R, Sylla, L. N., & Abbott, M. (2006). High-risk women's willingness to try a simulated vaginal microbicide: Results from a pilot study. *Women & Health, 42*(2), 71–88.

Moscicki, A. (2008). Vaginal microbicides: Where are we and where are we going? *Journal of Infection and Chemotherapy, 14*(5), 337–341.

Moscicki, A-B., Ma, Y., Holland C., & Vermund, S. H. (2001). Cervical ectopy in adolescent girls with and without human immunodeficiency virus infection. *The Journal of Infectious Diseases, 183*(6), 865–870.

Newman, P. A., Duan, N., Kakinami, L., & Roberts, K. (2008). What can HIV vaccine trials teach us about future HIV vaccine dissemination? *Vaccine, 26*(20), 2528–2536.

Newman, P. A, Duan, N., Rudy, E. T., & Johnston-Roberts, K. (2004). HIV risk and prevention in a post-vaccine context. *Vaccine, 22*(15–16), 1954–1963. Retrieved from www.guardian.co.uk/commentisfree/2010/aug/02/hiv-gel-men-abandon-safe-sex

Nicolosi, A., Correa Leite, M. L., Musicco, M., Arici, C., Gavazzeni, G., & Lazzarin A. (1994). The efficiency of male-to-female and female-to-male sexual transmission of the human immunodeficiency virus: A study of 730 stable couples. Italian Study Group on HIV Heterosexual Transmission. *Epidemiology, 5*(6), 570–575.

O'Brien, T. R., Busch, M. P., Donegan, E., Ward, J. W., Wong, L., Samson, S. M., … & Holmberg, S. D. (1994). Heterosexual transmission of human immunodeficiency virus type 1 from transfusion recipients to their sex partners. *Journal of Acquired Immune Deficiency Syndromes, 7*(7), 705–710.

Oltmans, A. E., & Hungerman, D. M. (2007). The power of the pill for the next generation. Working Paper 13402. Cambridge, MA: National Bureau of Economic Research. Retrieved from www.nber.org/papers/w13402.pdf

Oudshoorn, N. (2003). *The male pill: A biography of a technology in the making.* Durham, NC: Duke University Press.

Padian, N. S., Buvé, A., Balkus, J., Serwadda, D., & Ward, C. (2008). Biomedical interventions to prevent HIV infection: Evidence, challenges, and way forward. *The Lancet, 372*(9638), 585–599.

Patten, S. (2008). *The Canadian microbicides action plan.* Retrieved from www.cdnaids.ca/canadianmicrobicidesactionplan

Public Health Agency of Canada. (2010). *HIV/AIDS Epi Update: HIV/AIDS among women in Canada.* Retrieved from www.phac-aspc.gc.ca/aids-sida/publication/epi/2010/pdf/EN_Chapter5_Web.pdf

Public Health Agency of Canada. (2011, January/June). *The HIV epidemic in Canada over the next 25 years: Uncertainties, drivers and forerunners.* Unpublished Foresight Document. Ottawa: ON: Ministerial Advisory Council on the Federal Initiative to Address HIV/AIDS in Canada, Public Health Agency of Canada.

Pulerwitz, J., Gortmaker, S., & DeJong, W. (2000). Measuring sexual relationship power in HIV/STD research. *Sex Roles, 42*(7/8), 637–660.

Rudy, E. T., Newman, P. A., Duan, N., Kelly, E. M., Roberts, K. J., & Seiden, D. S. (2005). HIV vaccine acceptability among women at risk: Perceived barriers and facilitators to future HIV vaccine uptake. *AIDS Education and Prevention, 17*(3), 253–267.

Rupp, R. E., & Rosenthal, S. L. (2003). Vaginal microbicides and teenagers. *Current Opinion in Obstetrics and Gynecology, 15*(15), 371–375.

Sawires, S., Birnbaum, N., Abu-Raddad, L., Szekeres, G., & Gayle, J. (2009). Twenty-five years of HIV: Lessons for low prevalence scenarios. *Journal of Acquired Immune Deficiency Syndromes, 51*(Suppl. 3), S75–S82.

Severy, L. J., Tolley, E., Woodsong, C., & Guest, G. (2005). A framework for examining the sustained acceptability of microbicides. *AIDS and Behavior, 9*(1), 121–131.

Shannon, K., Kerr, T., Allinott, S., Chettiar, J., Shoveller, J., & Tyndall, M. (2008). Social and structural violence and power relations in mitigating HIV risk of drug-using women in survival sex work. *Social Science & Medicine, 66*(4), 911–921.

Short, M. B., Rosenthal, S. L., Auslander, B. A., & Succop, P. A. (2009). Relationship context associated with microbicide-like product use. *Journal of Pediatric and Adolescent Gynecology, 22*(5), 313–317.

Tanner, A. E., Fortenberry, J. D., Zimet, G. D., Reece, M., Graham, C. A., & Murray, M. (2010). Young women's use of a microbicide surrogate: The complex influence of relationship characteristics and perceived male partners' evaluations. *Archives of Sexual Behavior, 39*(3), 735–747.

Tharao, E., & Massaquoi, N. (2000). Black women and HIV/AIDS: Contextualizing their realities, their silence and proposing solutions. *Canadian Woman Studies/Les Cahiers de la Femme, 21*(2), 72–80.

Tolley, E. E., & Severy, L. J. (2006). Integrating behavioral and social science research into microbicide clinical trials: Challenges and opportunities. *American Journal of Public Health*, 96(1), 79–83.

United Nations Population Fund. (2007). *State of world population 2007: Unleashing the potential for urban growth.* Retrieved from www.unfpa.org/swp/swpmain.htm

Watkins, S. C., Rutenberg, N., & Wilkinson, D. (1997). Orderly theories, disorderly women. In G. W. Jones, R. M. Douglas, J. C. Caldwell, & R. M. D'Souza (Eds.), *The continuing demographic transition* (pp. 213–245). Oxford, UK: Clarendon Press.

Williams, C. C., Newman, P. A., Sakamoto, I., & Massaquoi, N. A. (2009). HIV prevention risks for Black women in Canada. *Social Science & Medicine*, 68(1), 12–20.

Williams, L. (1994). Determinants of couple agreement in US fertility decisions. *Family Planning Perspectives*, 26(4), 169–173.

Woodsong, C. (2004). Covert use of topical microbicides: Implications for acceptability and use. *Perspectives on Sexual and Reproductive Health*, 36(3), 127–131.

Woodsong, C., & Koo, H. (1999). Two good reasons: Women's and men's perspectives on dual contraceptive use. *Social Science & Medicine*, 49(5), 567–580.

Conclusion
ADDRESSING AND ADVANCING HIV PREVENTION EFFORTS FOR, BY, AND WITH WOMEN IN CANADA

Jacqueline Gahagan

As described in the various chapters contained in this book, both primary and secondary HIV prevention for, with, and by the diverse populations and communities of women in Canada remain significant public health and social justice challenges. Further, an understanding of the variable impact of intersecting and overlapping determinants of health, including gender, requires us to reframe our approaches to HIV prevention in a manner that allows us to remain open to more transdisciplinary methodologies, new perspectives, and novel prevention innovations. Without careful consideration of the unique ways in which women and girls, men and boys, experience HIV, we are unlikely to move beyond the current micro-level focused interventions, and we will simply continue to inadequately address the broader structural inequities fuelling HIV infection rates in Canada.

Informed by the preceding chapters, the following concluding comments further explore the utility of the research, policy, and programming nexus with specific regard to the way forward in addressing the next wave of HIV prevention interventions in Canada from a sex- and gender-based perspective. For example, bringing a sex- and gender-based analytic framework to the development and evaluation of current HIV prevention policies, programs, and related programmatic responses would assist us greatly in our efforts to understand the differential impact such responses have for both our primary and secondary prevention efforts for women, girls, men, and boys. At the same time, it is also essential that we recognize how biological factors *and* social factors cannot be simply disentangled for ease of prevention intervention development or evaluation purposes. We know that simply providing HIV policy analysts and prevention programmers with sex disaggregated HIV data alone will provide a limited perspective on how to address both the biological and social factors that synergistically inform contexts of HIV risk and HIV-related health outcomes.

In other words, a closer scrutiny of the differences of both biological (sex) *and* social (gender) determinants of health in terms of proximity to HIV infection for diverse populations of women, girls, men, and boys in Canada is critical in our efforts to develop novel prevention intervention and health promotion approaches (Low & Theriault, 2008). Clearly, this synergistic interaction between biological sex and socially informed, regulated, and enforced gender norms requires greater attention in our prevention efforts (Rubin & Herstad, 2009; Canadian Institutes of Health Research [CIHR], 2009; Status of Women Canada, 1998).

As indicated in many of the health equity perspectives brought forth in this book, we also need to ensure that the "evidence" we draw from to inform policy and programming responses comes from a deeper appreciation of the intersectionality of the determinants of health, as informed by gender, biological endowment, poverty, health services, and culture, among others. In a relational sense, our reconceptualizations of HIV prevention innovation for women and men, girls and boys, requires a more robust understanding of health as situated within broader social, political, and economic inequities (International Planned Parenthood Federation, 2010). As gender necessarily intersects and overlaps with other key determinants of health, from biology and genetic endowment to income and social status, we see the importance of these factors in shaping health and health outcomes (Public Health Agency of Canada [PHAC], 2010). The need for a gender and sex-based analytic framing becomes even more pressing as we continue to see high rates of HIV infection from heterosexual sex and yet limited inclusion of heterosexual men in the HIV prevention discourse (International Planned Parenthood Federation, 2010). Given that gender is generally understood as shared expectations and norms held by society about appropriate male and female behaviour, characteristics, and roles, such norms both influence and regulate social interactions, including HIV-related health-seeking behaviours (AIDS Accountability International, 2009; Gupta, 2000; Johnson, Greaves, & Repta, 2007). Further, we know that gender inequality refers to differential social opportunity and power based on gender, and those with less social opportunity and power are more likely to have their needs overlooked or marginalized (Armstrong, 2009; Commonwealth Secretariat & Atlantic Centre for Excellence in Women's Health, 2002; Nowatzki & Grant, 2011).

According to women's health researchers, women who are marginalized (firstly by gender and also potentially by race, culture, class, and sexual orientation) will have less access to social and health care systems and may be at higher risk of contracting communicable diseases, including HIV, than men (Arber & Khlat, 2002; Devries & Free, 2010; Johnson et al., 2007). An analysis of sex- and gender-based realities and expectations has the potential to contribute vital information to our understanding of HIV and its differential impact on men and women, and boys and girls. We know from previous HIV research that social stereotypes around women's sexuality and early misconceptions of women's HIV risk placed women at an increased risk for contracting HIV (Jenkins, 2000). Social norms, which sexualize women and girls yet vilify them for being sexual, condone male sexual promiscuity, place birth control responsibilities on females, dissuade public discourse on sex and sexuality, perpetuate uneven sexual dynamics, fuel stigma and discrimination, and exacerbate social exclusion, are harmful to women's health (International Planned Parenthood Federation, 2010). Additionally, gender-based barriers to health care often specific to women, such as lack of child care, respite care, or transportation, will impact women's ability to engage in health resource–seeking behaviours (Beadnell et al., 2003). For these reasons, gender- and sex-based analysis that explores the lived experiences of both men and women offers an important element to consider in the design, delivery, and evaluation of HIV prevention efforts (De Lay, 2004).

Given the utility of both sex- and gender-based analytic approaches in unpacking the complexities of HIV prevention, key questions remain, including why we do not see universal advocacy for the integration of both gender and sex analysis into research projects, and why prevention programming efforts and policy analytic frameworks neglect to include gender-based indicators in their evaluations. Although there has been variable success at ensuring the inclusion of gender in several key government working documents, often the centrality of gender does not filter down into program planning and policies at the various sectoral levels (Jurgens, 2004; CIHR, 2009). Despite the slow uptake within some sectors, there are signs of improvement, including the Departmental Action Plan on Gender-Based Analysis as put forth by the Privy Council Office in conjunction with the Treasury Board of Canada and Status of Women Canada in 2009. The purpose of this action plan was, in part, to respond to the recommendations put forth in the Auditor General of Canada's recommendation that gender-based analysis become standard practice across all federal government agencies and departments (Privy Council Office, Treasury Board of Canada Secretariat, & Status of Women Canada, 2009). The current approach fits well with two key Canadian HIV/AIDS guiding documents: *The Federal Initiative to Address HIV/ AIDS in Canada*, through key policy directions of partnership and engagement, integration, and accountability, and *Leading Together*, through a collaborative, shared, national response to the prevention of HIV and care, treatment, and support for those living with HIV/AIDS (Government of Canada, 2004; Canadian Public Health Association, 2006). Although neither document stresses the specific issue of greater attention to gender as a key driver of the epidemic in Canada, the hope is that as these key documents are updated, they will take a stronger stance on the utility of sex- and gender-based analytic frameworks in policy and programming as this approach becomes adopted and incorporated into government departmental action plans.

However, despite these potential advances, we must recognize that our national health care system is challenged by a variety of issues, ranging from resource constraints, to the federal, provincial, and territorial responsibility hubs, to mainstream health care systems that are still largely organized around the biomedical model of health care, and that within this mix, there remains an assumption that men and women are being equally, or at least adequately, addressed by a system originally designed for men (Jurgens, 2004; CIHR, 2009). In addition to recognizing how and why women and men's HIV prevention needs are different and how current mainstream health approaches may not adequately or equitably address these differences, we must also recognize that women are a highly heterogeneous group with vastly different experiences that serve to shape their HIV risk and HIV-related health outcomes (Native Women's Association of Canada, 2007). In particular, HIV-related health policies and programs must acknowledge and address how lesbian, bisexual, and trans women's health care needs may differ from heterosexual women's needs (i.e., safe-sex needs, pregnancy planning issues, hormone therapy) and how the lack of attention to such differences may have an impact on access and uptake to HIV prevention services and information. This is also true in relation to the unique needs of Aboriginal women, and of African, Caribbean, and Black women in Canada, as described by Peltier et al. (Chapter 4) and Tharao, Muchenje, and Mehes (Chapter 5) in this volume.

As indicated by the epidemiology of women and HIV/AIDS in Canada, the epidemic shows no signs of a reversal in infection rates. Beyond the epidemiological perspective, we see how framing these data from a determinants of health perspective can offer more insights into the contexts and intersecting factors that impact on primary and secondary prevention among diverse populations of women in Canada. Equally important is how such data are used to inform additional research, programming, and policy responses. This research-policy-programming nexus has important implications for how certain types of research findings are privileged over other types. The interface between the production of knowledge and the uptake of knowledge or "evidence" to inform policy and programming directions becomes potentially problematic in determining the underlying ideology that can drive this process. The focus on "evidence-informed" decision making can in turn lead to discussions of what constitutes policy-relevant evidence. In other words, these processes of knowledge generation and evidence-informed decision making are not static or apolitical but are nuanced through key stakeholders and their perceptions of the relevance of the stated problem, the research approach used, and the resultant data gleaned. In this way, separate strands of research, often disconnected from each other, create limitations in understanding and drawing from forms of knowledge outside our own area of expertise, which can stymie innovation in research methodology or lead to defaulting to a normative, reductionist epistemology (Santelli, 2006).

An alternative to this technocratic evidence-to-policy process is to regard the various knowledge users from government, academic, and community settings as co-producers of knowledge in a shifting away from a hierarchical positioning of levels of evidence related to perceptions of objectivity. Research paradigms based on a variety of assumptions, including ontological, epistemological, and methodological, among others, are used to frame our approach to our research—from the types of issues deemed research-worthy through to the types of research questions posed and forms of analysis and reporting utilized. Historically, the divide in these assumptions has tended to fall along the quantitative–qualitative schism with a privileging of particular types of expertise or levels of objectivity, often defaulting to more positivist, hypothetico-deductive approaches to research evidence and knowledge generation.

Given the ongoing HIV research, policy, and programming challenges we are facing in Canada, there is a need for more creative, transdisciplinary, culturally relevant approaches. Further, recognizing that the policy-research-programming nexus must be co-produced jointly by government, researchers/academics, and community, we require innovative mechanisms to make co-production possible. In an effort to achieve this, a coordinated national research agenda on HIV prevention by, for, and with women, trans women, and girls would help move this conversation forward. Such a national agenda would play a crucial role in knowledge generation and translation of research evidence to help inform policy and programming development by embracing greater horizontality in our efforts to mitigate the impact of HIV.

This book has provided many excellent examples of how greater coordination and sharing of our collective knowledge on, with, and by women, trans women, and girls and HIV prevention can yield better outcomes and greater traction on the evidence to policy and programming nexus. As we saw in Greene, Chambers, Masinde, and Mukandoli (Chapter 6), innovative approaches to housing policies for women can serve as an HIV prevention strategy to address structural inequities in access to safe and affordable housing. As indicated by Loutfy and Margolese (Chapter 10), programs related to preconception and pregnancy planning for women living with and affected by HIV requires consideration of both sex and gender analysis in HIV prevention and health outcomes for parents and their children. HIV prevention in Canadian prisons as described by Reece (Chapter 8) further illustrates the need to move beyond ideology to work collaboratively across sectors to ensure a gender-equitable approach to the provision of harm reduction strategies for women in prison. Meeting the HIV-related service needs of Aboriginal women as demonstrated by Peltier et al. (Chapter 4) speaks powerfully to the need to push for culturally relevant and appropriate approaches while recognizing the history of abuses experienced by Aboriginal peoples in Canada. These and the other authors in this book bring together a collective voice in furthering our understanding of the HIV prevention needs of diverse communities of women with a focus on issues of health equity in addressing the structural barriers faced. In this way, health as an issue of equity means more than simply changing individual behaviours; rather, it requires addressing the social environments that lead to sexism, racism, and stigma and discrimination and related inequities in research, policy, and programming that fuel the gender-based differential in HIV infection rates. By highlighting many of the creative, resilient, and painful journeys women encounter in trying to remain HIV negative, as well as the challenges and burdens they experience once found to be HIV positive, it is hoped that this book will serve as a call to action in setting our collective moral compass to address the primary and secondary HIV prevention needs of the diverse communities of women, trans women, and girls in Canada.

REFERENCES

AIDS Accountability International. (2009). *The AIDS accountability scorecard on women 2009.* Sweden: AIDS Accountability International.

Arber, S., & Khlat, M. (2002). Introduction to social and economic patterning of women's health in a changing world. *Social Science and Medicine, 54*(5), 643–647.

Armstrong, P. (2009). Public policy, gender and health. In D. Raphael (Ed.), *Social determinants of health* (2nd ed., pp. 350–361). Toronto, ON: Canadian Scholars' Press Inc.

Beadnell, B., Baker, S., Knox, K., Stielstra, S., Morrison, D. M., Degooyer, E., ... & Oxford, M. (2003). The influence of psychosocial difficulties on women's attrition in an HIV/STD prevention program. *AIDS Care, 15*(6), 807–820.

Canadian Institutes of Health Research. (2009). *Gender matters: Institute of gender and health strategic plan, 2009–2012.* Ottawa: Canadian Institutes of Health Research.

Canadian Public Health Association. (2006). *Leading together: Canada takes action on HIV/AIDS (2005–2010).* Condensed version. Ottawa, ON: Canadian Public Health Association.

Commonwealth Secretariat & Atlantic Centre for Excellence in Women's Health. (2002). *Gender mainstreaming in HIV/AIDS: Taking a multi-sectoral approach.* London, UK: Commonwealth Secretariat.

De Lay, P. (2004). Gender and monitoring the response to HIV/AIDS pandemic. *Emerging Infectious Diseases, 10*(11), 1979–1983.

Devries, K. M., & Free, C. (2010). "I told him not to use condoms": Masculinities, femininities and sexual health of Aboriginal Canadian young people. *Sociology of Health & Illness, 32*(6), 827–842.

Government of Canada. (2004). *The federal initiative to address HIV/AIDS in Canada: Strengthening the federal action in the Canadian response to HIV/AIDS.* Ottawa: Minister of Public Works and Government Services of Canada.

Gupta, G. R. (2000). *Gender, sexuality and HIV/AIDS: The what, the why, and the how.* Plenary address to the XIII International AIDS Conference, Durban, South Africa.

International Planned Parenthood Federation. (2010). *Men-streaming in sexual and reproductive health and HIV: A toolkit for policy development and advocacy.* London, UK: International Planned Parenthood Federation.

Jenkins, S. R. (2000). Toward theory development and measure evolution for studying women's relationships and HIV infection. *Sex Roles, 42*(7/8), 751–780.

Johnson, J. L., Greaves, L., & Repta, R. (2007). *Better science with sex and gender: A primer for health research.* Vancouver, BC: Women's Health Research Network.

Jurgens, R. (2004). *Deadly public policy: HIV/AIDS and government (in)action.* Arthur Kroger College Annual Lecture in Public Affairs and Civic Society, Carleton University, Ottawa.

Ottawa, ON: Canadian HIV/AIDS Legal Network.

Low, J., & Theriault, L. (2008). Health promotion policy in Canada: Lessons forgotten, lessons still to learn. *Health Promotion International, 23*(2), 200–206.

Native Women's Association of Canada. (2007). *Culturally relevant gender-based analysis: An issue paper.* Ottawa: Native Women's Association of Canada.

Nowatzki, N., & Grant, K. R. (2011). Sex is not enough: The need for gender-based analysis in health research. *Health Care for Women International, 32*(4), 263–277.

Privy Council Office, Treasury Board of Canada Secretariat, & Status of Women Canada. (2009). *Departmental action plan on gender-based analysis.* Retrieved from www.swc-cfc.gc.ca/pol/gba-acs/ap-pa/index-eng.html

Public Health Agency of Canada. (2010). *What determines health.* Retrieved from www.phac-aspc.gc.ca/ph-sp/determinants/index-eng.php

Rubin, D. S., & Herstad, B. (2009). *Integrating gender in policy implementation barriers analysis: A methodology.* Washington, DC.: Futures Health Group, Health Policy Initiative, Task Order 1.

Santelli, J. (2006). Ethical issues in health promotion research. In R. A. Crosby, R. DiClementa, & L. Salazar (Eds.), *Research methods in health promotion* (pp. 41–72). San Francisco, CA: John Wiley & Sons, Inc.

Status of Women Canada. (1998). *Gender-based analysis: A guide for policy-making.* Ottawa, ON: Status of Women Canada.

Contributors

Barry Adam is a Professor of Sociology at the University of Windsor, Windsor, Ontario.

Patricia Allard is the Deputy Director of Research and Policy with the Canadian HIV/AIDS Legal Network, Toronto, Ontario.

Chris Archibald is the Director of the HIV/AIDS Surveillance and Epidemiology Division with the Public Health Agency of Canada, Ottawa, Ontario.

Jacqueline Arthur is the Manager of Community Programs with the Public Health Agency of Canada, Ottawa, Ontario.

Greta Bauer is Associate Professor in the Department of Epidemiology and Biostatistics at the University of Western Ontario, London, Ontario.

Kristen Beausoleil is a Senior Policy Analyst in the Strategic Issues and Integrated Management Division with the Public Health Agency of Canada, Ottawa, Ontario.

Lori Chambers is the Research Coordinator at the Ontario HIV Treatment Network, Toronto, Ontario.

Monique Fong is the Executive Director of Healing Our Nations, Dartmouth, Nova Scotia.

Jacqueline Gahagan is Professor of Health Promotion at Dalhousie University, Halifax, Nova Scotia.

Saara Greene is an Assistant Professor in the School of Social Work at McMaster University, Hamilton, Ontario.

Jocelyne Guay is with the Centre for Communicable Disease and Infection Control, Public Health Agency of Canada, Ottawa, Ontario.

Jessica Halverson is the Manager of the HIV/AIDS and TB Surveillance Section with the Public Health Agency of Canada, Ottawa, Ontario.

Randy Jackson is a Ph.D. candidate in the School of Social Work at McMaster University, Hamilton, Ontario.

Cécile Kazatchkine is a Policy Analyst with the Canadian HIV/AIDS Legal Network, Toronto, Ontario.

Mona Loutfy is a scientist with the Women's College Research Institute, Toronto, Ontario.

Shari Margolese has served as the National Women's Representative of the Canadian Treatment Action Council and as a volunteer with Voice of Positive Women.

Renée Masching is the Research and Policy Manager at the Canadian Aboriginal AIDS Network, Vancouver, British Columbia.

Khatundi Masinde is the African and Caribbean Strategy Coordinator with the Ontario HIV Treatment Network, Toronto, Ontario.

Mira Mehes is the Research and Program Coordinator at Johns Hopkins University, Baltimore, Maryland.

Judy Mill is a Professor with the Faculty of Nursing at the University of Alberta, Edmonton, Alberta.

LaVerne Monette (deceased) was the Executive Director of the Ontario Aboriginal HIV/AIDS Strategy, Toronto, Ontario.

Marvelous Muchenje is the Project Coordinator at Women's Health in Women's Hands Community Health Centre, Toronto, Ontario.

Chantal Mukandoli is a member of Africans in Partnership Against AIDS, Toronto, Ontario.

San Patten is a Consultant with San Patten and Associates, Halifax, Nova Scotia.

Doris Peltier is an APHA Liaison with the Canadian Aboriginal AIDS Network, Vancouver, British Columbia.

Tracey Prentice is a Ph.D. candidate in Population Health at the University of Ottawa, Ottawa, Ontario.

Rai Reece is the Student Equity Program Advisor at the Toronto District School Board, Toronto, Ontario.

Christina Ricci is a Policy Analyst in the Senior Policy Unit with the Government of Alberta, Edmonton, Alberta.

Krista Shore is a Member at Large with the Board of Directors of the Canadian Aboriginal AIDS Network and Voices of Women Standing Committee member, Vancouver, British Columbia.

Alison Symington is the Senior Policy Analyst with the Canadian HIV/AIDS Legal Network, Toronto, Ontario.

Wangari Tharao is the Program and Research Manager at Women's Health in Women's Hands Community Health Centre, Toronto, Ontario.